AF598022

Current Clinical Pathology

Antonio Giordano, MD, PhD
Director, Sbarro Institute for Cancer Research and Molecular Medicine
and Center for Biotechnology
Temple University
Philadelphia, PA, USA

Series Editor

For further volumes:
http://www.springer.com/series/7632

Xichun Sun

Well-Differentiated Malignancies

New Perspectives

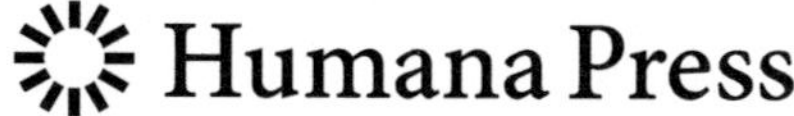

Xichun Sun, M.D, Ph.D.
Medical Director, Department of Pathology
Beckley Veterans Medical Center (West Virginia)
Staff Pathologist, McGuire Veterans Medical Center
Assistant Professor, Virginia Commonwealth University
Richmond, VA, USA

ISSN 2197-781X ISSN 2197-7828 (electronic)
ISBN 978-1-4939-1691-7 ISBN 978-1-4939-1692-4 (eBook)
DOI 10.1007/978-1-4939-1692-4
Springer New York Heidelberg Dordrecht London

Library of Congress Control Number: 2014946217

Printed on acid-free paper

Humana Press is a brand of Springer
Springer is part of Springer Science+Business Media (www.springer.com)

To Wei Wei, my beautiful, intelligent wife
Daniel W. Sun, my wonderful, beloved son
Isabella D. Sun, my creative, loving daughter

Preface

The conception of this book was inspired by the frequent encounters I had with lay friends and acquaintances when I felt pressed to describe the nature of my work primarily as a surgical pathologist. I often started the description by making an analogy to the process of verdict making in the court. The differentiation between benign and malignant lesions was frequently used as an example in order to give surgical pathologists their proper credit in patient care. The importance of the differentiation, I proclaimed, is analogous to separating petty criminals from desperados who wreaked havoc to the society. When further "confronted" by some inquisitive minds which were interested in how we make the calls, I oftentimes resorted to the citation of the basic features of malignancy (i.e., infiltrative growth pattern, cytological anaplasia) and benign lesions (i.e., encapsulation or circumscription) which medical students learn in their second year pathology course. However, in doing so I knew that I did not do enough justice to our trade.

It is well known that many malignancies, particularly the well differentiated (low grade is used interchangeably in this book), do not manifest the stereotypic morphological features. On the other hand, some benign lesions can appear to be infiltrative and even possess marked cytological atypia. For instance, renal and pulmonary non–small cell carcinomas usually lack an infiltrative growth pattern. Instead, they show well circumscription. Renal papillary carcinoma is actually encapsulated in most cases. Paradoxically, papillary adenoma of the kidney, the premalignant counterpart of papillary carcinoma, lacks encapsulation. In thyroid pathology, capsular (or vascular) invasion becomes the yardstick in the differential diagnosis of follicular tumors. In the benign realm, mammary radial scar and nipple adenoma can be easily over-diagnosed as invasive carcinoma by the unwary since they have an appearance of infiltrative growth pattern. Furthermore, due to the robust epithelial/stromal interactions and/or histological arrangements of the organs, some benign cutaneous and ovarian epithelial lesions are seemingly deeply infiltrative and additional features are needed to avoid over-diagnosis. Moreover, a nodular growth pattern should not be deemed as invasive in salivary gland tumors, whereas it is one of the key characteristics of myxofibrosarcoma of the soft tissue.

Each tissue and organ in this miraculous super-machine we call human body is ingeniously and specifically designed and crafted to perform unique functions. This ingeniousness and uniqueness dictate that all the constituent cells be masterfully regulated and coordinated. Neoplasm occurs when the mechanisms are undermined with malignancy representing a total meltdown of the regulation and coordination. Tissue/organ specific morphological clues, even subtle (not the salient stereotypic features), should manifest not only just at molecular levels, but also at cellular and histological levels when a total meltdown of the mechanisms occurs. Thus, if a tissue/organ specific approach is used in lieu of the universal stereotypic criteria, many dreadful consequences of under-diagnosing malignancies could be significantly reduced.

Three years ago I embarked on an ambitious mission of immersing myself in the enormously rich literature of surgical pathology, oncology, developmental biology, histology and physiology. As I dug deeper along the way, it started to dawn on me that a tissue/organ specific criteria approach is feasible. In the inceptive stage of the book, I keenly contemplated on proposing a new term "malignant atypia" to call attention to the key morphological features of different well-differentiated malignancies. The fear that it might alienate many people by sounding presumptuous led to its dropping out in the final draft. In retrospect, it might not be a bad idea at all, if the introduction could help raise the awareness of the key morphological features of different malignancies, and therefore contributing to the de-dogmatization of stereotypic malignant features in practicing surgical pathologists.

The second task for me was to come up with some explanation for the tissue/organ specific criteria as pedagogic teaching and personal experience constantly reminded me that if we understand the "why," we tend to retain the "what" longer and to practice it more dexterously. To my encouragement, the "whys," at least plausible ones, are not difficult to come by.

In this book, I made attempts to compile an exhaustive list of well differentiated malignancy in most of the body organs/tissues. Conspicuously, the hematopoietic and lymphoid system, however, is conspicuously left out mainly because of the current trend toward heavy dependence on immunohistochemical and molecular studies in the diagnosis, and the author's limited experience and knowledge. A new section could be added in the second edition of this book if it makes to it. This book is divided into ten chapters, each of which begins with a review of pertinent development biology, histology and physiology. This constitutes the basis for further discussion of the key morphological features for each malignancy which follows. Those key morphological features are highlighted in a different light (angle) in the differential diagnosis in which mostly the benign masqueraders are compared and contrasted with the malignancy.

I wish to thank the Springer Publishing staff for espousing this project and their patience with the progress of the manuscript. Special thanks go to Dr. William Frable, Professor Emeritus at Department of Pathology, Virginia Commonwealth University. His encouraging remarks dispelled many self-doubts I had during this endeavor. I am also deeply indebted to my family for their never-wavering support, sacrifice and suffering. It is therefore befitting to dedicate this book to them.

Richmond, USA Xichun Sun

Contents

1 Cutaneous Tissue

Review of Pertinent Physiology and Histology of the Skin

Keratinocytes

The important barrier function of the epidermis is supported by the epidermal appendages such as the hair follicles and sebaceous and sweat glands. The epidermis contains a basal layer of proliferative keratinocytes that adhere to the underlying basement membrane. In the process of differentiation, the committed basal cells detach from the basement membrane and progress through different stages and form three distinctive layers: the spinous, the granular, and the stratum corneum. The molecular mechanism underlying this complex process is still poorly understood [1, 2].

Three pools of keratinocyte stem cells have been identified. They are located in the interfollicular basal layer, the hair follicle bulge, and the sebaceous gland. Under normal circumstance, they are responsible for the homeostasis of their respective home structures. However, each of them has the potential to produce the other two structures [2–5]. Furthermore, recent data indicate the existence of a fourth source of keratinocyte stem cells in the sweat glands [3, 4].

Dermal Fibroblasts

The epidermal appendages are generated through a complex inductive influence of the dermis which determines the nature of the ectodermal differentiation. The adult dermal stroma contains at least three different types of fibroblasts in the adults [6–8]. They include the CD10-positive, CD34-positive, and factor XIII-positive fibroblasts. The CD10-positive cells are present in the periadnexal stroma. The CD34-positive cells are probably bone marrow derived, located perivascularly. They probably form a complex network as the intestinal pericryptal fibroblasts and play an important role in antigen presentation and host immune reactions. Similar in what is seen in the GI surgical pathology I which loss of the pericryptal cells is indicative for malignancy, loss of CD34-positive cells is an important feature of invasive cutaneous malignancies including squamous cell carcinoma, basal cell carcinoma, and malignant melanoma. It signifies the destruction of the dermal immune barrier.

Factor XIII-positive fibroblasts are predominantly present in the papillary dermis surrounding the vasculature and sweat glands. Dermatofibroma cells show reactivity for factor XIII, whereas tumor cells in dermatofibrosarcoma protuberans

X. Sun, *Well-Differentiated Malignancies: New Perspectives*, Current Clinical Pathology,
DOI 10.1007/978-1-4939-1692-4_1, © Springer Science+Business Media New York 2015

are positive for CD34. The characteristic storiform pattern of the latter might reflect the cells' property to form a three-dimensional immunological meshwork.

Melanocytes

Melanocytes are charged with the important task of shielding the organism from injurious UV lights. They are derived from the neural crest which migrates to the dermis before settling down in the epidermis and hair follicles. This important migratory property is reflected in many melanocytic lesions, both benign and malignant.

In the epidermis, they form a symbiotic relationship with the keratinocytes in the form of so-called melanokeratinocyte units [9, 10]. In the unit, the differentiated melanocytes are located in the basal layer (in a ratio of 1:5 with the basal cells), and through their cellular processes, each interacts with proximately 36 keratinocytes. In contrast to keratinocytes which are rapidly replaced, normal melanocytes have a slow turnover rate which is tightly controlled by the keratinocytes through various mechanisms.

Stromal Invasion in the Context of Cutaneous Dermis

Due to the unique histological arrangement of the dermal appendages, most of benign epithelial lesions are surrounded by dermal tissue. Benign melanocytic nevoid cells also have the natural propensity to penetrate the dermis. Therefore, the criteria for dermal invasion need to be strengthened if the concept is to remain diagnostically relevant.

In this chapter, we propose a set of key features for dermal invasion for four major categories of cutaneous malignancy: squamous cell carcinoma, basal cell carcinoma, eccrine carcinoma, and melanoma. Importantly, the lack of CD34 fibroblasts might represent a universal yardstick in cutaneous surgical pathology [11, 12].

Key Morphological Features of Well-Differentiated Squamous Cell Carcinoma

- Dyskeratosis
- Stromal Invasion (Figs. 1.1 and 1.2)

Discussion

Dissimilar to mucosal squamous cell carcinomas, cutaneous squamous carcinomas are mostly UV light related. Even though the stem cells in the adnexal structures have the potential to give rise to epidermis, the adnexal structures apparently manage to prevent the involvement by the dysplastic squamous cells. This is in contrast to the situation in the squamous mucosa in which dysplastic cell frequently involves the underlying glandular structures mimicking invasive carcinoma.

The bland squamous cells of well-differentiated squamous cells demonstrate dyskeratosis which is characterized by early keratinization (keratin pearls in the basal and parabasal layers) and excessive cytoplasmic keratinization. It is not to be confused with squamous eddies and horn cysts which are present in seborrheic keratosis and trichilemmal or trichoblastic lesions, respectively.

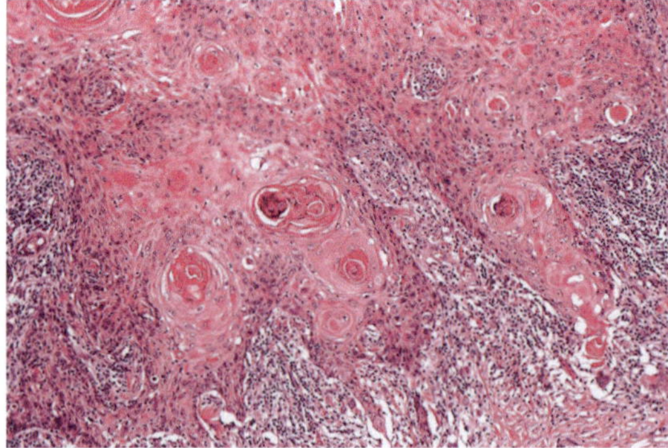

Fig. 1.1 Well-differentiated squamous cell carcinoma. Stromal invasion by irregular nests (Pathology of the Skin, *Elsevier/Mosby*, 2005; Dermatology, *Elsevier/Saunders*, 2011 with permission)

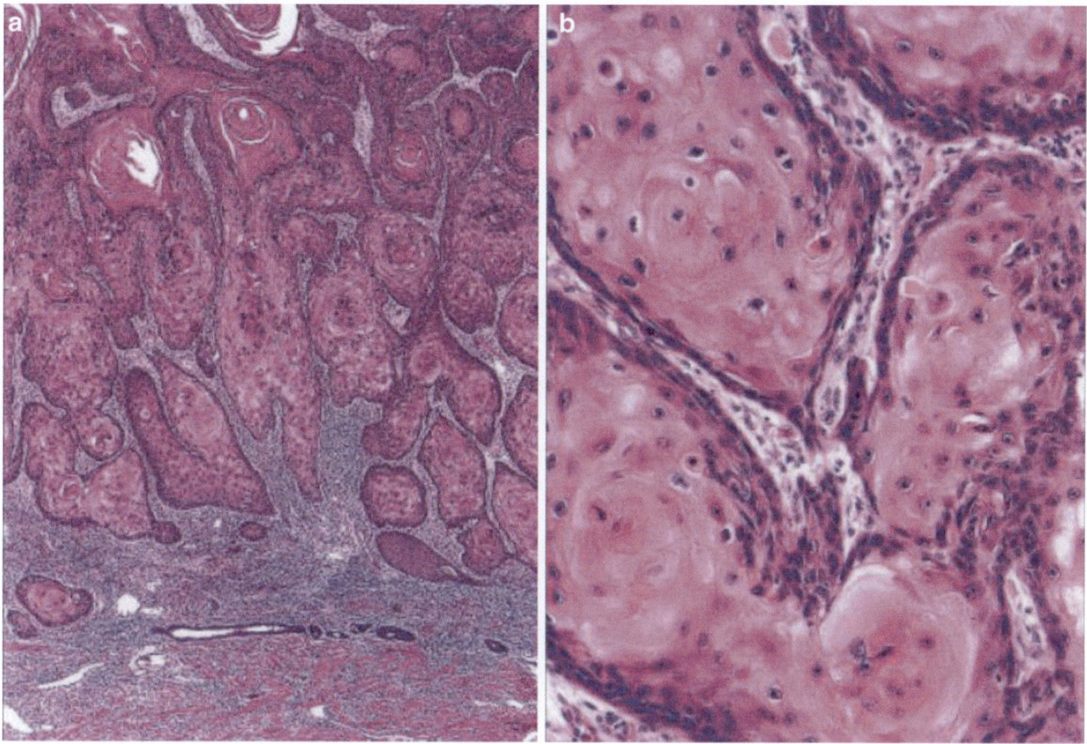

Fig. 1.2 Well-differentiated squamous cell carcinoma. Note dyskeratotic cells (Pathology of the Skin, *Elsevier/Mosby*, 2005 with permission)

Identification of stromal invasion of the squamous cell carcinoma can be tricky. On the one hand, verrucous and keratoacanthoma variants have a well-circumscribed contour. On the other hand, several benign squamous proliferations appear to invade the dermis. Familiarity with their histological presentations is valuable in avoiding overdiagnosis. Like in other locations, a panel of immunostainings (p53, MMMp-1, and ki67) may be useful. Recent evidence indicates that the stroma of squamous cell carcinoma lacks CD34 fibroblasts (Fig. 1.3). Instead, it has increased expression of SMA-positive myofibroblasts (Fig. 1.4).

Differential Diagnosis

Pseudoepitheliomatous Hyperplasia

Pseudoepitheliomatous hyperplasia typically involves both the epidermis and the follicular infundibular and even acrosyringia. In fact, the acanthotic downgrowths have been thought to represent expanded follicular infundibula. Appropriate differentiation from well-differentiated squamous cell carcinoma would require the appreciation of the underlying inflammatory process and shape of the invasive components and their connection to the surface and shape (jagged pointed tips and a broad base connected to the surface) (Fig. 1.5). In addition to the usual immunostaining panel (p53, MMP-1, and Ki67), immunostainings for CD34 and SMA seems to be valuable [13–15]. The stromal cells of invasive squamous carcinoma lack reactivity for CD34, whereas SMA stain lights up haphazardly arranged myofibroblasts (desmoplasia).

Prurigo Nodularis

It shows hyperkeratosis with acanthosis in addition to the accompanying pseudoepitheliomatous proliferation. Helpful clues include spongiosis, inflammatory cells, and prominence of blood vessels and nerve endings.

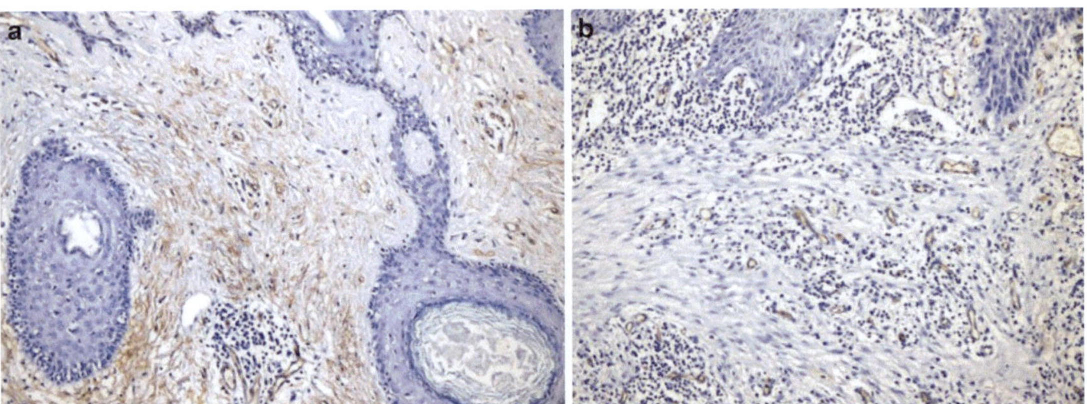

Fig. 1.3 Stroma of squamous cell carcinoma lacks CD34+ fibroblasts (**b**). Benign dermis contains abundant CD34+ fibroblasts (**a**)

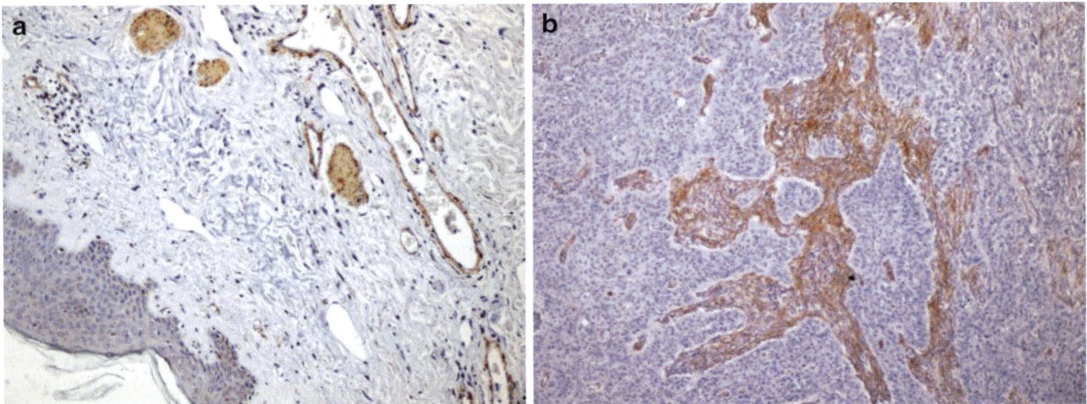

Fig. 1.4 Stroma of squamous cell carcinoma contains SMA-positive fibroblast (**b**). Benign dermis lacks SMA-positive fibroblasts (**a**)

Irritated Seborrheic Keratosis (Inverted Follicular Keratosis)

The lesion presents as an endophytic proliferation of squamous and basaloid cells. Characteristically, it contains many squamous eddies which are different from the horn pearls of well-differentiated squamous cells in that they are well circumscribed, small in size, and numerous in number. Frequently, the downgrowth can be seen to originate in the vicinity of a follicle.

Tricholemmoma and Desmoplastic Tricholemmoma

Desmoplastic tricholemmomas can have irregular downgrowth of bland epithelial cells into a sclerotic or desmoplastic stroma. Attention to the superficial portion usually reveals changes typical of a tricholemmoma. Tricholemmomas present as lobules with peripheral columnar cell palisading and a distinct thick basement membrane. Cytoplasmic clearing involves variable number of cells.

Pilar Sheath Acanthoma (Proliferating Pilar Tumor)

The proliferating squamous lobules show glassy eosinophilic cytoplasm. Portion of the tumor can show peripheral palisading, a thickened basement membrane, and cytoplasmic clearing. Abrupt change into keratin production is another feature of the central cells. Sometimes, squamous proliferations are seen to radiate from the wall of

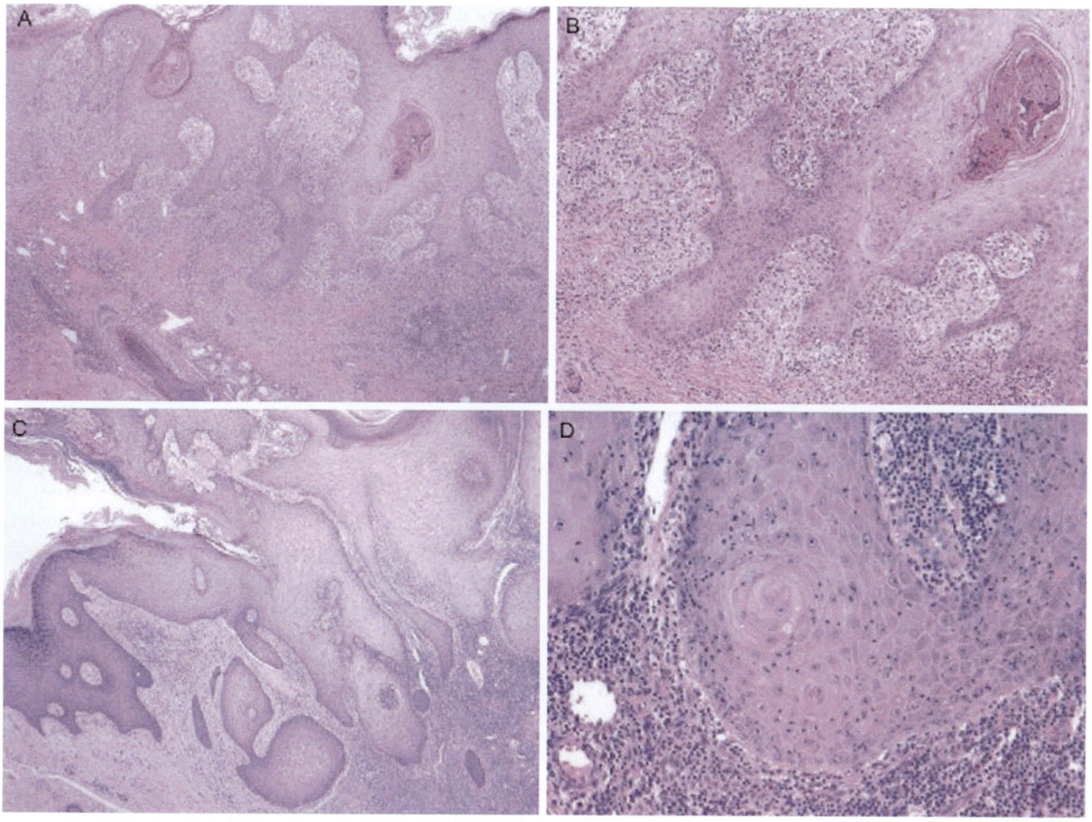

Fig. 1.5 Pseudoepitheliomatous hyperplasia. Note broad bases and lack of dyskeratosis (American Journal of Dermatopathology, *Wolters Kluwer/Lippincott Williams & Wilkins*, 2012 with permission)

the pilar cysts into the dermis and subcutaneous tissue. Some degree of cytological atypia as well as individual cell keratinization can be seen.

Key Morphological Features of Basal Cell Carcinoma

- Basaloid cell morphology
- Peripheral palisading and clefts (Fig. 1.6)

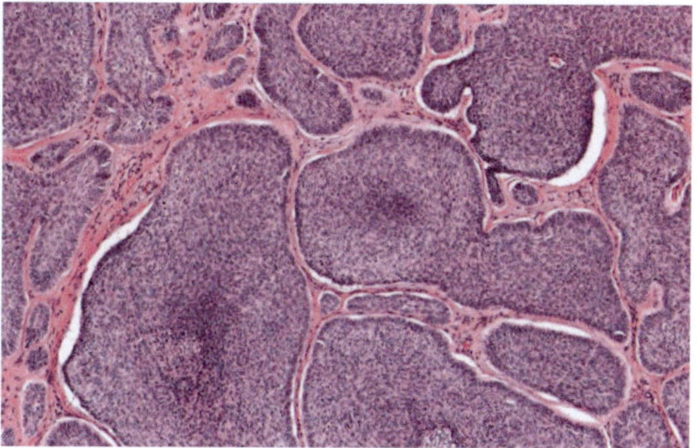

Fig. 1.6 Basal cell carcinoma with basaloid cells with peripheral palisading and clefting

Discussion

Even though there is evidence for its interfollicular origin, cutaneous basal cell carcinomas have been shown to manifest histochemical differentiation to hair follicles. Actually, the 2006 WHO Classification has placed it under the adnexal tumor category.

Basal cell carcinomas can be divided into two major subcategories: differentiated and undifferentiated. The differentiation is frequently toward adnexal components. Even in the keratotic subtype, the keratinization shows pilar differentiation in the form of parakeratosis and horn cysts.

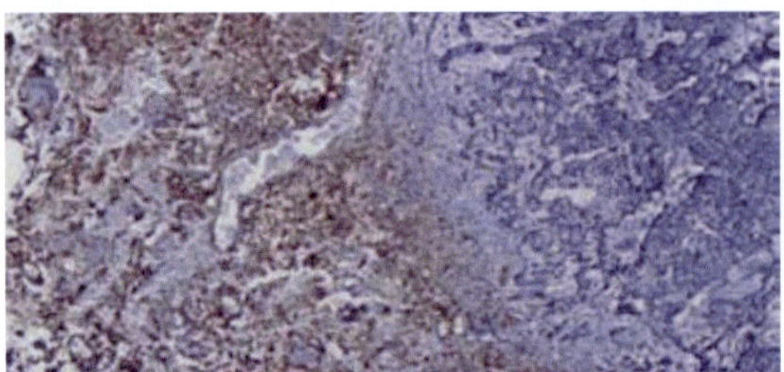

Fig. 1.7 Stroma of basal cell carcinoma lacks CD34+ fibroblasts

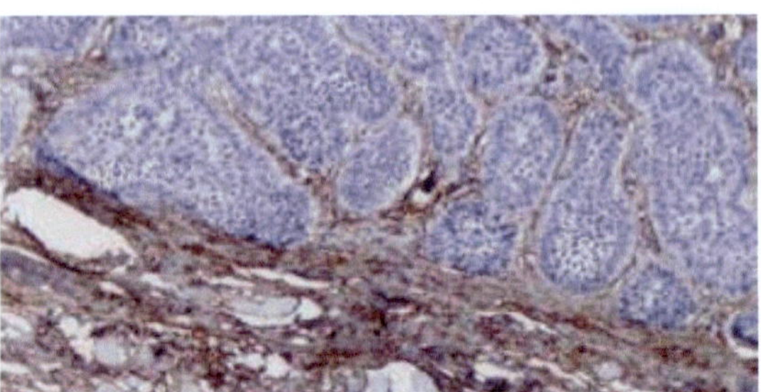

Fig. 1.8 Stroma of trichoepithelioma contains CD34+ fibroblasts

At microscopic level, the basaloid cells resemble the normal epidermal basal cells and basal cells in squamous cell carcinoma. Significant differences are, however, evident at the ultrastructural level. The basaloid tumor cells have defective expressions of hemidesmosomes, anchoring filaments and integrins, as well as bullous pemphigoid antigen [16–18]. These changes might be the underlying mechanism for the characteristic clefting around the tumor clusters. This characteristic clefting has long been discounted as a processing artifact. However, recent evidence shows that the clefts correspond to the low-refractility areas seen in vivo by reflectance confocal microscopy [19]. These ultrastructural defects indicates that the basal cell carcinoma cells have problem in establishing close attachments with the stromal components and are consistent with the inability of the tumor to metastasize.

Basal cell carcinoma cells seem to induce a parallel proliferation of spindle cells around the tumor nests, and the spindle cells show partial differentiation toward the follicular connective sheath [20]. However, the cells seem to lack CD10 and CD34 reactivity (Fig. 1.7). Instead, the malignant epithelial cells demonstrate diffuse staining for CD10 [18]. This important feature can be very useful in the differential diagnosis.

Differential Diagnosis

Trichoepithelioma, Trichoblastoma

Trichoepitheliomas are composed of well-circumscribed, symmetrical lesions composed of basaloid cells and horn cysts with trichilemmal keratinization. Even though peripheral palisading is evident, there is no stromal clefting. The epithelial cells are positive for CK20. In contrast to the diffuse Bcl-2 staining in basal cell carcinoma, only the peripheral cells show reactivity. The surrounding stroma is typically cellular and CD34 positive (Fig. 1.8).

Trichoblastomas differ from trichoepitheliomas by their small size, location, and lack of keratinizing horn cysts.

Seborrheic Keratosis

Seborrheic keratosis is composed of basaloid and squamous cells and can manifest in six different histological patterns. They all lack peripheral palisading and stromal clefting.

Eccrine Poroma

Eccrine poromas consist of uniform basaloid cells in cords and columns extending down to the dermis. Occasional narrow ductal and cytoplasmic lumen formation and cytoplasmic clearing are evident. There is neither peripheral palisading nor clefting. The intracytoplasmic lumina and ducts are positive for CEA, EMA, and PAS.

Basaloid Follicular Infundibulum Tumor and Basaloid Follicular Hamartoma

Basaloid follicular infundibulum tumors present as horizontal, fenestrated, pale squamous cell proliferation with multiple connections to the epidermis. There is peripheral palisading. However, the tumor cells have more cytoplasm and lack stromal clefting.

Basaloid hamartoma has both basaloid and squamous proliferations with interconnecting narrow bands emanating from the hair follicle infundibula. Occasional horn cysts can be seen. The cells show peripheral palisading, but lack clefting.

Key Morphological Features of Well-Differentiated Eccrine Carcinoma

- Silhouette of asymmetry
- Epithelial–stromal clefting, ill circumscription, non-vertical orientation (Figs. 1.9, 1.10, 1.11, and 1.12)

Discussion

This set of criteria was first proposed by Dr. Ackerman for the differentiation of malignant melanoma from Spitz nevus and later expanded to include adnexal tumors [21, 22]. The validity of the criteria has recently been confirmed in a study of eccrine tumors [23].

Benign adnexal tumors are symmetrical and well circumscribed with smooth borders (Fig. 1.12). They tend to form V-shaped, uniform nests which are oriented vertical to the epidermal surface (in resemblance to the orientation of normal adnexal structures) (Fig. 1.13). Importantly, the tumor cells seem to be able to attract a rim of condensed fibrous tissue which separates them from the dermal stroma by a cleft, probably reflective of the important epithelial–stromal interaction in the adnexal genesis (Fig. 1.14). Presumably, the fibrous cells are CD10-positive fibroblasts.

On the contrary, malignant adnexal tumors are asymmetrical and poorly circumscribed. The variably sized, non-V-shaped nests are arranged in a non-vertical fashion. When clefts are present, the epithelial cells are separated from altered stroma which probably lacks CD10- and/or CD 34-positive fibroblasts.

Thus, the contrasting silhouettes between the benign and malignant adnexal tumors might reflect the loss of a healthy epithelial–stromal interaction in adnexal malignancy.

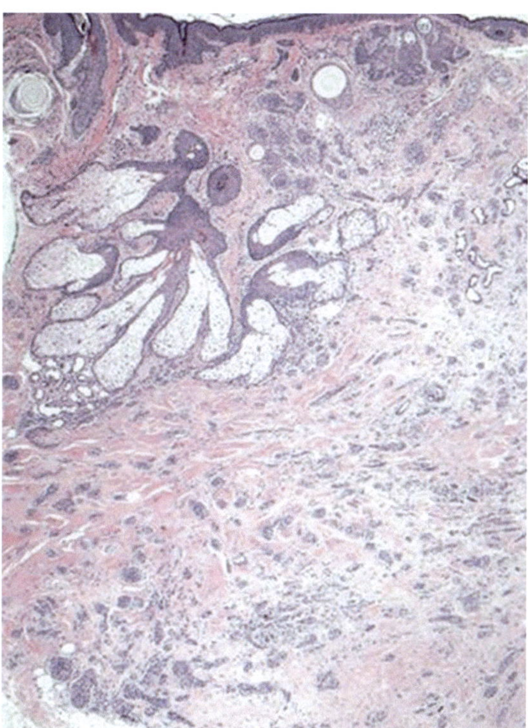

Fig. 1.9 Microcystic carcinoma. Silhouette of asymmetry (Dermatology, *Elsevier/Saunders*, 2011 with permission)

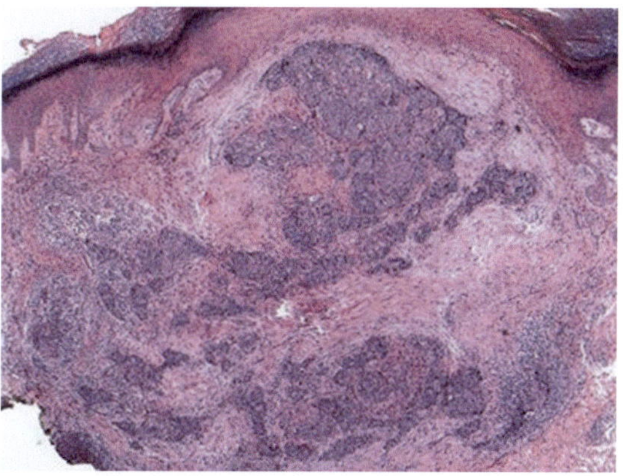

Fig. 1.10 Porocarcinoma. Silhouette of asymmetry and poor circumscription (Modern Pathology, *Nature Publishing Group*, 2006 with permission)

Another useful feature for eccrine tumors is that many of the benign sweat gland tumors have two populations of cells with one of them showing myoepithelial differentiation.

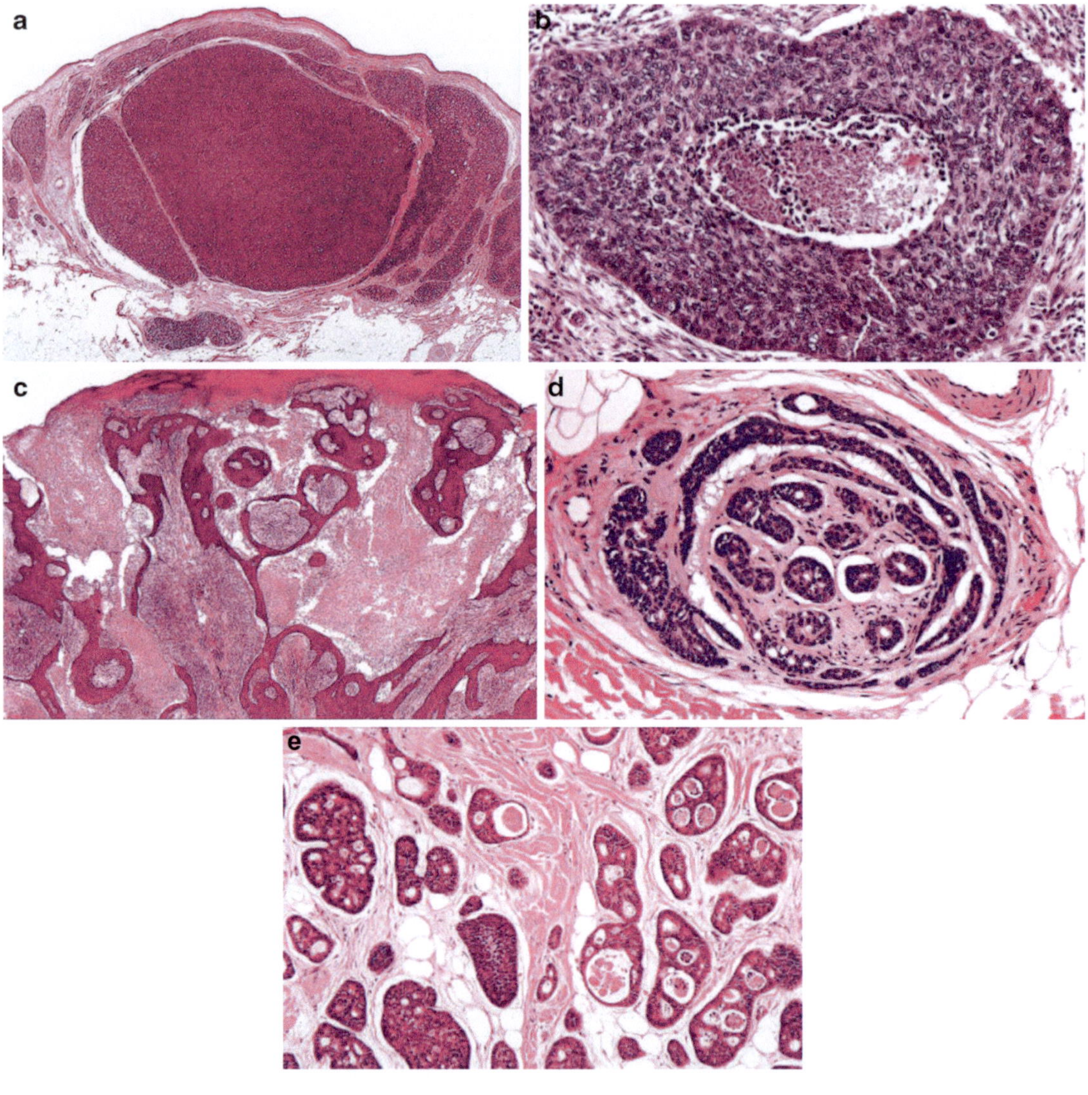

Fig. 1.11 Adnexal carcinoma. Epithelial–stromal clefting (Pathology of the Skin, *Elsevier/Mosby*, 2005 with permission)

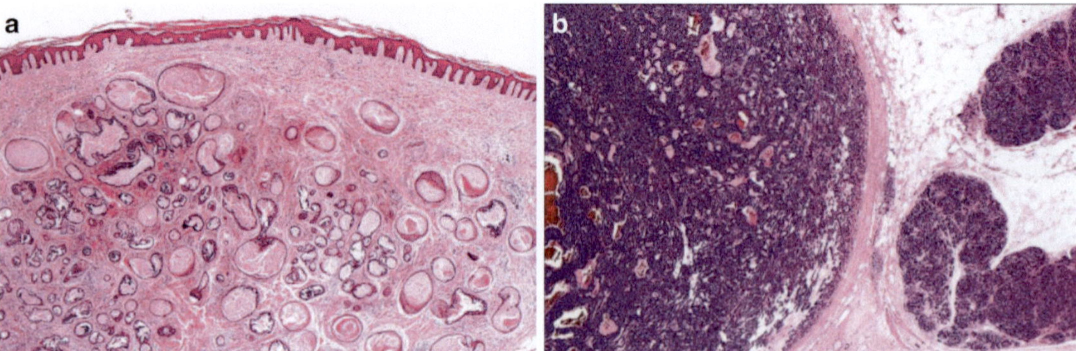

Fig. 1.12 Benign adnexal tumor. Note well circumscription, symmetry, and V-shaped contours (Pathology of the Skin, *Elsevier/Mosby*, 2005 with permission)

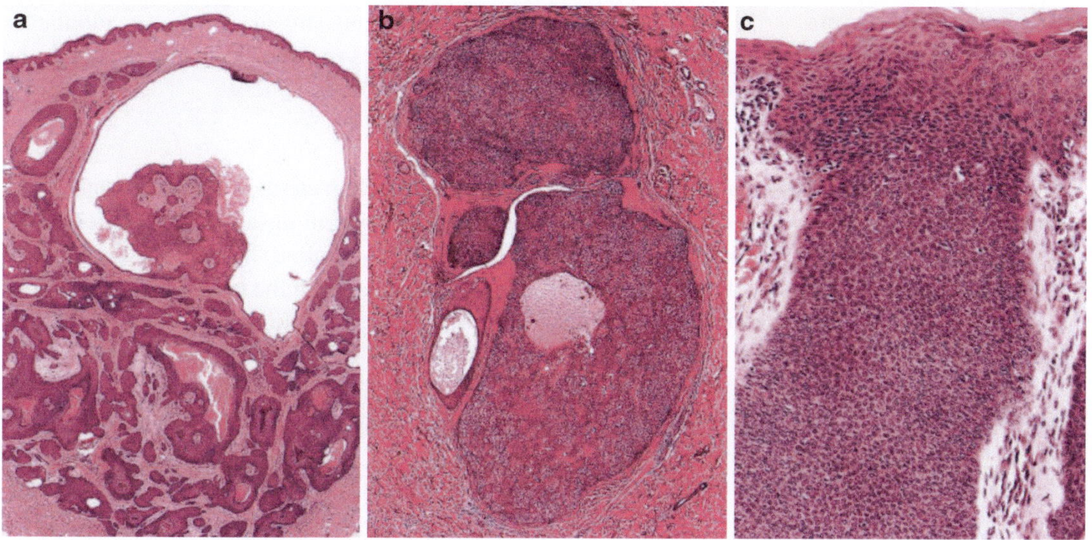

Fig. 1.13 Benign adnexal tumor. Vertical orientation (Pathology of the Skin, *Elsevier/Mosby*, 2005 with permission)

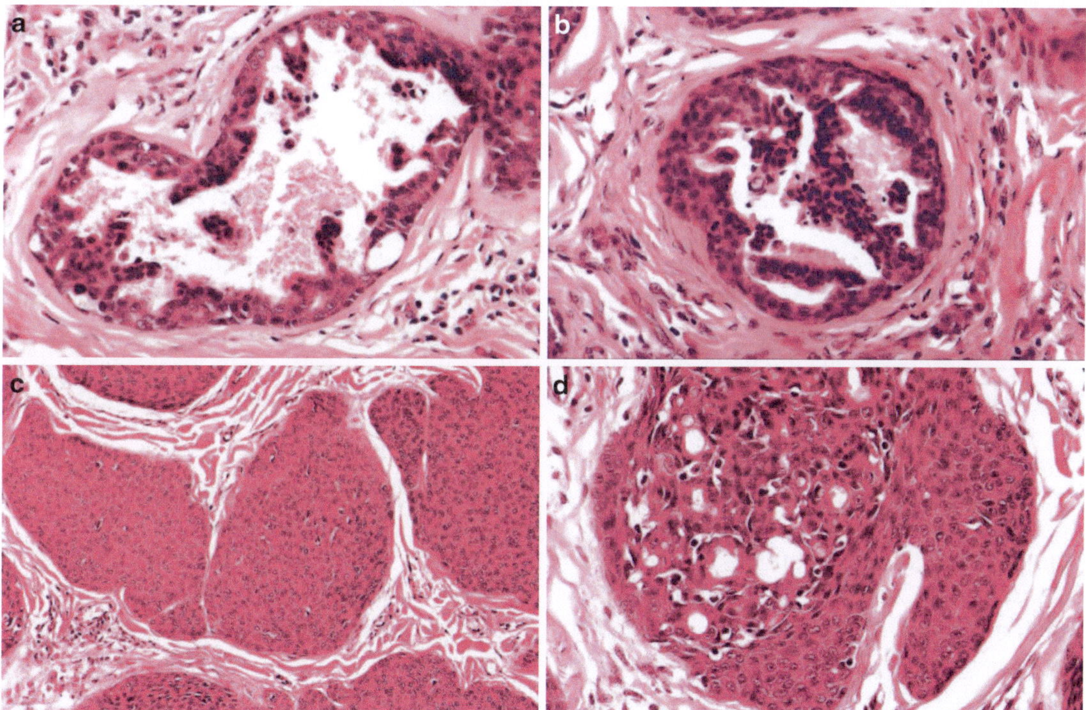

Fig. 1.14 Benign adnexal tumors. Stromal–stromal clefts. The stromal cells close to the tumor are presumably CD10+ (Pathology of the Skin, *Elsevier/Mosby*, 2005; Dermatology, *Elsevier/Saunders*, 2011with permission)

Differential Diagnosis

Hidradenoma Papilliferum

Hidradenoma papilliferum is well circumscribed with a fibrous capsule. It is composed of papillae, cysts, and tubules of cells with apocrine differentiation. Typical structures are composed of two layers of cells with the outer layer being myoepithelial cells. Occasionally only one layer of columnar cells is noted.

Nodular Hidradenoma

Nodular hidradenoma is thought to be a tumor intermediate between eccrine poroma and eccrine spiradenoma. It is lobulated and well circumscribed even though it might extend into the subcutaneous tissue. Immature poroma like epithelial cell can show occasional keratinization. The tubular lumina can vary in size. Occasionally, wide cystic structures lined by a layer of columnar cells are seen. However, more often than not they contain degenerative cells with no polarity. Even though some tumor cells show positivity for S100 and vimentin, no clear-cut myoepithelial cells are present. The ductal cells are also positive for EMA, CEA, and cytokeratin [24–26].

Syringocystadenoma Papilliferum

This tumor is characterized by an exophytic proliferation of papillary fronds with cystic penetration into the deep dermis. The lining cells are usually two layers thick with the outer layer being myoepithelial cells. The tumor shows both apocrine and eccrine differentiation, and the deeper cystic portion can have squamous metaplasia. The stroma is featured by a dense plasma cell infiltration.

Papillary Eccrine Adenoma, Tubular Apocrine Adenoma

The tumors are well circumscribed even though the tubules can be irregular, branching, and even show intraluminal papillary projection and cribriform features. The two entities share similar morphological features with the only difference being the lack of apocrine differentiation in the former. Typically they contain well-formed tubular structures with occasional cystic dilation and intracystic papillary structures. The tubules are characteristically lined by double to multiple layers of cells. Myoepithelial differentiation is present in the peripheral layer.

Eccrine Spiradenoma

The tumor is lobular and often encapsulated. The tumor cells typically present in intervening cords composed of dual cell types. The undifferentiated cells located at the periphery have small dark nuclei. The secretory cells are larger with pale nuclei, and many are arranged into tubular or ductal structures in which myoepithelial cells are identifiable at the periphery.

Cylindroma

The tumor is characterized by islands of epithelial cells arranged in jigsaw puzzle pieces which are shrouded by hyaline sheaths. The small undifferentiated cells are at the periphery and manifest palisading. Larger pale cells are located in the center and participate in lumen formation. The tumor is thought to differentiate into the intradermal coiled ductal region with myoepithelial cells.

Syringoma

This tumor is characterized by small comma-like tails present in a fibrous stroma. Even though the ductal structures often contain two layers of cells, there is no myoepithelial differentiation. Cuboidal, flat cells and intracytoplasmic lumina are frequently seen. The tumor is believed to show differentiation toward the epidermal eccrine duct. The luminal cells are positive for CEA and EMA.

Desmoplastic Trichoepithelioma

Desmoplastic trichoepithelioma resembles microcystic adnexal carcinoma in that it contains comma-like epithelial clusters in a markedly fibrotic stroma. The tumor however appears to be symmetrical and lacks deep involvement, perineural invasion, as well as ductal differentiation.

Key Morphological Features of Malignant Melanoma

- Silhouette of asymmetrical growth pattern
- Altered stroma (lymphoid-like) (Figs. 1.15 and 1.16)

Discussion

Under normal circumstances, the melanocyte proliferation is under the tight control of keratinocytes in the so-called melanokeratinocyte unit. Deregulation of the unit as a result of cell injury leads to continuous proliferation of

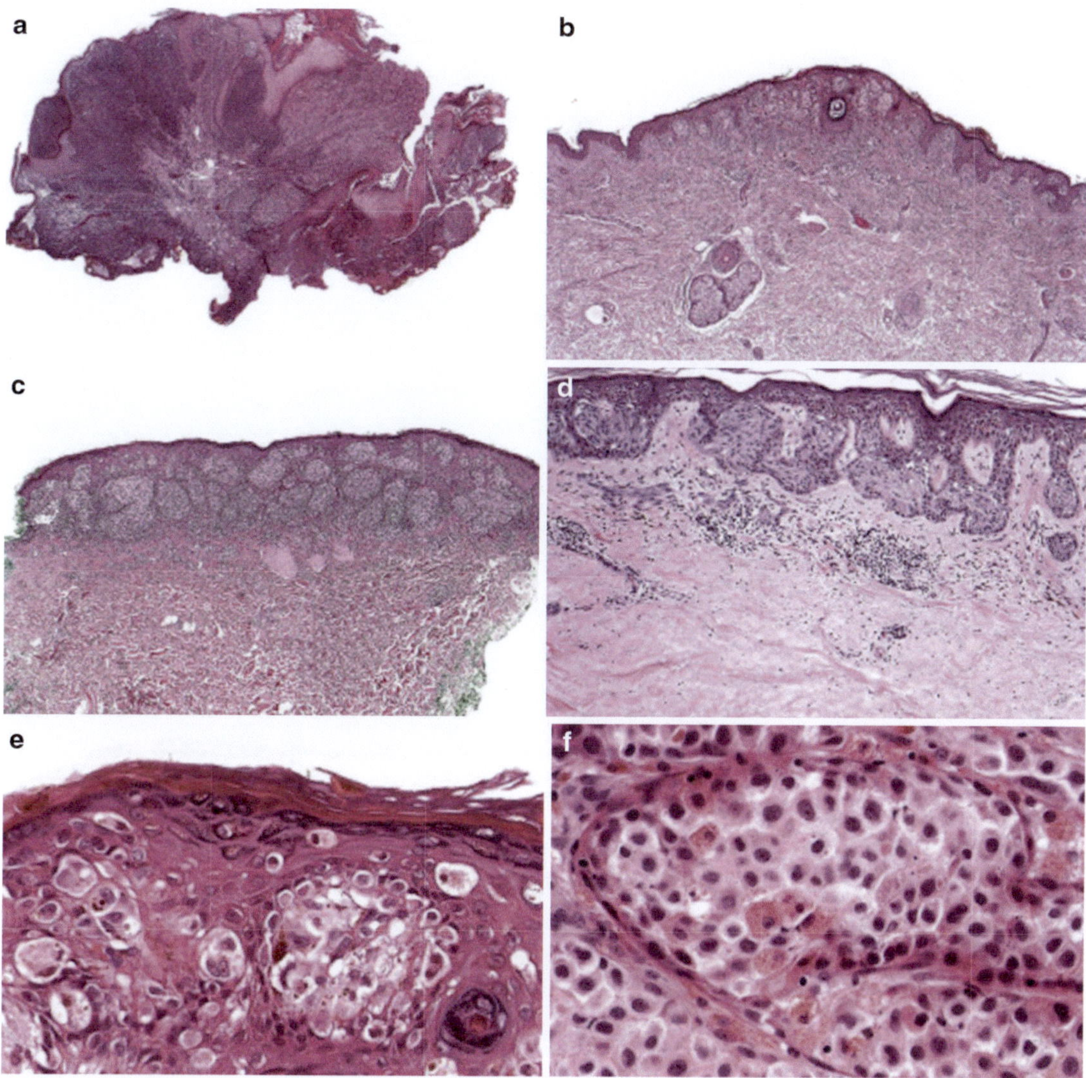

Fig. 1.15 Histological features of Melanoma. Asymmetrical growth (**a**), poor circumscription (**b**), irregular and confluent nests (**c**, **d**), pagetoid spread (**e**), lack of maturation (**f**)

melanocytes [9, 10, 27, 28]. Melanomagenesis requires the perpetuation of the initial injury by an inflammatory process which induces additional mutational changes [29]. Injured melanocytes seem to be able to self- perpetuate an inflammatory process through the production of a plethora of cytokines and chemokines. Recent evidence indicates that aging stromal fibroblasts might play a very important role in the process. Aging (p53 null) fibroblasts promote tumor progression through the expansion of lymphoid-like stromal network [30, 31]. Probably through the production of SPARC and other factors, the melanoma stroma loses CD34 fibroblasts [32–34]. Instead, the stromal cells assume the phenotype of myofibroblasts (SMA positivity) (Fig. 1.17).

In contrast to benign nevi which are clonal, malignant melanomas are heterogeneous. This heterogeneity of malignant melanoma is likely to manifest in multiple ways. Importantly, different subclones of malignant cells have differential expressions of adhesion and motility factors

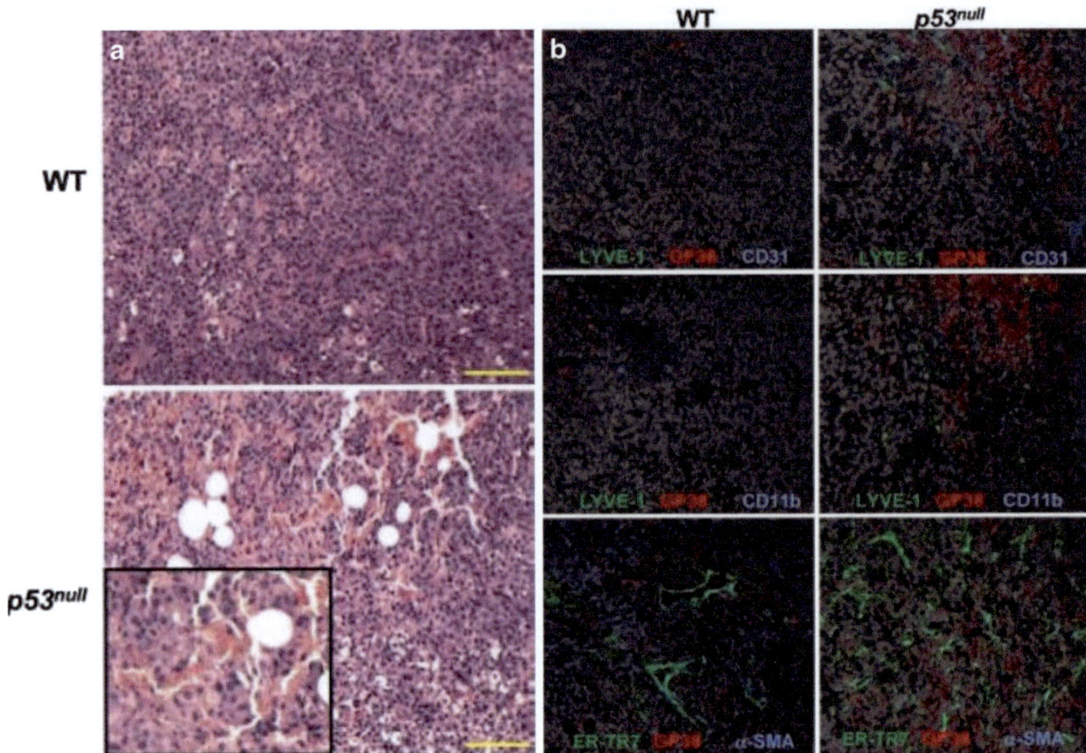

Fig. 1.16 Expansion of lymphoid stroma of malignant melanoma in B16F1 melanoma inoculated subcutaneously (panel **a**). Immunohistochemical stains confirm the lymphoid nature of the stroma (panel **b**). This feature might become diagnostically useful (Cancer Research, *American Association of Cancer Research*, 2013; Melanoma Research, *Wolters Kluwer/Lippincott Williams & Wilkins*, 2013 with permission)

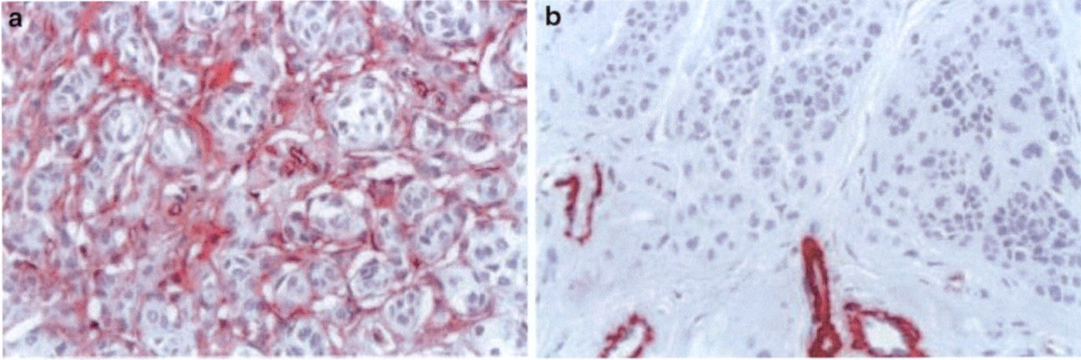

Fig. 1.17 Stroma of malignant melanoma lacks CD34+fibroblasts (**a**). The stroma of benign nevus contains CD34+ fibroblasts (**b**)

allowing for variations in their negotiations with the dermal and epidermal components. Thus, the variations underlie the asymmetrical growth pattern characteristic of melanoma. Apparently, the asymmetrical growth pattern manifests in more aspects than seen in eccrine tumors to include lateral borders, epidermal alterations, cytological details, nest and pigment distribution, and even the distribution of inflammatory cells [35–37]. This asymmetrical growth pattern can be expanded to include even expansive nodular formation and pagetoid spread. The former represents the presence of a subclone with selective growth advantage over the others. The latter

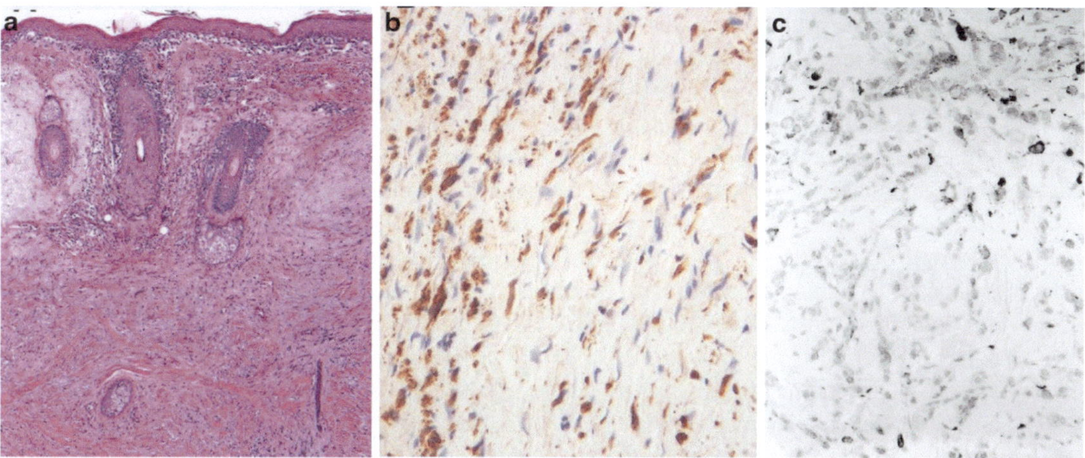

Fig. 1.18 Desmoplastic melanoma. Diffuse S100 positivity and loss of HMB45 in deep levels (**c**) (American Journal of Surgical Pathology, *Wolters Kluwer/Lippincott Williams & Wilkins*, 1999 with permission)

might reflect the absence of proper adhesion molecules for dermal infiltration.

Another feature of malignant melanocytic cells is the loss of senescence (gain of immortality) [38–40]. Benign nevi generally retain the capability to senescence, and because of their monoclonality, the cells seem to show uniformity in maturation in that cells at the depth have the same degree of maturation. This maturation can be illustrated by an HMB45 stain which shows decreasing reactivity with descent in the dermis (Fig. 1.18).

Differential Diagnosis

Spitz Nevus

Spitz nevus resembles malignant melanoma in many aspects. The cells can show diffuse pleomorphism and even pagetoid spread. Important features include well circumscription, symmetry, vertical orientation of nests, and presence of Kamino bodies. There is also a healthy melanocyte–keratinocyte relationship in the form of epithelial hyperplasia and elongation of rete ridges.

Spindle Cell Nevus (Nevus of Reed)

Spindle cell nevus shares many morphological similarities with Spitz nevus. The major differences include a spindle cell shape and heavy pigmentation.

Dysplastic Nevus

Dysplastic nevus manifests as lentiginous and nested proliferation of cytologically atypical cells. The cytological atypia is typically spotty (random atypia) and ranges from minor to severe (melanoma in situ) in degree. The lesion is typically symmetrical and the involved rete ridges are elongated with nests near their tips or sides. Frequently the nests form a bridge between adjacent rete ridges. The cells in the nests are usually spindle in shape and arranged with their long axis in parallel to the epidermal surface. There is no pagetoid growth pattern. When a dermal component is present, maturation is evident.

Desmoplastic Nevus

Desplastic nevus is generally well circumscribed and symmetric. It may contain Spitz nevus like cells, scattered cytological atypia, and even intranuclear pseudoinclusions. The associated epidermis often shows acanthosis. When a junctional component is present, a broad shoulder effect is evident. It lacks pagetoid spread, lentigo malignum-like proliferation. Maturation is evident in the dermal component.

Desmoplastic melanoma is characterized by spindle cells dispersed in a dense stroma and can be easily missed. The tumor cells show differentiation toward fibroblast and schwannian differentiation and thus are negative for Melan A and

HMB45 (superficial cells can be positive). Their melanocytic nature can only be picked up by diffuse S100 reactivity. Neurotropism and dense lymphocytic infiltration as well as associated lentigo malignum or atypical melanocytic hyperplasia are important clues.

Deep Penetrating Nevus

This entity has some features of blue nevus, Spitz nevus, and combined nevus. The penetration of fat and collagen, lack of maturation, cytological atypia, and even nuclear pseudoinclusions can cause confusion with melanoma. However, the lesion typically presents in a well-circumscribed, pyramid shape with vertical orientation of cells. Instead of destroying the structures in the path, the nevus cells tend to surround the hair follicles, sweat glands, and nerves. The cellular atypia is also random even though it can reach a high level with open chromatin and prominent nucleoli. Mitotic activities are low (ki67 < 5 % vs 25 to 75 % in melanoma).

Acral Nevus, Nevus of Special Anatomical Site

The melanokeratinocyte units are probably regulated/affected differently in these special anatomical sites as such the acral, genital areas, as well as skin flexures. Nevi in these areas are poorly circumscribed and asymmetrical. Histologically, they usually are more cellular and manifest a lentiginous growth pattern (vs nested patterns). Central pagetoid spread can be present. They are differentiated from the acrolentiginous melanoma by their small size, presence of dermal maturation, low mitotic activity, as well as lack of lateral pagetoid spread and lack of diffuse high-grade atypia.

Recurrent Nevus and Congenital Nevus

Apparently related to the wound healing process, recurrent nevi can occasionally show cytological and architectural atypia. The nevoid nests can be irregular and confluent, and sometimes, pagetoid spread is evident. Useful clues include a low mitotic rate, horizontal fibrosis in the superficial dermis, and a history of biopsy.

Congenital nevi typically show bland melanocytic cells infiltrating into the deep reticular dermis, sometimes even into the septae of the subcutaneous fat in an Indian file pattern. Frequently, they involve adnexal structures, blood vessels, and nerves. Furthermore, the nevi have poor circumscription and asymmetry (band-like), increased number of single cells, and confluence of nests. To make things worse, the proliferative nodules can show diffuse infiltration of atypical cells with mitotic activity and prominent nucleoli. However, congenital nevi can be diagnosed based on the presence of maturation and lack of necrosis, uniform high-grade atypia, brisk mitotic activity, and destructive expansile growth pattern. (Nevi in neonates are known to show marked cytological atypia and pagetoid spread.)

Halo Nevus

Halo nevus is characterized by prominent inflammatory infiltration with resultant loss of melanocytes. The lesion is largely delimited and symmetrical. The inflammatory infiltrate is predominantly composed of lymphohistiocytes which tend to be distributed in a homogenous fashion throughout the lesion and leaves the rete ridges largely intact. There is maturation and mitotic activities are low. In melanoma undergoing regression, the inflammatory infiltration is patchy and there is fibrosis at different stages. Pagetoid and expansile growth patterns are incompatible with halo nevus.

References

1. Sotiropoulou PA, Blanpain C. Development and homeostasis of the skin epidermis. Cold Spring Harb Perspect Biol. 2012;4(7):a008383.
2. Doupe DP, Jones PH. Interfollicular epidermal homeostasis: dicing with differentiation. Exp Dermatol. 2012;21(4):249–53.
3. Biedermann T, et al. Human eccrine sweat gland cells can reconstitute a stratified epidermis. J Invest Dermatol. 2010;130(8):1996–2009.
4. Lu CP, et al. Identification of stem cell populations in sweat glands and ducts reveals roles in homeostasis and wound repair. Cell. 2012;150(1):136–50.

5. Pincelli C, Marconi A. Keratinocyte stem cells: friends and foes. J Cell Physiol. 2010;225(2):310–5.
6. Velazquz EF, Ming GE. Chapter 3. Histology of the skin. In: Elder DE et al., editors. Lever's histopathology of the skin. Philadelphia: Lippincott Williams & Wilkins/a Wolters Kluwer business; 2009. p. 7–66.
7. Sorrell JM, Caplan AI. Fibroblasts-a diverse population at the center of it all. Int Rev Cell Mol Biol. 2009;276:161–214.
8. Sorrell JM, Caplan AI. Fibroblast heterogeneity: more than skin deep. J Cell Sci. 2004;117(Pt 5):667–75.
9. Haass NK, Herlyn M. Normal human melanocyte homeostasis as a paradigm for understanding melanoma. J Investig Dermatol Symp Proc. 2005;10(2):153–63.
10. Haass NK, et al. Adhesion, migration and communication in melanocytes and melanoma. Pigment Cell Res. 2005;18(3):150–9.
11. Wessel C, et al. CD34(+) fibrocytes in melanocytic nevi and malignant melanomas of the skin. Virchows Arch. 2008;453(5):485–9.
12. Kacar A, et al. Stromal expression of CD34, alpha-smooth muscle actin and CD26/DPPIV in squamous cell carcinoma of the skin: a comparative immunohistochemical study. Pathol Oncol Res. 2012;18(1):25–31.
13. El-Khoury J, Kibbi AG, Abbas O. Mucocutaneous pseudoepitheliomatous hyperplasia: a review. Am J Dermatopathol. 2012;34(2):165–75.
14. Zayour M, Lazova R. Pseudoepitheliomatous hyperplasia: a review. Am J Dermatopathol. 2011;33(2):112–22. quiz 123–6.
15. Kacar A, et al. Stromal expression of CD34, alpha-smooth muscle actin and CD26/DPPIV in squamous cell carcinoma of the skin: a comparative immunohistochemical study. Pathol Oncol Res. 2011;18(1):25–31.
16. Korman NJ, Hrabovsky SL. Basal cell carcinomas display extensive abnormalities in the hemidesmosome anchoring fibril complex. Exp Dermatol. 1993;2(3):139–44.
17. Bahadoran P, et al. Altered expression of the hemidesmosome-anchoring filament complex proteins in basal cell carcinoma: possible role in the origin of peritumoral lacunae. Br J Dermatol. 1997;136(1):35–42.
18. Kirkham N. Tumors and cysts of the epidermis. In: Elder DE et al., editors. Lever's histopathology of the skin. Philadelphia: Lippincott Williams & Wilkins/a Wolters Kluwer business; 2009. p. 791–851.
19. Ulrich M, et al. Peritumoral clefting in basal cell carcinoma: correlation of in vivo reflectance confocal microscopy and routine histology. J Cutan Pathol. 2011;38(2):190–5.
20. Sellheyer K, Krahl D. Does the peritumoral stroma of basal cell carcinoma recapitulate the follicular connective tissue sheath? J Cutan Pathol. 2011;38(7):551–9.
21. Ackerman AB. Differentiation of benign from malignant neoplasms by silhouette. Am J Dermatopathol. 1989;11(4):297–300.
22. Ackerman AB, Böer A. Histopathologic diagnosis of adnexal epithelial neoplasms atlas and text. New York: Ardor Scribendi; 2008.
23. Tirumalae R, Roopa M. Benign vs. malignant skin adnexal neoplasms: how useful are silhouettes? Indian J Dermatol. 2013;58(1):30–3.
24. Hoang MP. Role of immunohistochemistry in diagnosing tumors of cutaneous appendages. Am J Dermatopathol. 2011;33(8):765–71. quiz 772–4.
25. Obaidat NA, Alsaad KO, Ghazarian D. Skin adnexal neoplasms–part 2: an approach to tumours of cutaneous sweat glands. J Clin Pathol. 2007;60(2):145–59.
26. Crowson AN, Magro CM, Mihm MC. Malignant adnexal neoplasms. Mod Pathol. 2006;19 Suppl 2:S93–126.
27. Schatton T, Frank MH. Cancer stem cells and human malignant melanoma. Pigment Cell Melanoma Res. 2008;21(1):39–55.
28. Epstein JI, Netto GJ. Biopsy interpretation of the prostate. Philadelphia: Lippincott Williams & Wilkins/a Wolters Kluwer business; 2008.
29. Umansky V, Sevko A. Melanoma-induced immunosuppression and its neutralization. Semin Cancer Biol. 2012;22(4):319–26.
30. Guo G, et al. Trp53 inactivation in the tumor microenvironment promotes tumor progression by expanding the immunosuppressive lymphoid-like stromal network. Cancer Res. 2013;73(6):1668–75.
31. Huang Y, et al. p53 regulates mesenchymal stem cell-mediated tumor suppression in a tumor microenvironment through immune modulation. Oncogene. 2014;33(29):3830–8.
32. Brandner JM, Haass NK. Melanoma's connections to the tumour microenvironment. Pathology. 2013;45(5):443–52.
33. Box NF, Vukmer TO, Terzian T. Targeting p53 in melanoma. Pigment Cell Melanoma Res. 2014;27(1):8–10.
34. Pierard GE, Pierard-Franchimont C, Delvenne P. Malignant melanoma and its stromal nonimmune microecosystem. J Oncol. 2012;2012:584219.
35. Mooi WJ, Krausz T. Chapter 9. Melanoma: general features. In: Pathology of melanocytic disorders. London: Hodder Arnold; 2007. p. 251–84.
36. Urso C, et al. Histological features used in the diagnosis of melanoma are frequently found in benign melanocytic nevi. J Clin Pathol. 2005;58(4):409–12.
37. Massi G, Leboit PE. Chapter 25. Criteria for the diagnosis of malignant melanoma. In: Histological diagnosis of nevi and melanoma. Darmstadt: Springer; 2004. p. 385–402.
38. Soo JK, et al. Malignancy without immortality? Cellular immortalization as a possible late event in melanoma progression. Pigment Cell Melanoma Res. 2011;24(3):490–503.
39. Bansal R, Nikiforov MA. Pathways of oncogene-induced senescence in human melanocytic cells. Cell Cycle. 2010;9(14):2782–8.
40. Bandyopadhyay D, et al. Dynamic assembly of chromatin complexes during cellular senescence: implications for the growth arrest of human melanocytic nevi. Aging Cell. 2007;6(4):577–91.

2 Soft Tissues

Key Morphological Features of Low-Grade Fibromyxoid Sarcoma

- Alternating fibrous and myxoid areas
- Random or whorled growth pattern (Figs. 2.1 and 2.2)

Discussion

Typically the tumor presents as well-circumscribed masses even though microscopic infiltration into the adjacent tissue is frequently present. Many cases of low-grade fibromyxoid sarcoma are located in the skeletal muscles indicating a possible derivation from the fibroblasts in the muscle associated fascia. As discussed in the skin and kidney sections, fibroblast heterogeneity is likely to a universal phenomenon as each tissue or organ has its unique mechanical and functional needs [1, 2].

In fact, the tumor is composed of bland spindle cells with low mitotic figures and no necrosis. The spindle cells are arranged in an alternating fibrous and myxoid pattern. The fibrous areas resemble the distribution of normal fibroblasts in the normal endomysium, whereas the myxoid areas correspond to the spaces occupied by muscle fibers in a muscle bundle. Ultrastructurally, the tumor cells show perineurial and myofibroblastic differentiation [3, 4]. Many cases are positive for EMA and cytokeratins [5, 6].

Differential Diagnosis

Myxoid Neurofibroma and Perineuroma

Myxoid neurofibroma cells are more spindly and wavy. The tumor cells are diffusely S100 positive. Perineuriomas typically lack myxoid areas, and the tumor cells are diffusely SMA positive.

Nodular Fasciitis

Nodular fasciitis is characterized by tissue culture fibroblasts, cleftlike spaces, and extravasation of red blood cells as well as a rapid clinical course.

Myxofibrosarcoma, Malignant Peripheral Nerve Sheath Tumor

Myxofibrosarcomas typically occur in the subcutaneous tissue in the old. The cells are more atypical and present in a uniform myxoid stroma.

Malignant peripheral nerve sheath tumor cells are more elongated and wavy. They are arranged in hypercellular fascicles and sheets.

Myxoma, Myxoid Liposarcoma, and Spindle Cell Liposarcoma

Myxomas lack the alternating fibrous and myxoid pattern as well as plexiform vessels. Myxoid and spindle cell liposarcomas have lipoblasts and lipoid background.

Myxoid DFSP

Dermatofibrosarcoma protuberans presents in superficial locations and contains storiform

X. Sun, *Well-Differentiated Malignancies: New Perspectives*, Current Clinical Pathology,
DOI 10.1007/978-1-4939-1692-4_2,

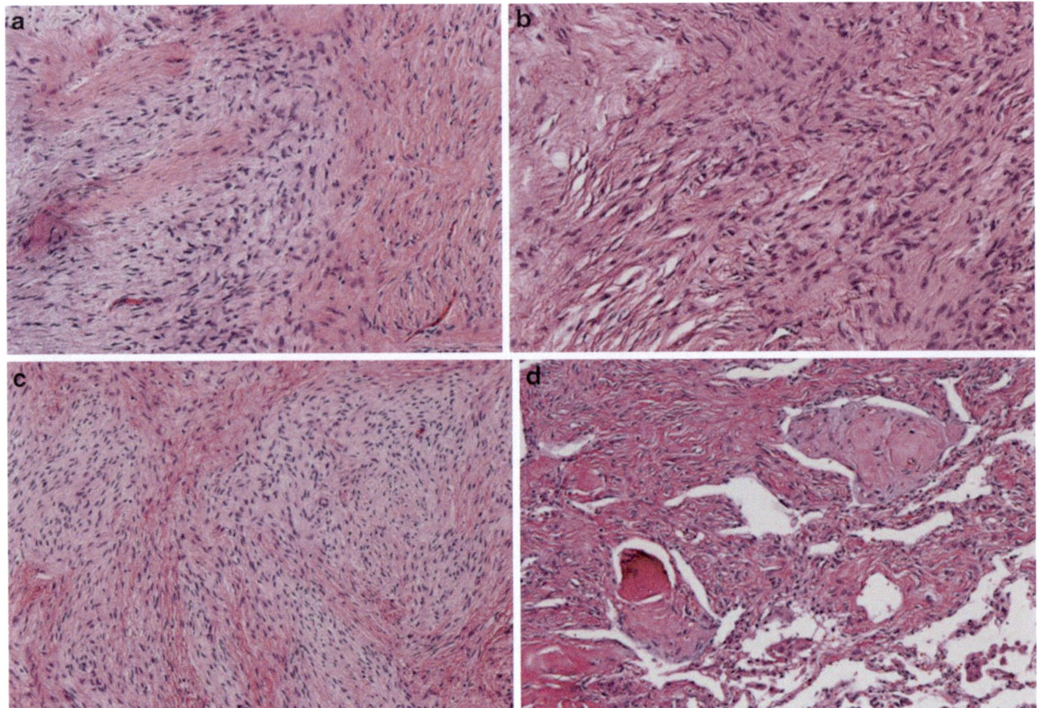

Fig. 2.1 Fibromyxoid sarcoma showing alternating fibrous and myxoid areas (American Journal of Surgical Pathology, *Wolters Kluwer/Lippincott Williams & Wilkins*, 2011 with permission)

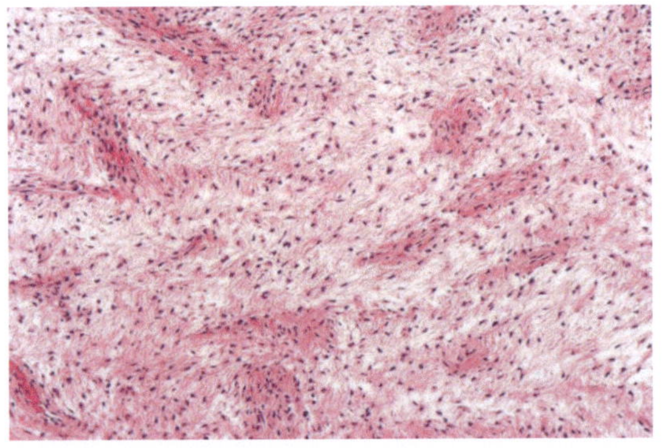

Fig. 2.2 Fibromyxoid sarcoma with random or whorled growth pattern and perivascular condensation (Enzinger & Weiss's Soft Tissue Tumors, *Elsevier/Saunders*, 2008 with permission)

arrangement of spindle cells which show CD34 positivity.

Key Morphological Features of Myxofibrosarcoma

- Multinodular pattern of spindle or stellate cells
- Diffuse Myxoid stroma with curvilinear vessels (Figs. 2.3, 2.4, and 2.5)

Discussion

Myxofibrosarcomas typically present in the subcutaneous tissue in the extremities of the elderly and manifest as vague nodules composed of spindle cells distributed in a myxoid stroma. In this myxoid background, elongated curvilinear capillaries are prominent. The tumor cells are frequently CD34 positive and show tendency to perivascular condensation. It is thus indicated that the tumor cells are probably related to the vascular adventitial cells [7, 8]. At ultrastructural level, myofibroblastic differentiation is evident [6].

Differential Diagnosis

Nodular Fasciitis

Nodular fasciitis has tissue culture-like fibroblastic and myofibroblastic proliferation. Although mitotic figures are readily evident, there is no cytological atypia. In addition, there are slitlike spaces, extravasation of red blood cells, and keloid-like collage bundles.

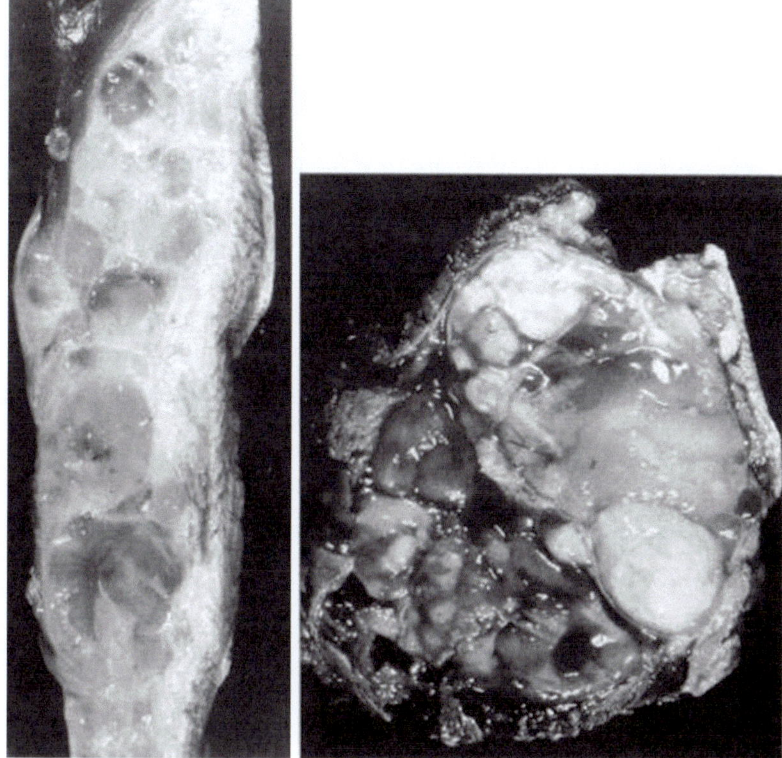

Fig. 2.3 Myxofibrosarcoma. Multinodular growth pattern (Enzinger & Weiss's Soft Tissue Tumors, *Elsevier/Saunders*, 2008; American Journal of Surgical Pathology, *Wolters Kluwer/Lippincott Williams & Wilkins*, 1996 with permission)

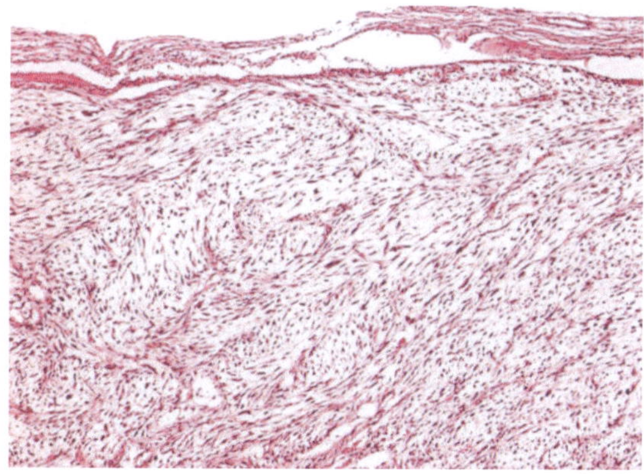

Fig. 2.4 Myxofibrosarcoma. Bland spindle or stellate cells (Enzinger & Weiss's Soft Tissue Tumors, *Elsevier/Saunders*, 2008 with permission)

Myxoid Liposarcoma

The tumor cells are more ovoid and the capillaries are more developed in myxoid liposarcoma. The tumor is usually deep seated and contains characteristic lipoblasts.

Myxoma, Nerve Sheath Myxoma, Myxoid Chondrosarcoma

Myxomas show less cellular atypia and mitotic activity and lack typical curvilinear vessels and perivascular condensation.

Myxoid chondrosarcomas also lack curvilinear capillaries. The tumor cells are round. The stroma is more chondroid with prominent hemorrhage.

Fibromyxoid Sarcoma

See differential diagnosis for fibromyxoid sarcoma.

Key Morphological Feature of Dermatofibrosarcoma Protuberans

- Monomorphic slender cells in a storiform pattern
- Diffuse infiltrative border (Figs. 2.6 and 2.7)

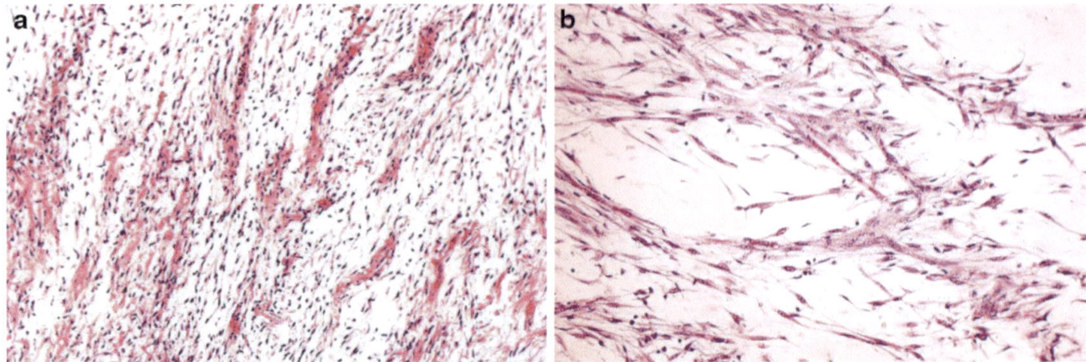

Fig. 2.5 Myxofibrosarcoma. Curvilinear vessels with perivascular condensation of tumor cells and myxoid stroma (Enzinger & Weiss's Soft Tissue Tumors, *Elsevier/Saunders*, 2008 with permission)

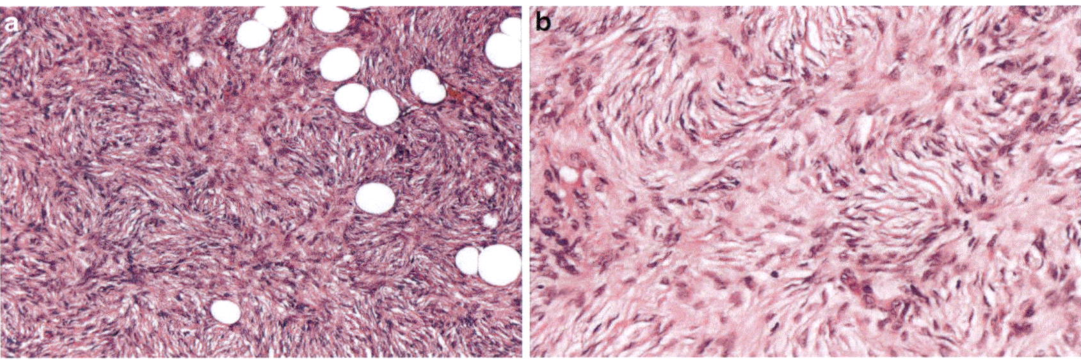

Fig. 2.6 Dermatofibrosarcoma protuberans. Monomorphic spindle cells in a storiform pattern (Enzinger & Weiss's Soft Tissue Tumors, *Elsevier/Saunders*, 2008 with permission)

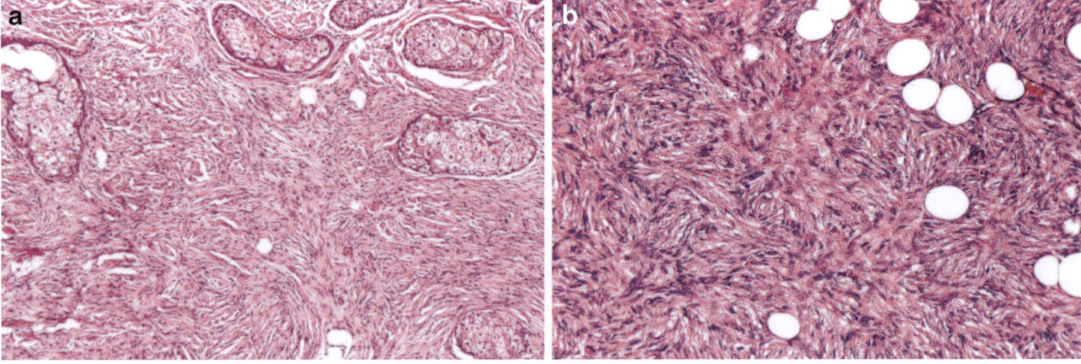

Fig. 2.7 Dermatofibrosarcoma protuberans. Infiltrative pattern (Enzinger & Weiss's Soft Tissue Tumors, *Elsevier/Saunders*, 2008 with permission)

Discussion

Whereas benign fibrohistiocytoma is related to the XIII- and CD10-positive dermal fibroblasts, dermatofibrosarcoma protuberans is derived from the CD34-positive dermal fibroblasts which manifest perineurial differentiation. The characteristic cartwheel (storiform) arrangement of tumor cells probably reflects the inherent cellular property to form a 3D mesh-like immunological barrier for the dermis.

Also included in the intermediate malignancy category of fibrohistiocytic tumors are angiomatoid fibrohistiocytoma and plexiform histiocytoma [9, 10]. The former actually represents a tumor of the lymph node stromal cell with characteristic cystic areas and chronic inflammatory infiltration. The intimate relationship between the fibroblasts and histiocytic cells in plexiform histiocytoma is different from that seen in most of other fibrohistiocytomas. Instead of having an admixture of both cellular components, the tumor is featured by nodules of histiocytic cells surrounded by fibroblastic fascicles.

Differential Diagnosis

Benign Fibrohistiocytoma

Typical benign fibrohistiocytomas are composed of admixed fibroblasts and xanthoma-like histiocytes with entrapped collagen and hemosiderin. This admixture indicates a unique relationship between these two phenotypic different cell types (through differentiation or attraction). The fibroblastic component is arranged in short, crisscrossing short fascicules. Multinucleated cells, chronic inflammatory cells, as well as cystic hemorrhage and associated changes are common features. Tentacular extensions can be seen at deep margin, but is focal.

Deep fibrohistiocytomas, however, are more cellular. Not only can they manifest a focal storiform pattern; there are also increased mitotic activities (up to 10/10HPF), a zone of necrosis, and even fat infiltration. In this case, immunostaining for factor XIII, CD10, and CD34 is very helpful in making the distinction.

Neurofibroma

The diffuse form of neurofibroma usually has areas showing neural differentiation. It lacks a storiform growth pattern, an infiltrative border, as well as high cellularity, mitotic index.

Key Morphological Features of Desmoid-Type Fibromatosis

- Bland-looking spindle cells in longitudinal fascicles in a nodular growth pattern
- Infiltrative border (Figs. 2.8 and 2.9)

Discussion

Deep fibromatosis has characteristic somatic beta-catenin or adenomatous polyposis coli (HPC) mutations which allow intranuclear accumulation of beta-catenin with resultant cell proliferation [11]. This important feature can be diagnostically useful.

Deep fibromatosis appears to be a tumor of the fibroblasts in the deep fascia. The typical long sweeping fascicules are composed of bland fibroblasts and are less cellular with less defined cell borders than the V-shaped fascicules characteristic of fibrosarcoma. These differences are probably a reflection of the different mechanical stresses in which fascia and tendons are programmed to withstand. Deep fascia tissue binds the muscle tissue with the adjacent tissue, and in doing so, it diffuses mechanical stress over a large area. Long sweeping fascicules are more suitable than herringbone-like structures for this purpose. The main function of a tendon is to concentrate the force generated by skeletal muscle tissue and transmit it to the bone. A V-shaped pattern seems to suit the purpose.

Differential Diagnosis

Reactive Fibroblastic/Myofibroblastic Lesions

The reactive lesions have less regularity in the arrangement of spindle cells and lack an infiltrative border. Frequently, they show focal hemorrhage and hemosiderin deposition.

Fibrosarcoma

Fibrosarcoma has become a rare diagnosis and one of exclusion. Typically it is composed of uniform spindle cells in a distinctive herringbone pattern. The nuclei are hyperchromatic with frequent overlapping.

Solitary Fibrous Tumor

Solitary fibrous tumor has the classical patternless pattern and high cellularity as well as hemangiopericytoma-like areas. The tumor cells are CD34 positive.

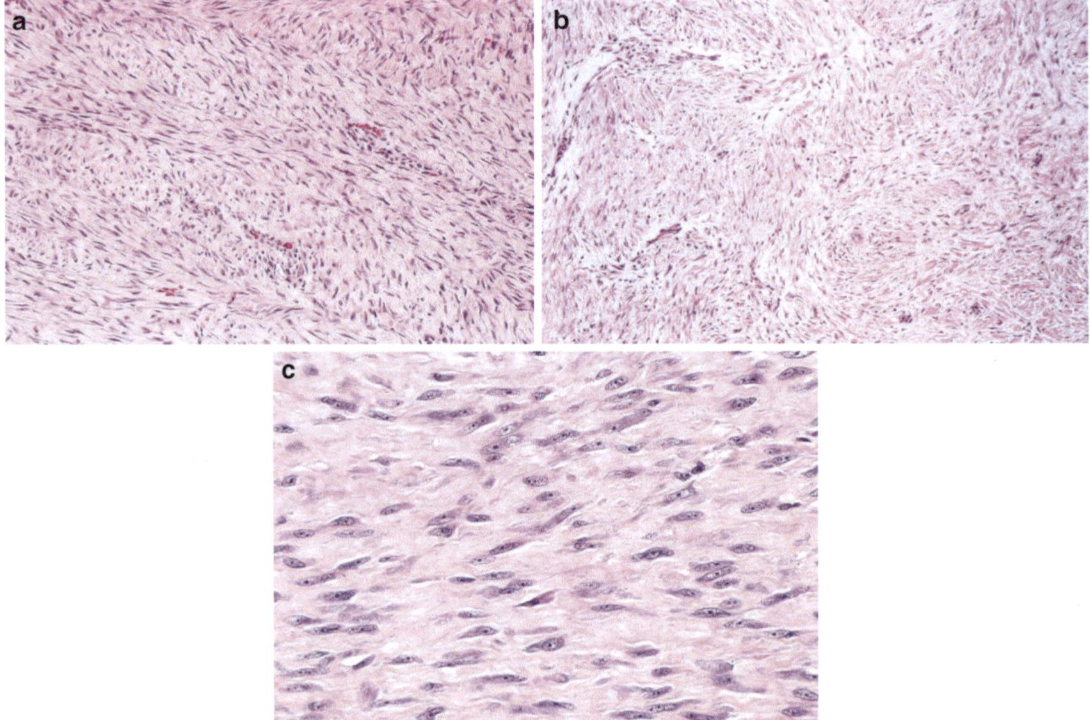

Fig. 2.8 Fibromatosis. Bland spindle cells in longitudinal fascicles (Enzinger & Weiss's Soft Tissue Tumors, *Elsevier/Saunders*, 2008 with permission)

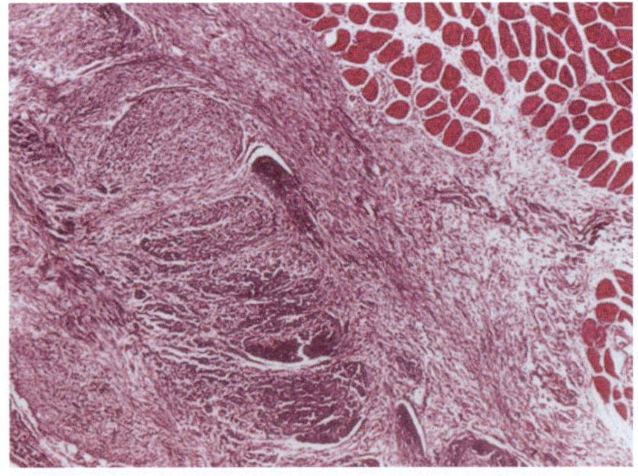

Fig. 2.9 Fibromatosis. Infiltrative border (Enzinger & Weiss's Soft Tissue Tumors, *Elsevier/Saunders*, 2008 with permission)

Desmoplastic Fibroma of Bone

Radiological information indicating the location in a bone is most helpful as it shares the morphological features with fibromatosis.

Morphological Features of Well-Differentiated Rhabdomyosarcoma

- Diffuse spindle cell lesion
- Presence of rhabdomyoblasts (Figs. 2.10 and 2.11)

Discussion

Primarily a pediatric sarcoma, rhabdomyosarcomas are far more common than rhabdomyomas. One unique feature of the sarcoma is that it often arises at sites where skeletal muscle is not a normal component or only scant.

In an analogy to lipogenesis, rhabdomyogenesis is a complex multistage process during which dramatic metamorphogenesis occurs. Stuck at various differentiation stages as a result of botched execution of the metamorphogenic drama.

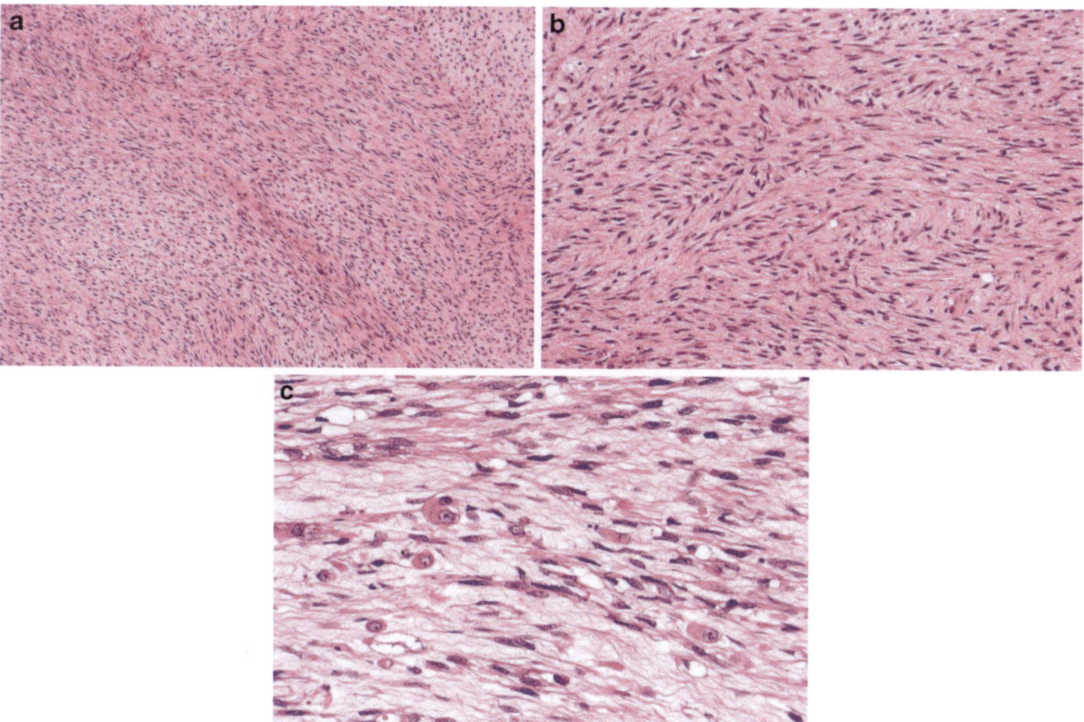

Fig. 2.10 Rhabdomyosarcoma. Spindle cells (**a**, **b**). Rhabdoblasts (**c**) (Enzinger & Weiss's Soft Tissue Tumors, *Elsevier/Saunders*, 2008 with permission)

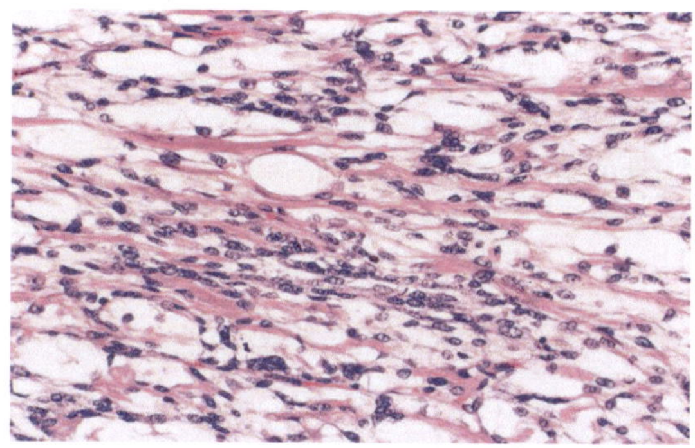

Fig. 2.11 Rhabdomyosarcoma. Rhabdoblasts (Enzinger & Weiss's Soft Tissue Tumors, *Elsevier/Saunders*, 2008 with permission)

Low-grade rhabdomyosarcoma includes the spindle cell and botryoid variants which bear resemblance to late-stage fetal myoblasts [12, 13].

In low-grade rhabdomyosarcoma (to some extent, embryonal variant also), identification of rhabdomyoblasts constitutes the most important aspect of making the diagnosis. There is a wide range of morphological variations for rhabdomyoblasts which might reflect the dramatic metamorphism in rhabdomyogenesis [14, 15]. Typically, they are spindle to plump cells with eosinophilic cytoplasm, cigar-shaped nuclei, and prominent nucleoli. Cross striations can be present, but is not required. Other shapes include ribbonlike, tadpole, racquet, spider, and broken straw.

Benign mimickers of rhabdomyoblasts are legion. They include macrophages, squamous cells, crystal-containing cells, and rhabdoid cells. Sometimes, immunostainings might be needed to ascertain the cell nature. To avoid confusing apoptotic cells for rhabdoblasts, the cell nuclei should be viable. To avoid calling entrapped muscle cells as rhabdoblasts, attention to the striation and nuclear feature offers help. In rhabdomyoblasts, the striation usually traverses only part of the cell which contains moderate to severe atypical nuclei with prominent nucleoli.

The botryoid variant is characterized by a cambium layer underneath a mucosa. The tumor cells range from primitive to stellate cells, to cells with clear-cut myoblastic differentiation and are distributed in a loosely cellular, myxoid stroma. The cambium layer is featured by the condensation of tumor cells which are separated from the mucosa by a zone of hypocellular stroma.

Differential Diagnosis

Fetal and Juvenile Rhabdomas

They are generally small, well-circumscribed, superficial lesions. The arrays of spindle cells interweave and form myxoid tubules. There is lack of rhabdomyoblasts.

Genital Rhabdomyoma

Genital rhabdomyoma presents as a polypoid mass covered by epithelium. It is differentiated from the botryoid variant sarcoma by the lack of a cambium layer, cytological atypia, and rhabdomyoblasts.

Leiomyomatous Lesion and Fibrosarcoma

These entities may be mimicked by spindle cell rhabdomyosarcoma. Typically, they lack rhabdomyoblasts. Sometimes, the differentiation can be revealed only with immunohistochemical stains.

Inflammatory Myofibroblastic Tumor

Inflammatory myofibroblastic tumor is usually vascular with a conspicuous inflammatory component. The tumor cells are spindle to stellar with a tissue culture-like appearance. They are ALK positive and in many cases show reactivity for AE1/AE3. There is lack of rhabdoblasts.

Reactive Spindle Cell Lesions

Pseudosarcomatous myofibroblastic proliferation occurs mainly in the genitourinary tract in patients who has had a history of recent procedure in the system. The lack of a cambium layer and rhabdomyoblasts helps make the distinction.

Proliferative Fasciitis and Myositis

These two closely related entities are characterized by proliferating spindle cells and large basophilic ganglion-like cells which might even be mitotically active. The ganglion-like cells lack striation and cytoplasmic basophilia. In questionable cases, immunostainings might be needed in differentiating them from rhabdomyoblasts. Rapid clinical history is another important clue to their benign nature.

Key Morphological Feature of Well-Differentiated Leiomyosarcoma

- Mild Cytological atypia
- Mitotic activity (>1/10 HPF) (Fig. 2.12)

Discussion

The histocytological features of leiomyomatous tumors reflect the fundamental function of the smooth muscle tissue: generation of

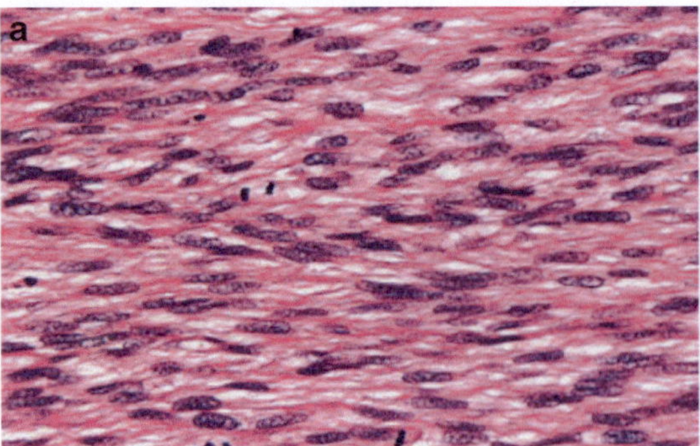

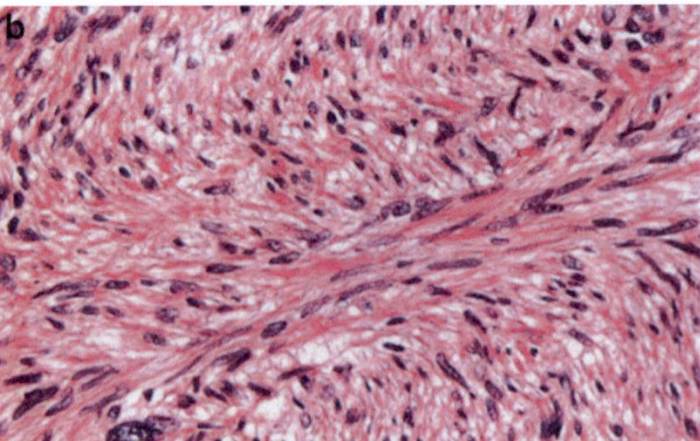

Fig. 2.12 Leiomyosarcoma. Mitotic figures and cytological atypia (Modern Pathology, *Nature Publishing Group*, 2014 with permission)

continuous, diffuse contraction of low force. The tumor cells are fusiform with centrally located cigar-shaped nuclei. Frequently, they show longitudinal striation and clumped myofilamentous material in the cytoplasm. Another important feature which may reveal the tumor's leiomyomatous nature is the presence of perinuclear glycogen vacuoles which might indent the nucleus. In well-differentiated tumors, the cells are typically arranged in fascicles intersecting at right angles, reminiscent of the longitudinal and circular layers in luminal organs.

In stark contrast to the criteria used for uterine leiomyosarcoma, the degree of atypia and mitotic activities for nonuterine leiomyosarcoma is much lower [16, 17]. Well-differentiated leiomyosarcoma might show mild cytological atypia, and the mitotic activity can be as low as 1/10 HPF. Necrosis is not a common feature of leiomyosarcoma except for the one in the retroperitoneal location where significant coagulative necrosis can occur.

Differential Diagnosis

Fibrosarcoma, Malignant Peripheral Nerve Sheath Tumor

Even though at low power, these spindle cells might resemble leiomyosarcoma, their cytological morphologies usually reveal their nonleiomyomatous nature. Fibrosarcomatous cells are tapered and arranged in a typical herringbone-like pattern. Cells in malignant peripheral nerve sheath tumor are wavy. Both types of tumor cells lack either longitudinal striation or clumped myofibrillar material.

Reactive Myofibroblastic Lesion

These reactive lesions are composed of poorly arranged bipolar or stellate cells with basophilic cytoplasm. Inflammatory infiltrates and sometimes bizzare nuclei are present.

Leiomyoma

Benign leiomyoma is differentiated from sarcoma by the lack of cytological atypia and rare mitotic activity (usually less than 1/50 HPF).

Key Morphological Features of Well-Differentiated Liposarcoma

- Lipoblasts or atypical stromal cells
- Mature adipose tissue (Figs. 2.13 and 2.14)

Discussion

Lipogenesis resembles rhabdomyogenesis in that both processes involve multiple stages during which dramatic morphological changes occur. The cellular stages include adipose stem cell, committed preadipocyte, lipoblast, and mature white adipocyte. The adult adipose tissue also contains multipotent stem cells which can differentiate into

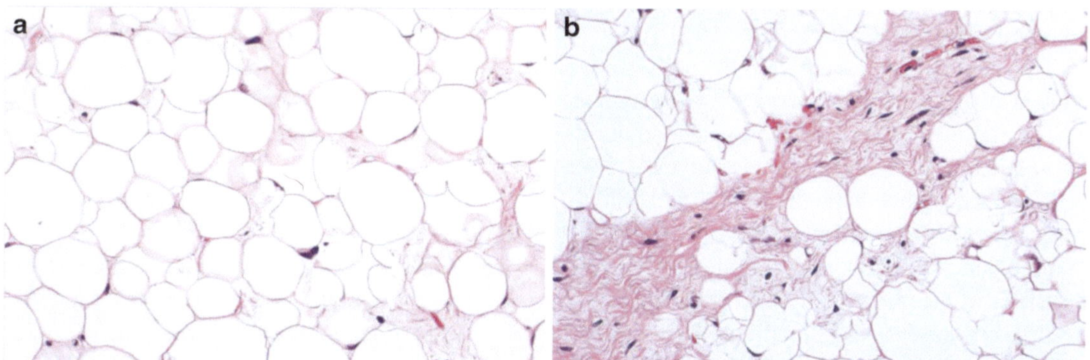

Fig. 2.13 Well-differentiated liposarcoma. Mature fat tissue, lipoblasts, and atypical stromal cells. Note variation in size of mature lipocytes (Enzinger & Weiss's Soft Tissue Tumors, *Elsevier/Saunders*, 2008 with permission)

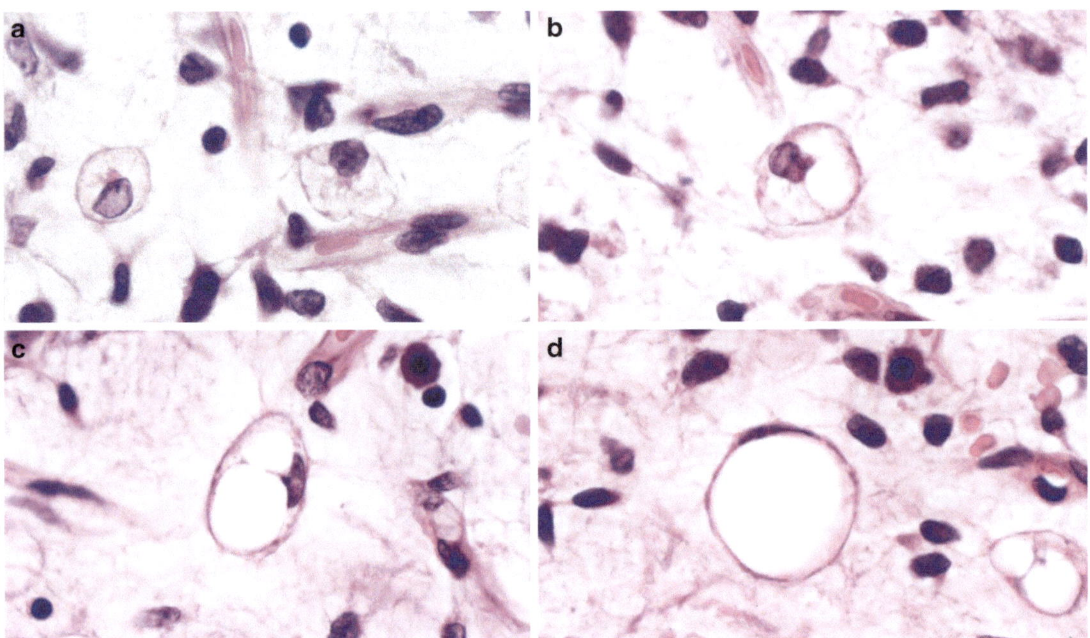

Fig. 2.14 Lipoblasts (Enzinger & Weiss's Soft Tissue Tumors, *Elsevier/Saunders*, 2008 with permission)

many other mesenchymal cell types [18, 19]. Even mature adipocytes could undergo dedifferentiation and transdifferentiation.

Analogous to the situation in rhabdomyosarcoma, the diagnosis of liposarcoma relies heavily on the identification of lipoblasts and/or atypical stromal cells (preadipocytes). The lipoblast criteria proposed by Dr. Weiss are very useful, and their strict application sorts out many mimickers which all have bubbly or vacuolar cytoplasm [20]. Basically, the criteria require the presence of (1) a hyperchromatic or sharply scalloped nucleus; (2) lipid drops in the cytoplasm; and (3) an appropriate histological context.

The nuclear atypia for spindle cells in the context of a lipomatous lesion needs to be specifically defined to exclude multinucleated floret-like cells and multinucleated histiocytes. These cells can be highly hyperchromatic and mitotically active. Multinucleated floret-like cells are the hallmark of pleomorphic lipoma. To make a diagnosis of pleomorphic liposarcoma, lipoblasts need to be present. The spindle cells in spindle cell lipoma are bland and produce ropy collagen. Lack of cytological atypia and lipoblasts separates it from spindle cell liposarcoma.

In difficult cases, immunostainings for CD34, CDk4, and MDM2 can be helpful. Lipoblast and atypical spindle cells are positive for CD34, whereas CDk4 and MDM2 stains help light up the atypical spindle cells [20, 21].

Differential Diagnosis

Benign Lipomas

(Hibernoma spindle cell lipoma, pleomorphic lipoma, chondroid lipoma intramuscular lipoma)

These benign entities can be easily differentiated from liposarcoma if the lipoblast criteria are applied strictly and the multinucleated cells are left out of the picture in the evaluation of cytological atypia for spindle cells.

Fat Necrosis, Lipogranuloma, Reactive Fatty Changes

These reactive entities may produce cells mimicking both lipoblasts and atypical spindle cells. Thus, strict application of the criteria is key. The right histological context such as superficial location, inflammatory cells, and granuloma might provide a clue to their benignity. However, it is helpful to know that lipomatous lesions can also be superimposed by reactive changes.

Key Morphological Features of Well-Differentiated Angiosarcoma

- Anastomosing and dissecting irregular vascular proliferation
- Lack of pericytes (Fig. 2.15)

Key Morphological Features of Epithelioid Hemangioendothelioma

- Vascular proliferation with intracytoplasmic lumen formation (Fig. 2.16)

Key Morphological Features of Kaposi Sarcoma

- Irregular-shaped slit-like spaces
- Spindle cells and lymphocytes (Fig.. 2.17)

Discussion

Vasculogenesis and Angiogenesis

Vasculogenesis and angiogenesis are complex processes which involve two mechanisms in the lumen formation: cord hollowing and cell hollowing [22–25]. In both mechanisms, a functional and architectural coupling between the endothelial cells and pericytes is essential. Not only do the pericytes facilitate endothelial cell proliferation, survival, and stabilization; they also exert inhibitory effects on the growth, migration, and other functions of the endothelial cells [26]. Lymphangiogenesis involves seemingly different mechanisms from the blood vessels in that the lymphatic endothelial cells interact directly with the extracellular matrix [27–29]. As a result, no pericytes nor basement membrane is present in capillary lymphatics.

Angiosarcoma

In angiosarcoma, the malignant endothelial cells lose the ability to couple with pericytes with resultant unbridled cellular proliferation and migration. Well-differentiated angiosarcoma

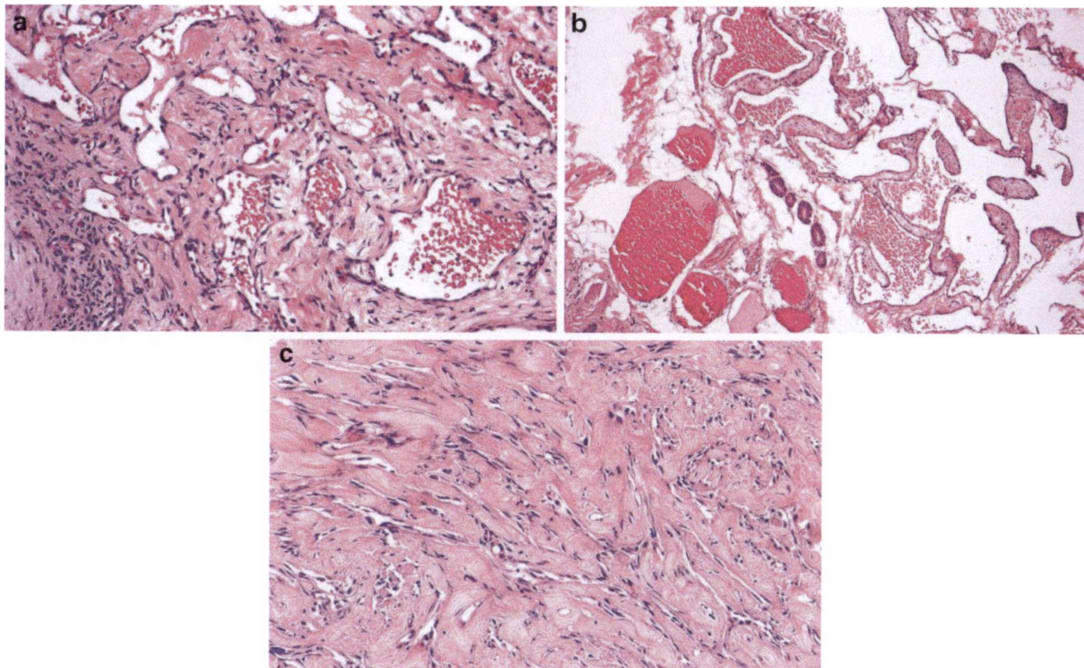

Fig. 2.15 Well-differentiated angiosarcoma. Anastomosing vessel channels with no pericytes (Enzinger & Weiss's Soft Tissue Tumors, *Elsevier/Saunders*, 2008 with permission)

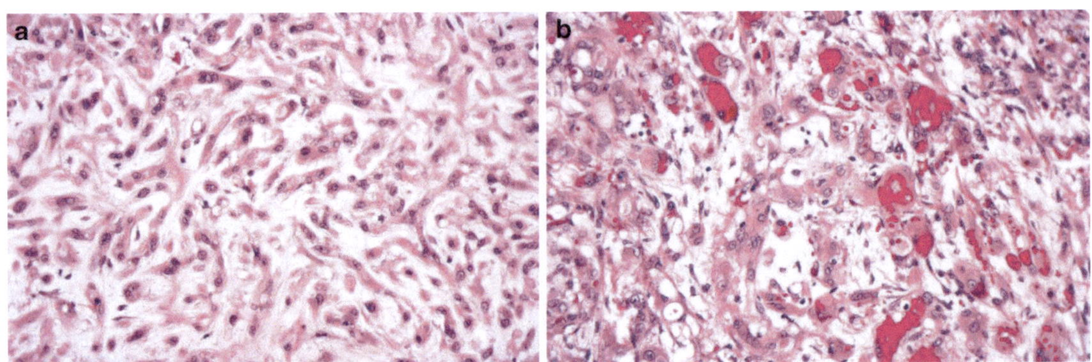

Fig. 2.16 Epithelioid hemangioendothelioma. Intracytoplasmic lumens (Enzinger & Weiss's Soft Tissue Tumors, *Elsevier/Saunders*, 2008 with permission)

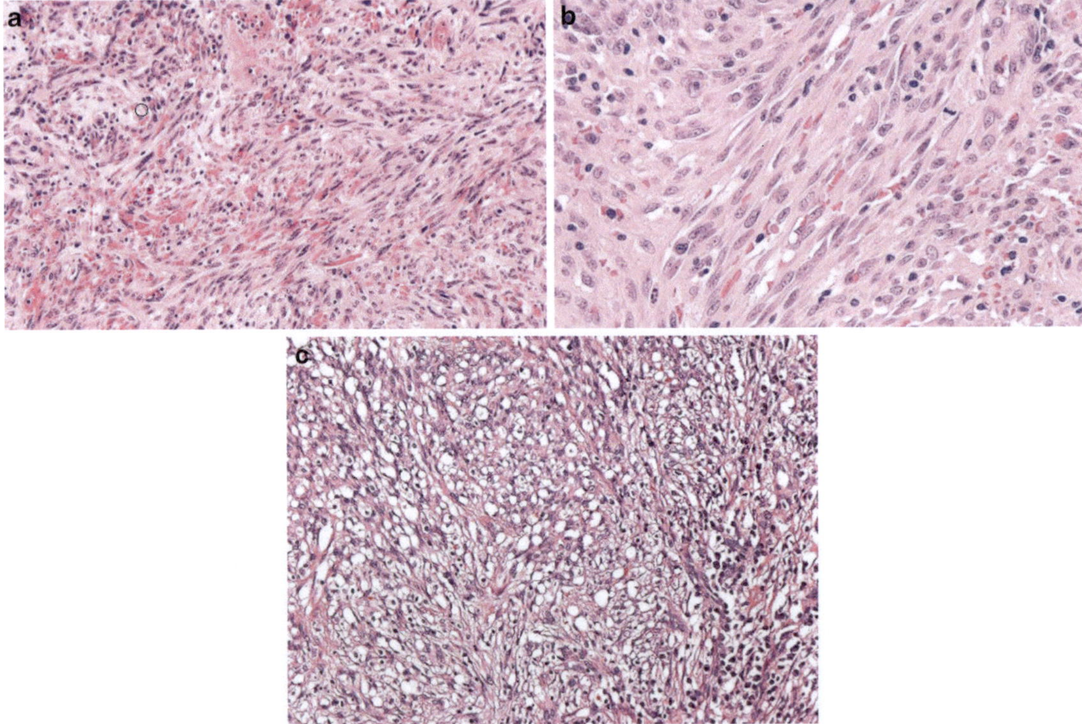

Fig. 2.17 Kaposi sarcoma. Spindle cells, slit-like spaces, and lymphocytes (Enzinger & Weiss's Soft Tissue Tumors, *Elsevier/Saunders*, 2008 with permission)

contains vascular structures which are irregular and haphazardly arranged. The vascular channels interconnect and dissect into the connective or fat tissue. The endothelial cells are invested by minimal basement membrane material and lack accompanying pericytes. Even though pericytes have been reported in poorly differentiated angiosarcoma, they are focal and lack the normal apposition as evidenced in normal vessels [30–33].

Hemangioendothelioma

Hemangioendothelioma includes several histological variants which might be reflective of endothelial heterogeneity, a phenomenon which has gained steady recognition [28, 34]. Apparently, the cell hollowing mechanism is activated in the tumor pathogenesis without much participation of pericytes. Typical epithelioid hemangioendothelioma consists of cord and nests of endothelial cells with intracytoplasmic vacuoles (lumens). Even though the Dabska–retiform variant often seems to show an intraluminal growth pattern, the lack of pericytes, lymphocytic infiltration, and even lymphatic markers indicate a lymphatic differentiation. The lack of pericytes (with exception of kaposiform hemangioendothelioma) probably plays a role in the formation of papillary intravascular proliferations with matchstick arrangement of endothelial cells and gaping retiform vessels lined by hobnail cells. Occasional intracytoplasmic vacuoles and hobnail cells are consistent with the involvement of both mechanisms

Kaposi Sarcoma

Kaposi sarcoma represents reprogramming of blood vessel endothelium toward lymphatic endothelial phenotype by the Kaposi sarcoma virus [31, 33]. This reprogramming lacks the involvement of pericytes and probably involves the activation of both lumen-forming mechanisms. The lack of pericyte involvement and proper extracellular matrix results in the slit- like vascular lumens formed by spindle cells. The characteristic hyaline globules represent intracytoplasmic red blood cells that are incompletely digested.

Differential Diagnosis

For Angiosarcoma

Hemangioma

Under this umbrella of hemangioma, many overlapping categories exist based on different parameters such as the vessel type, cell morphology, location, and the nature of the proliferation. In general, it is composed of well-formed blood vessels containing both endothelial cells and pericytes. It lacks the dissecting and anastomosing growth pattern characteristic of well-differentiated angiosarcoma.

Papillary Endothelial Hyperplasia

Papillary endothelial hyperplasia contains many small papillae projecting a vascular lumen as a result of endothelial proliferation into an organizing thrombus. The presence of numerous small papillae and their subsequent fusion and clumping can result in an anastomosing pattern. However, its intravascular nature and lack of endothelial layering point to the right diagnosis. In cases where the proliferation extends outside of the vessel or presents entirely outside of vessel lumen as a result of organizing hematoma, an immunostaining for pericytes (SMA) may offer some help.

For Hemangioendothelioma

Hobnail Hemangioma

It contains dilated vessels lined by hobnail endothelial cell with occasional intraluminal papillary tufts. The deeper portions may contain slitlike vessels which ramify in the dermis. Hemorrhage and hemosiderin deposits as well as lymphocytes and dermal sclerosis are important clues to the lesion. The endothelial cells are positive for D2-40 and VEGFR3.

Epithelioid Hemangioma

This lesion has large number of capillary vessels, many of which are composed of endothelial cells with abundant cytoplasm. The epithelioid cells can form intraluminal clusters or solid structures. It can be differentiated from epithelioid hemangioendothelioma by well-formed vascular lumens, the presence of pericytes, and lack of intracellular vacuoles. Prominent inflammatory component is another feature. The inflammatory component can form germinal centers and contain increased number of eosinophils.

For Kaposi Sarcoma

Spindle Cell Hemangioma

Spindle cell hemangioma contains cavernous vessels lined by flat endothelial cells. The intervening stroma is interspersed by spindle and epithelioid cells. The spindle areas might represent occluded vessels. Vacuoles or intracytoplasmic lumens can be seen in the epithelioid cells.

Fibrosarcoma

Fibrosarcoma can resemble the highly cellular form of Kaposi sarcoma. However, it lacks the slitlike vessels and a frequent inflammatory infiltration. In addition, the spindle cells are arranged in a characteristic V-shaped pattern instead of curvilinear fascicles. There is no hyaline globules nor intracytoplasmic vacuoles.

Kaposiform Hemangioendothelioma

This tumor occurs primarily in the children and adolescents and contains alternating areas resembling Kaposi sarcoma and hemangioma. It also has characteristic glomeruloid structures which are surrounded by pericytes. In difficult cases, an immunostaining for HHV-8 can be employed.

Vascular Transformation of Lymph Nodes

In vascular transformation of lymph nodes, there is expansion of capillary vessels in the subcapsular and medullary sinuses. There is neither cellular spindling nor slitlike vessels.

References

1. Sorrell JM, Caplan AI. Fibroblast heterogeneity: more than skin deep. J Cell Sci. 2004;117(Pt 5):667–75.
2. Sorrell JM, Caplan AI. Fibroblasts-a diverse population at the center of it all. Int Rev Cell Mol Biol. 2009;276:161–214.
3. Zamecnik M, Michal M. Low-grade fibromyxoid sarcoma: a report of eight cases with histologic, immunohistochemical, and ultrastructural study. Ann Diagn Pathol. 2000;4(4):207–17.
4. Antonescu CR, Baren A. Spectrum of low-grade fibrosarcomas: a comparative ultrastructural analysis of low-grade myxofibrosarcoma and fibromyxoid sarcoma. Ultrastruct Pathol. 2004;28(5–6):321–32.
5. Weiss SW, Goldblum JR. Chapter 11. Fibrosarcoma. In: Enzinger & Weiss's soft tissue tumors. Philadelphia: Mosby/Elsevier; 2008. p. 303–30.
6. Miettinen M. Chapter 13. Fibroblastic and myofibroblastic neoplasms with malignant potential. In: Miettinen M, editor. Modern soft tissue pathology: tumors and non-neoplastic conditions. New York: Cambridge University Press; 2010. p. 348–92.
7. Crisan M, et al. Perivascular cells for regenerative medicine. J Cell Mol Med. 2012;16(12):2851–60.
8. Armulik A, Genove G, Betsholtz C. Pericytes: developmental, physiological, and pathological perspectives, problems, and promises. Dev Cell. 2011;21(2): 193–215.
9. Fanburg-Smith JC, Miettinen M. Angiomatoid "malignant" fibrous histiocytoma: a clinicopathologic study of 158 cases and further exploration of the myoid phenotype. Hum Pathol. 1999;30(11): 1336–43.
10. Hollowood K, Holley MP, Fletcher CD. Plexiform fibrohistiocytic tumour: clinicopathological, immunohistochemical and ultrastructural analysis in favour of a myofibroblastic lesion. Histopathology. 1991;19(6): 503–13.
11. Weiss SW, Goldblum JR. Chapter 9. Fibromatosis. In: Enzinger & Weiss's soft tissue tumors. Philadelphia: Mosby/Elsevier; 2008. p. 227–56.
12. De Giovanni C, et al. Molecular and cellular biology of rhabdomyosarcoma. Future Oncol. 2009;5(9): 1449–75.
13. Saab R, Spunt SL, Skapek SX. Myogenesis and rhabdomyosarcoma the Jekyll and Hyde of skeletal muscle. Curr Top Dev Biol. 2011;94:197–234.
14. Weiss SW, Goldblum JR. Chapter 21. Rhabdomyosarcoma. In: Enzinger & Weiss's soft tissue tumors. Philadelphia: Mosby/Elsevier; 2008. p. 595–632.
15. Prasad V, et al. Chapter 20. Rhabdoma and rhabdomyosarcoma. In: Miettinen M, editor. Modern soft tissue pathology: tumors and non-neoplastic conditions. New York: Cambridge University Press; 2010. p. 546–73.
16. Prasad V. Chapter 16. Smooth muscle tumors. In: Miettinen M, editor. Modern soft tissue pathology: tumors and non-neoplastic conditions. New York: Cambridge University Press; 2010. p. 460–90.
17. Weiss SW, Goldblum JR. Chapter 18. Leiomyosarcoma. In: Enzinger & Weiss's soft tissue tumors. Philadelphia: Mosby/Elsevier; 2008. p. 545–64.
18. Cawthorn WP, Scheller EL, MacDougald OA. Adipose tissue stem cells meet preadipocyte commitment: going back to the future. J Lipid Res. 2012;53(2): 227–46.
19. Sarjeant K, Stephens JM. Adipogenesis. Cold Spring Harb Perspect Biol. 2012;4(9):a008417.
20. Weiss SW, Goldblum JR. Chapter 16. Liposaroma. In: Enzinger & Weiss's soft tissue tumors. Philadelphia: Mosby/Elsevier; 2008. p. 477–516.
21. Miettinen M. Chapter 15. Atypical lipomatous tumor and liposarcoma. In: Miettinen M, editor. Modern soft tissue pathology: tumors and non-neoplastic conditions. New York: Cambridge University Press; 2010. p. 432–59.
22. Kassmeyer S, et al. New insights in vascular development: vasculogenesis and endothelial progenitor cells. Anat Histol Embryol. 2009;38(1):1–11.
23. Davis GE, et al. Molecular basis for endothelial lumen formation and tubulogenesis during vasculogenesis and angiogenic sprouting. Int Rev Cell Mol Biol. 2011;288:101–65.
24. Lammert E, Axnick J. Vascular lumen formation. Cold Spring Harb Perspect Med. 2012;2(4):a006619.
25. Kamei M, et al. Endothelial tubes assemble from intracellular vacuoles in vivo. Nature. 2006;442 (7101):453–6.
26. Ribatti D, Nico B, Crivellato E. The role of pericytes in angiogenesis. Int J Dev Biol. 2011;55(3):261–8.

27. Tammela T, Alitalo K. Lymphangiogenesis: molecular mechanisms and future promise. Cell. 2010;140(4): 460–76.
28. Aird WC. Endothelial cell heterogeneity. Cold Spring Harb Perspect Med. 2012;2(1):a006429.
29. Choi I, Lee S, Hong YK. The new era of the lymphatic system: no longer secondary to the blood vascular system. Cold Spring Harb Perspect Med. 2012;2(4): a006445.
30. Meis-Kindblom JM, Kindblom LG. Angiosarcoma of soft tissue: a study of 80 cases. Am J Surg Pathol. 1998;22(6):683–97.
31. Miettinen M. Chapter 22. Hemangioendotheliomas, angiosarcomas and Kaposi sarcoma. In: Miettinen M, editor. Modern soft tissue pathology: tumors and non-neoplastic conditions. New York: Cambridge University Press; 2010. p. 617–47.
32. Weiss SW, Goldblum JR. Chapter 23. Hemangioendothelioma: vascular tumors of intermediate malignancy. In: Enzinger & Weiss's soft tissue tumors. Philadelphia: Mosby/Elsevier; 2008. p. 681–702.
33. Weiss SW, Goldblum JR. Chapter 24. Malignant vascular lesions. In: Enzinger & Weiss's soft tissue tumors. Philadelphia: Mosby/Elsevier; 2008. p. 703–32.
34. Requena L, Kutzner H. Hemangioendothelioma. Semin Diagn Pathol. 2013;30(1):29–44.

Skeletal System

3

Overview

During the embryonal stage, two types of ossification mechanism are involved. In the endochondral process, ossification starts on the framework of prefabricated chondroid tissue. This type of ossification also forms the basis for bone elongation and callus formation. The osteogenic and chondrogenic processes are so intricately connected that both osteoid and chondroid components are often seen in osteoid forming and chondroid tumors, benign or malignant.

The normal bone homeostasis features constant modeling and remodeling which is a result of concerted efforts of the three key elements (osteogenic progenitors, osteoclasts, and sinusoids) of the hematopoietic microenvironment [1–3]. Benign bone-forming tissue (also chondroid tissue) respects the sinusoid stroma as well as the adjacent benign trabeculae. Malignant osteoid (also chondroid) tissue gains bone matrix absorbing capability which is normally the domain of osteoclasts [4, 5]. This gain of function gives rise to the permeative growth pattern characteristic of malignant osteosarcoma and chondrosarcoma. In permeative growth pattern, the malignant matrix-forming tissue fills the bone marrow cavity and occasionally entraps and destroys preexisting benign trabeculae.

Malignant osteoid is defined as osteoid tissue that is rimmed by stromal cells and/or layers of osteoblasts [6] (Fig. 3.1). When chondroid component is present, the malignant nature of the osteoid can be revealed by the altered interaction pattern. Malignant osteoid is randomly distributed in chondroid lobules (Fig. 3.2). This is in contrast to the peripheral arrangement evidenced in benign tissue. This important feature can be very useful in the differentiation of chondrosarcoma and chondroblastic osteosarcoma. In the former, the reactive (benign) bone formation is in the form of attenuated semicircles which surround the malignant chondroid tissue (Fig. 3.3). In the latter, the chondroid lobules are in direct contact with sheets of spindle cells which produce lacelike osteoid. The lacelike osteoid tissue is scattered throughout the chondroid lobule.

Morphological Features of Low-Grade Osteosarcoma

- Bone trabeculae lined by interlacing fascicles of spindle cells
- Permeative growth pattern (Figs. 3.4 and 3.5)

Discussion

Low-grade osteosarcoma is characterized by a permeative growth pattern of well-formed bony trabeculae which are rimmed by spindle cells [6].

Surface osteosarcomas are apparently derived from osteogenic stromal cells located outside the medullary cavity [6]. Strictly speaking, periosteal

X. Sun, *Well-Differentiated Malignancies: New Perspectives*, Current Clinical Pathology,
DOI 10.1007/978-1-4939-1692-4_3,

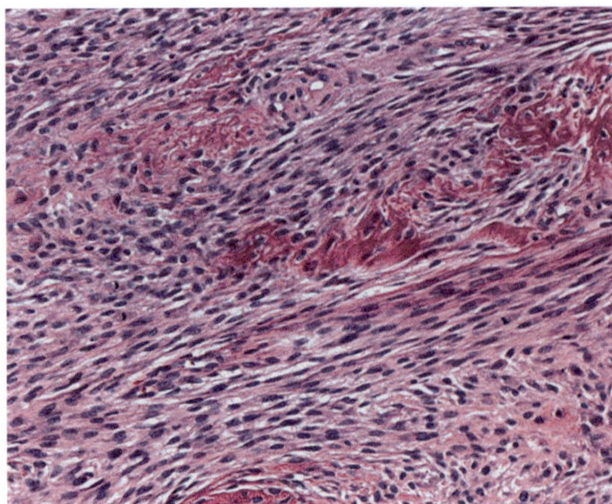

Fig 3.1 Malignant osteoid. Note the rimming by spindle stromal cells (Tumors of the Bones and Joints, *Armed Force Institute of Pathology/American Registry of Pathology*, 2005 with permission)

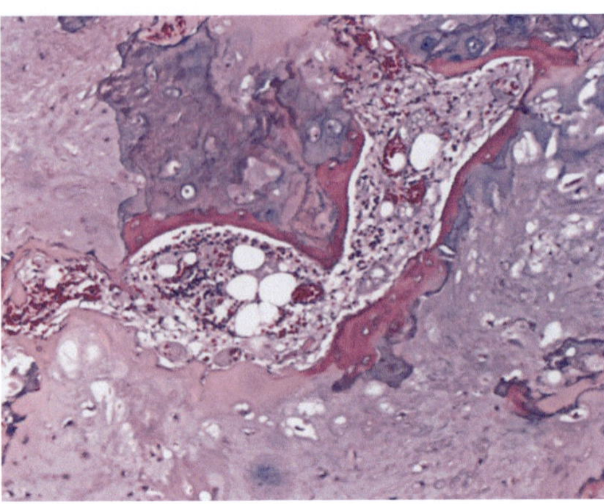

Fig 3.3 Reactive bone (osteoid). Attenuated semicircles surround malignant chondroid tissue (Tumors of the Bones and Joints, *Armed Force Institute of Pathology/ American Registry of Pathology*, 2005 with permission)

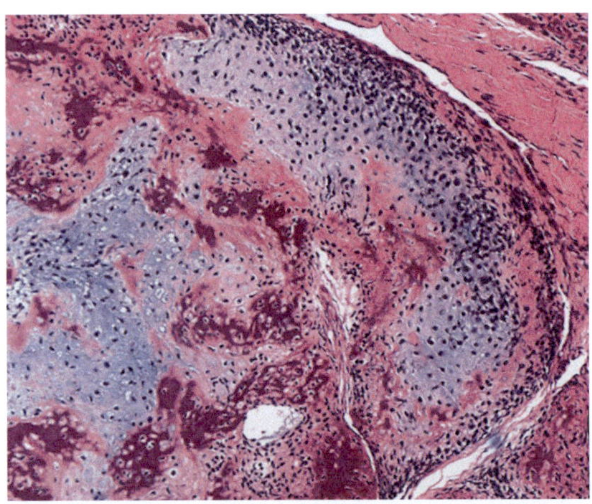

Fig 3.2 Malignant osteoid. Note randomness in the distribution of osteoid material in a chondroid lobule (Tumors of the Bones and Joints, *Armed Force Institute of Pathology/ American Registry of Pathology*, 2005 with permission)

osteosarcoma is considered moderately differentiated. It is included in this book along with parosteal osteosarcoma. These two entities have some differences from the medullary osteosarcoma which reflects their respective stem cell location and properties. Therefore, the criteria for medullary osteosarcoma need to be modified. For instance, the tumor stroma is usually less cellular in parosteal variant, whereas periosteal osteosarcoma has no medullary involvement at all.

Periosteal osteosarcoma involves the diaphysis and has no medullary involvement (Fig. 3.6). It represents as a well-circumscribed chondroid mass with limited capability to erode the underlying cortical bone. The malignant osteoid presents in the center of chondroid lobules in a feather-like pattern rather than rimming them as in reactive bone formation [6] (Fig. 3.7). The chondroblastic cell shows peripheral condensation and spindling. This tumor probably arises from an osteogenic stem cell located at periosteum. This is in contrast to the arrangement in osteochondroma in which the orderly benign chondroid–osteoid relationship is maintained. The chondrocytes at the tumor base are arranged in columns resembling the normal growth plate.

Parosteal osteosarcoma typically involves the metaphysis of long bones (Fig. 3.8). It is lobulated with occasional cartilage nodules. However, invasion into the adjacent muscles and the medullary cavity is frequently seen. In those cases with no gross medullary involvement, microscopic involvement can be identified. The chondroid nodules are interspersed by osteoid trabeculae which are broad and in parallel to each other [7]. In some cases, a cartilaginous cap might be present. The cells, however, are randomly distributed and lack the columnar arrangement as seen in osteochondroma. The tumor

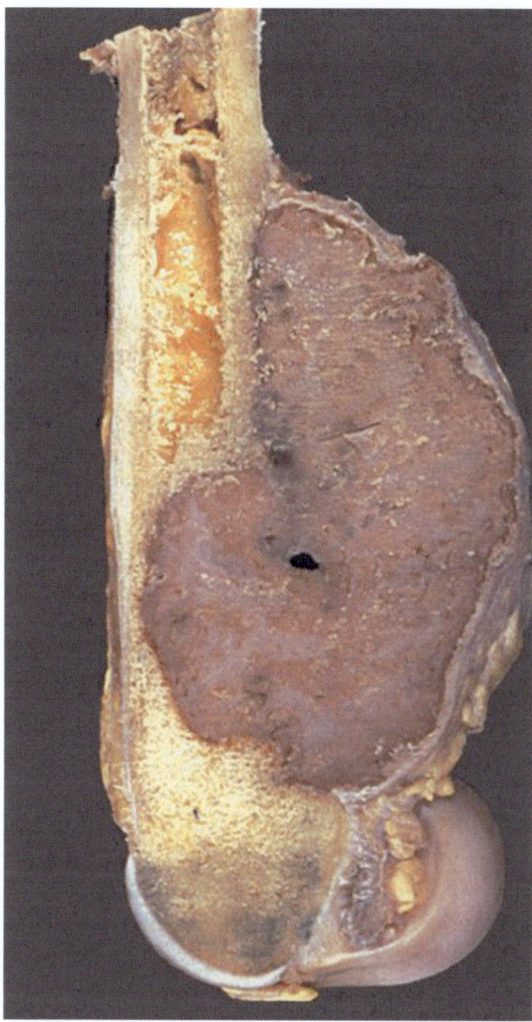

Fig. 3.4 Low-grade osteosarcoma (Tumors of the Bones and Joints, *Armed Force Institute of Pathology/American Registry of Pathology*, 2005 with permission)

stroma is less cellular than that of medullary osteosarcoma (Fig. 3.9). This tumor is likely to have its derivation from an osteogenic stem cell located in the growth plate.

Differential Diagnosis

Osteoid Osteoma, Osteoblastoma

These two entities have similar histological presentations, with tumor size being the only difference. Their anastomosing bony trabeculae are rimmed by one layer of osteoblasts and loose stroma. Permeative growth pattern is lacking. Probably because of the long duration of benign osteoid tumors, chondroid tissue is infrequently seen. However, when it is present, the chondroid lobules tend to be rimmed by osteoid trabeculae.

Osteochondroma

Osteochondroma maintains the benign chondroid–osteoid relationship evident in normal endochondral ossification. In addition, the chondrocytes at the tumor base show orderly columnar arrangement. The cavities between the bony trabeculae are filled with normal bone marrow tissue.

Desmoplastic Fibroma and Fibrous Dysplasia

Desmoplastic fibroma is a spindle cell lesion which produces no osteoid matrix. Instead, abundant collagen material is evident. The tumor stroma is less cellular and lacks fasciculation.

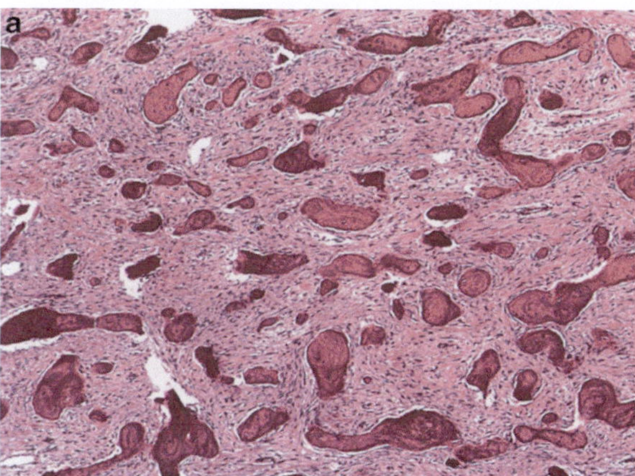

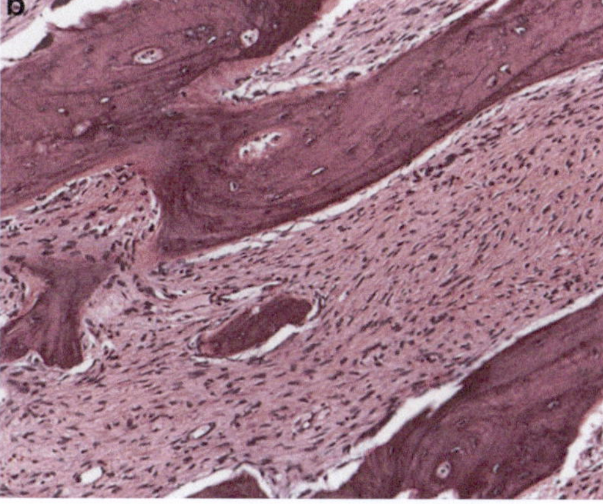

Fig. 3.5 Low-grade osteosarcoma. Permeative growth pattern by interlacing fascicles of spindle cells (Tumors of the Bones and Joints, *Armed Force Institute of Pathology/American Registry of Pathology*, 2005 with permission)

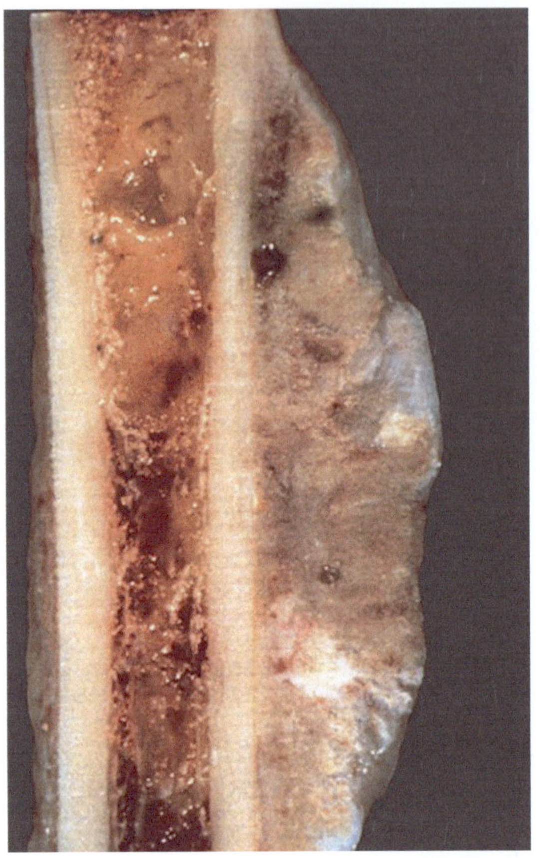

Fig. 3.6 Periosteal osteosarcoma. Tumor involves the diaphysis with no medullary involvement (Tumors of the Bones and Joints, *Armed Force Institute of Pathology/American Registry of Pathology*, 2005 with permission)

Fibrous dysplasia is osteoid producing; however, the stroma is also hypocellular. The bony spicules are well circumscribed and nonpermeative. Rimming osteoblasts are lacking.

Chondrosarcoma

Chondrosarcoma differs from osteosarcoma by the lack of malignant osteoid tissue. The permeative material is malignant chondroid lobules. Reactive bone formation should not be interpreted as malignant osteoid.

Key Morphological Features of Low-Grade Chondrosarcoma

- Increased cellularity, binucleation
- Permeation of medullary cavity (Figs. 3.10 and 3.11)

Discussion

Low-grade chondrosarcoma can be diagnosed by increased cellularity, binucleation, and a permeative growth pattern. A permeative growth pattern needs to be emphasized as increased cellularity is a quite objective index. Moreover, enchondromas in small bones can have increased cellularity and

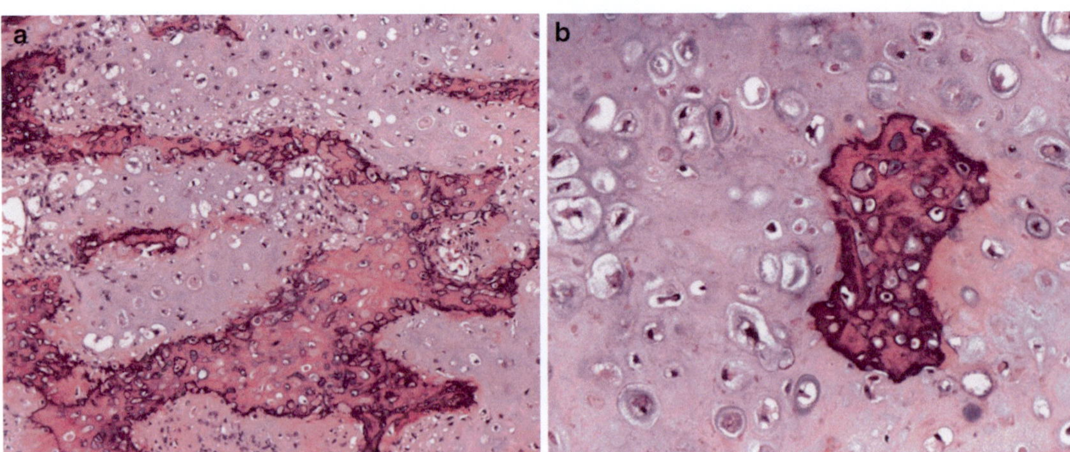

Fig. 3.7 Periosteal osteosarcoma. Chondroid material is studied with malignant osteoid material (Tumors of the Bones and Joints, *Armed Force Institute of Pathology/American Registry of Pathology*, 2005 with permission)

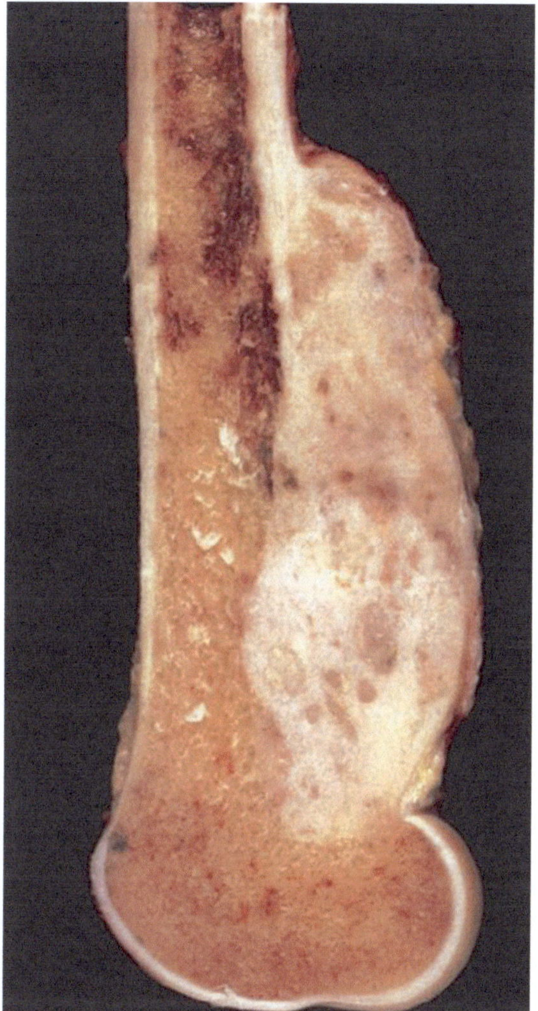

Fig. 3.8 Parosteal osteosarcoma. Tumor involves the metaphysis with medullary involvement (Tumors of the Bones and Joints, *Armed Force Institute of Pathology/American Registry of Pathology*, 2005 with permission)

significant cytological atypia [7]. To make a diagnosis of periosteal chondrosarcoma, permeation of the surrounding soft tissue is needed.

Both calcification and reactive ossification are common for chondroid tumors, benign or malignant (exception: chondroid fibroma contains only calcification). Reactive bone formation is to be differentiated from malignant osteoid in that it typically contains only one layer of osteoblasts and is not rimmed by a cellular stroma.

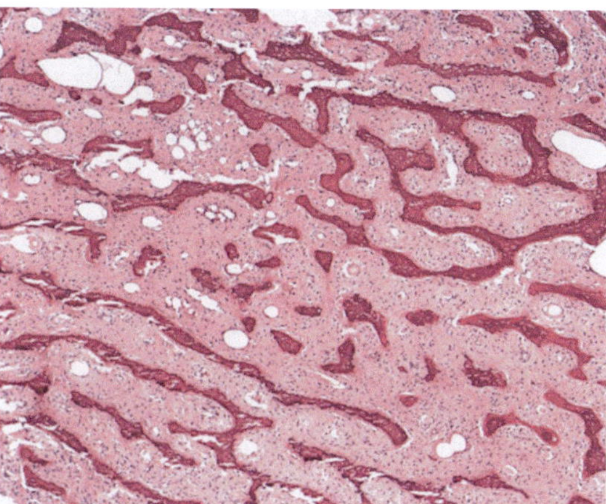

Fig. 3.9 Parosteal osteosarcoma. Parallel osteoid trabeculae with less cellular stroma than that of classical osteosarcoma (Tumors of the Bones and Joints, *Armed Force Institute of Pathology/American Registry of Pathology*, 2005 with permission)

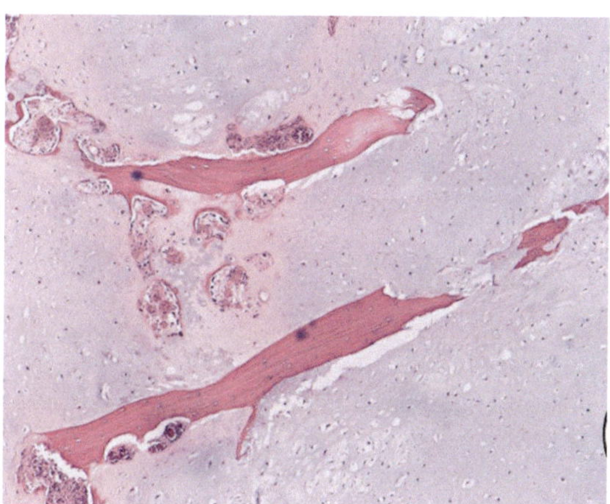

Fig. 3.10 Chondrosarcoma. Permeative growth pattern (Tumors of the Bones and Joints, *Armed Force Institute of Pathology/American Registry of Pathology*, 2005 with permission)

Differential Diagnosis

Enchondroma

Even though enchondroma in small bones can have increased cellularity, significant atypia, and binucleation, there is lack of a permeative growth pattern. Instead, normal bone marrow elements are interspersed among chondroid lobules.

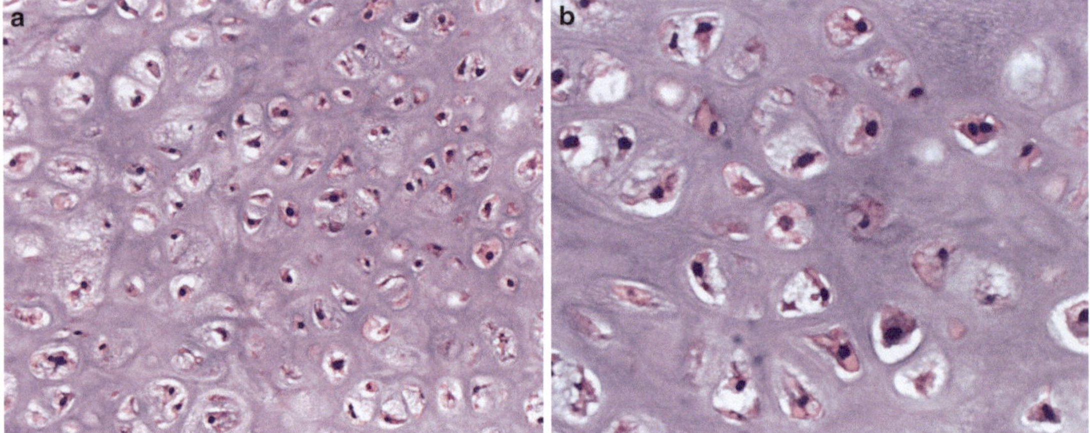

Fig. 3.11 Chondrosarcoma. Note hypercellularity and binucleation of malignant chondroid tissue (Tumors of the Bones and Joints, *Armed Force Institute of Pathology/American Registry of Pathology*, 2005 with permission)

Chondroblastoma

Chondroblastoma can have hypercellularity; however, the mononuclear cells contain longitudinal grooves and characteristic pericellular calcification. Even though chondroid matrix material, lacuna formation is not as evident as in other chondroid tumors. There is no medullary permeation.

Osteochondroma

Osteochondroma maintains the benign chondroid–osteoid relationship evident in normal endochondral ossification. In addition, the chondrocytes at the tumor base show orderly columnar arrangement. The cavities between the bony trabeculae are filled with normal bone marrow tissue.

Osteosarcoma

Osteosarcoma can contain both osteoid and chondroid tissues and manifests a permeative growth pattern. This is in contrast to the reactive bone formation in chondrosarcoma. The reactive bony tissue tends to form semicircles around malignant chondroid lobules rather than infiltrating the lobules as manifested in osteosarcoma.

References

1. Rosenberg AE, Roth SI. Chapter 4. Bone. In: Mills SE, editor. Histology for pathologists. Philadelphia: Lippincott Williams & Wilkins/Wolters Kluwer; 2007. p. 75–96.
2. Bianco P, Sacchetti B, Riminucci M. Osteoprogenitors and the hematopoietic microenvironment. Best Pract Res Clin Haematol. 2011;24(1):37–47.
3. Schaffler MB, et al. Osteocytes: master orchestrators of bone. Calcif Tissue Int. 2014;94(1):5–24.
4. Toledo SR et al. Bone deposition, bone resorption, and osteosarcoma. J Orthop Res. 2010;28(9):1142–8.
5. Power PF et al. ETV5 as a regulator of matrix metalloproteinase 2 in human chondrosarcoma. J Orthop Res. 2012;31(3):493–501.
6. Unni KK. Chapter 5. Bone forming lesions. In: Tumors of the bones and joints. Silver Spring: ARP press; 2005. p. 119–92.
7. Unni KK. Chapter 4. Cartilaginous lesions. In: Tumors of the bones and joints. Silver Spring: ARP press; 2005. p. 37–118.

4 Nervous System

Review of Pertinent Histology and Physiology of Peripheral Nerve Sheath

Schwann cells play a very important role in the many aspects of the peripheral nervous system. Schwann cells have well-developed cellular processes which allow to wrap around axons and form tight junctions with each other [1–3]. Each axon is sheathed by one layer of Schwann cells which connect to each other at the node of Ranvier. This wrapping property might underlie the wavy appearance of nuclei seen in nerve sheath tumors. If one visions the Schwann cell arrangement in a nerve fascicle, the resemblance to the Verocay body characteristic of schwannomas becomes evident. Apparently, the neoplastic cells are polarized and supported by basal laminin on both sides.

The nerve sheath also contains mast cells which probably play a role in the angiogenesis and formation and maintenance of the blood–nerve barrier. The interaction between mast cells and Schwann cells is through the production of paracrine factors [4]. Through the production of TGF beta, mast cells influence the collagen production of nerve sheath cells. Mast cells are frequently seen in neurofibromas, less so in schwannomas.

Key Morphological Feature of Well-Differentiated Malignant Peripheral Nerve Sheath Tumors

- Hypercellular fascicles, sheets
- Diffuse nuclear enlargement, hyperchromasia (Fig. 4.1)

Discussion

Corresponding to decreased SOX10 and S100 expression, most malignant peripheral nerve sheath tumor cells show little schwannian or perineurial differentiation [3, 5]. Only at ultrastructural level, some schwannian differentiation manifests in some low-grade tumors. Instead, fibroblastic differentiation becomes evident. The tumor cells have underdeveloped cellular processes and cell junctions. Along with the absence of long spacing collagen and diminished basal laminin material, the cell process underdevelopment allows cells to unfold to form fascicular and sheet structures [2, 6–9].

The diffuse nuclear atypia manifests as nuclear enlargement and hyperchromasia. It should not be confused with the focal degenerative atypia which is common in benign nerve sheath tumors.

X. Sun, *Well-Differentiated Malignancies: New Perspectives*, Current Clinical Pathology,
DOI 10.1007/978-1-4939-1692-4_4, © Springer Science+Business Media New York 2015

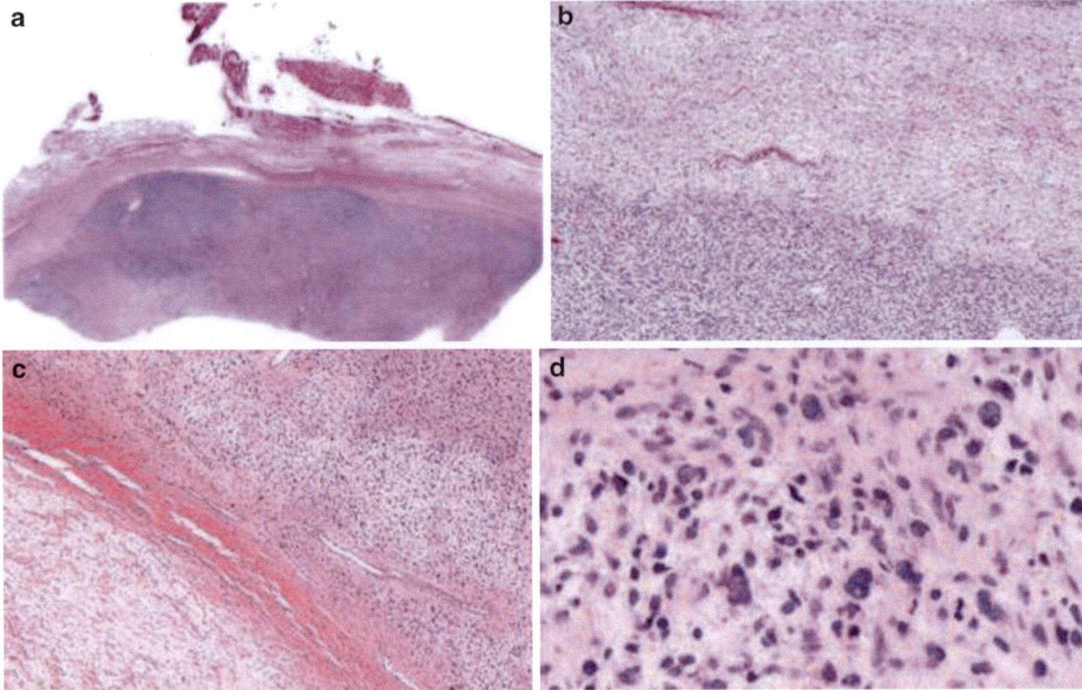

Fig. 4.1 Low-grade malignant peripheral nerve sheath tumor. Note cellular crowding, nuclear enlargement, and hyperchromasia

Differential Diagnosis

Neurofibroma

Typically, neurofibromas have the characteristic wavy nuclei and shredded carrot-type collagen which prevent the cells to form well-formed cellular fascicules or sheets. Focal atypia is degenerative in nature (bizarre nuclei with smudgy texture). In cellular neurofibromas, the cells tend to have more cytoplasm with or without well-formed fascicles. The plexiform variant might form fascicles. The fascicles however, are less cellular (more fibrous and mucinous).

Schwannoma

Schwannomas are usually easy to diagnose due to their characteristic Antonin A and B areas. They also are encapsulated and contain hyalinized blood vessels. Cellular schwannomas can form fascicles, contain focal necrosis, and even show significant bone erosion. The fascicles are however less cellular and are composed of bland cells. Additional features include encapsulation, subcapsular lymphocytic infiltration, as well as hyalinized vessels. The plexiform variant may also show fasciculation and even lack encapsulation. The fascicles are also hypocellular and composed of bland cells.

In difficult cases, a panel of immunostainings might help. Benign nerve sheath tumors are positive for p16 and p27 and show low reactivity for p53 and Ki6 [10, 11]. In general, they have a mitotic rate less than 4/10 HPF. Also, they show diffuse S100 reactivity in contrast to the weak and focal staining seen in malignant cells.

Review of Pertinent Histology and Physiology of Astrocyte

Astrocytes

Astrocytes are the key player in the central nervous system. They are involved in virtually every aspect of the business of the system. Importantly, through their highly specialized cellular processes and cell junctions, they provide a highly sophisticated framework for the system allowing the formation of different functional domains, the blood–brain barrier [12–15]. Moreover, through the non-overlapping arrangement of the exuberant arborization of cellular processes, each cell has its distinctive cellular domain which can be brought out with a GFAP stain.

Not only are astrocytes an important component of the blood–brain barrier; they also control the angiogenic/vasculogenic process in the system [16–18]. Probably as a check and balance mechanism in order to prevent oxidative stress in this highly metabolically active system, glial cells also are equipped with means to rein in the angiogenic/vasculogenic process. This mechanism is likely to be powerful and preserved in gliomas. As circumstantial evidence, microvascular hyperplasia characteristic of grade IV gliomas represents ineffective angiogenesis probably as a result of compromise between high levels of counteracting factors. To circumvent it, glioma cells develop multiple mechanisms for neovascularization [16, 18].

Astrocytes are heterogeneous and the extended family members express common astrocytic markers but have morphological and functional differences to accommodate specific structural and physiological needs.

Key Morphological Features for Diffuse Gliomas (WHO Grade II)

- Increased cellularity due to cell domain disruption
- Infiltrative nature (Fig. 4.2)

Discussion

The infiltrative gliomas represent a spectrum of malignant glial cell tumors characterized by well-defined morphological features. Grade II tumors are characterized by moderately increased cellularity. Tumors of higher grades have increased mitotic activity and cytological anaplasia (grade III) and necrosis or microvascular hyperplasia (grade IV). Localized gliomas are a group of benign glial tumors which have distinct molecular, histological, and anatomical features, reflecting astrocyte heterogeneity.

Corresponding to decreasing expression of GFAP, glioma cells have decreased development of cellular processes and GAP junctions. Importantly there is a grade-dependent decrease in the expression of GAP junction protein connexin 43 [19–21]. This important protein plays an essential role in glial morphology, proliferation, and motility. Underdeveloped cellular processes and cell junctions allow cells to get close (hypercellularity in a fixed bony cavity) and migrate (infiltration of normal tissue). This is in contrast to the hypercellularity in reactive gliosis. In mild to moderate gliosis, the characteristic cellular domain is maintained by the non-overlapping arrangement of the exuberant process arborization [12, 22]. Only in severe diffuse gliosis the orderly cellular domain is disrupted probably through overexpression of GFAP and connexin 43 which bring cells closer to each other by allowing intermingling and overlapping of cellular processes (Fig. 4.3). Therefore, the contrasting morphological differences can be highlighted by a GFAP stain. With the stain, even the difference between reactive and neoplastic gemistocytic cells can be appreciated.

The infiltrative nature of malignant gliomas can be appreciated by the presence of entrapped axons and neurons, haphazard arrangement of atypical cells, edematous splaying of neuropil, microcyst formation, as well as microcalcifications [22, 23]. Cellular condensation around vessels and axons and underneath the pia is also an indication of malignancy. Only malignant glial cells with poorly developed cellular processes and cellular junctions can form clusters around those structures.

In difficult cases where the infiltrative nature is not evident due to the small size or location of the specimen, a panel of immunostainings might be helpful. Reactive glial cells are negative for WT-1 and low mitotic activity and p53 reactivity.

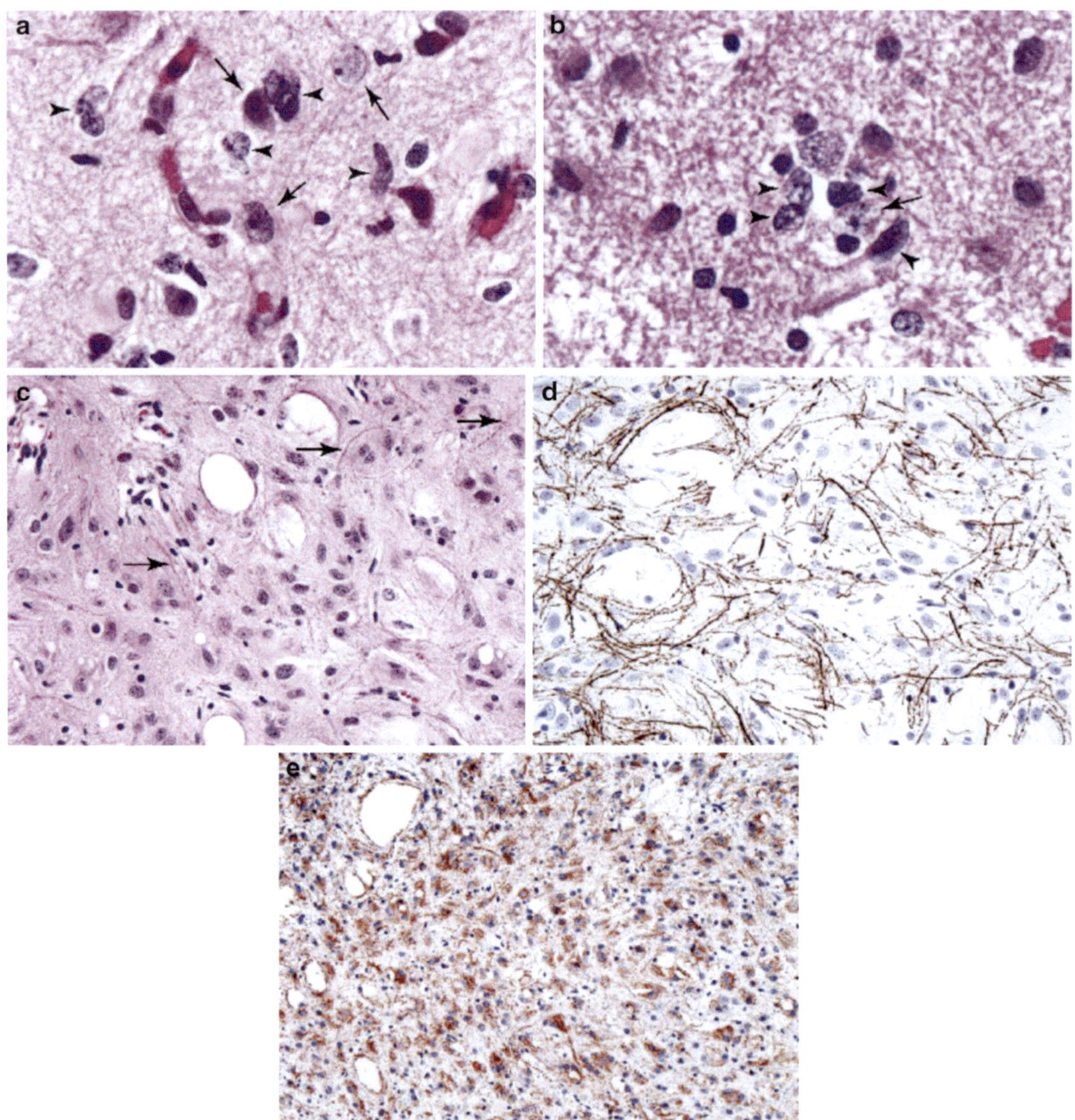

Fig. 4.2 Infiltrative astrocytoma, WHO grade II. Note infiltrative border with cortical neurons (**a**, **b**; *arrows*, cortical neurons; *arrowheads*, tumor cells). Microcystic changes (**c**). Neurofilament protein immunostaining highlights axons (**d**). Glial fibrillary acid protein stain lights up neoplastic astrocytes with poorly developed cellular processes (**e**) (Practical Surgical Neuropathology, *Elsevier/Churchill Livingstone*, 2010 with permission)

Differential Diagnosis

Reactive Gliosis

Reactive gliosis manifests a spectrum of atypical changes and can mimic gliomas to perfection. Reactive astrocytes usually demonstrate extensive arborization of processes and show orientation to the inciting injury. They appear evenly distributed and the radial arrangement of fibrillar processes can be brought out by GFAP staining.

Even in severe diffuse gliosis where the cellular domain is disrupted, the reactive nature of the cells can be appreciated by the exuberant proliferation of the cellular processes in contrast to the poorly developed cellular processes in diffuse astrocytomas.

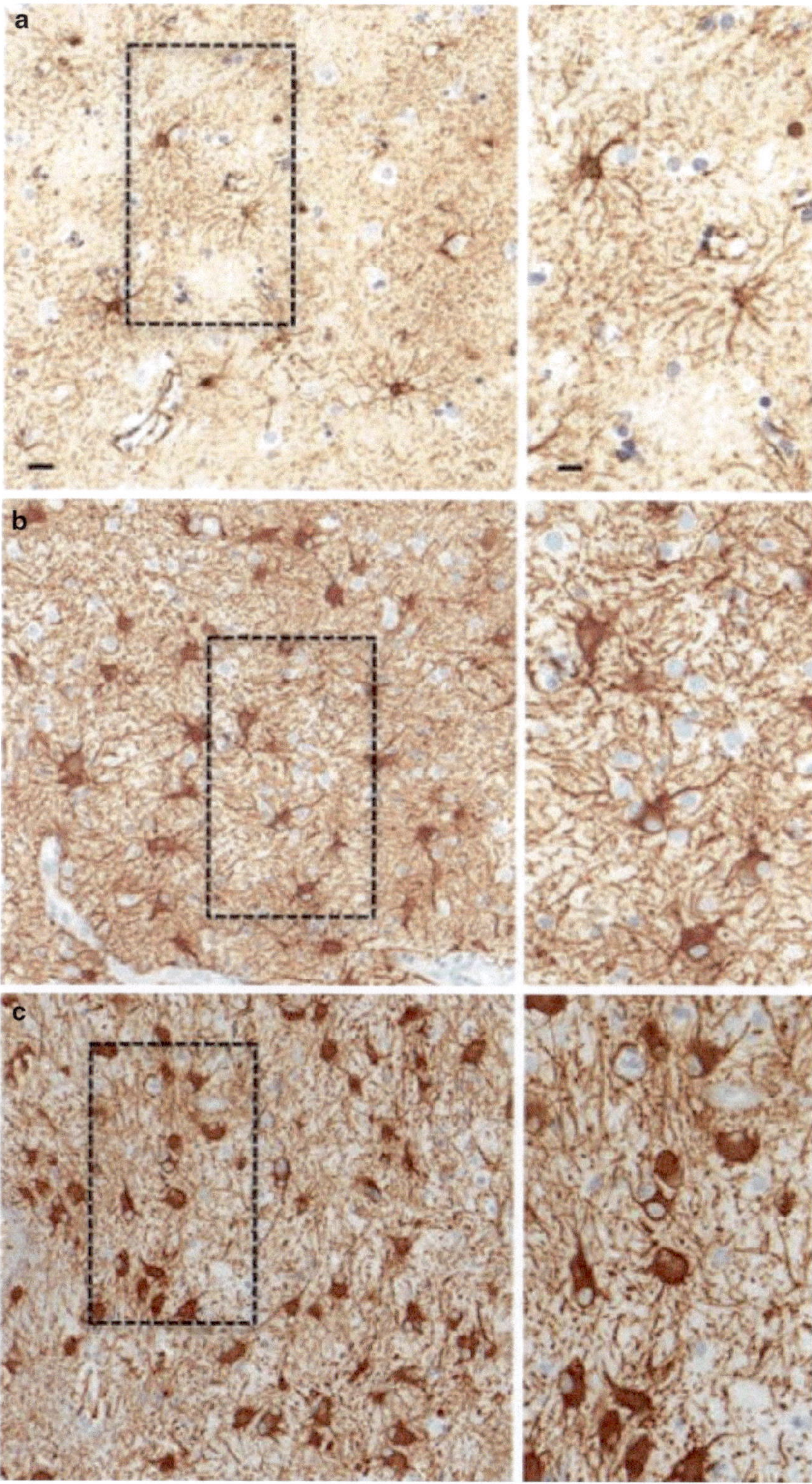

Fig. 4.3 Reactive gliosis. Glial fibrillary acid protein stain. Mild gliosis (**a**) and moderate gliosis (**b**). Note that even in severe gliosis (**c**), reactive astrocytes are dispersed and contain more cellular processes than neoplastic cells (Practical Surgical Neuropathology, *Elsevier/Churchill Livingstone*, 2010 with permission)

Localized Gliomas

Localized gliomas might be confused with grade 2 and higher-grade diffuse gliomas. Typically, their localized feature can be readily evident by radiological studies even though microscopic infiltration can be present at the tumor periphery. Morphologically, they can be differentiated from the diffuse gliomas by their characteristic cytological and histological presentations and/or anatomical locations [22–25].

Pilocytic astrocytomas are characterized by extensive microcystic changes, hair-like fibrillated processes, and Rosenthal fibers.

Despite marked cellularity and polymorphism, pleomorphic xanthoastrocytomas lack brisk mitotic figures, necrosis, and vascular hyperplasia. The tumor cells are occasionally arranged in fascicles cells, vacuolated. Other features include superficial location, abundant reticulin, eosinophilic granular bodies, and perivascular lymphocytes.

Subependymal giant cells astrocytomas arise from the lateral ventricles and are composed of large atypical cells with neuronal differentiation.

References

1. Ross MH, Pawlina W. Chapter 12. Nerve system. In: Histology: a text and atlas with correlated cell and molecular biology. Philadelphia: Lippincott Williams & Wilkins; 2006. p. 318–63.
2. Pummi KP et al. Tight junction proteins and perineurial cells in neurofibromas. J Histochem Cytochem. 2006;54(1):53–61.
3. Flaiz C et al. Impaired intercellular adhesion and immature adherens junctions in merlin-deficient human primary schwannoma cells. Glia. 2008;56(5): 506–15.
4. Doddrell RD et al. Loss of SOX10 function contributes to the phenotype of human Merlin-null schwannoma cells. Brain. 2013;136(Pt 2):549–63.
5. Flaiz C et al. Altered adhesive structures and their relation to RhoGTPase activation in merlin-deficient Schwannoma. Brain Pathol. 2009;19(1): 27–38.
6. Miettinen M. Chapter 24. Nerve sheath tumors. In: Miettinen M, editor. Modern soft tissue pathology: tumors and non-neoplastic conditions. New York: Cambridge University Press; 2010. p. 660–723.
7. Staser K, Yang FC, Clapp DW. Mast cells and the neurofibroma microenvironment. Blood. 2010;116(2): 157–64.
8. Kirkpatrick CJ, Curry A. Interaction between mast cells and perineurial fibroblasts in neurofibroma. New insights into mast cell function. Pathol Res Pract. 1988;183(4):453–61.
9. Ushigome S et al. Perineurial cell tumor and the significance of the perineurial cells in neurofibroma. Acta Pathol Jpn. 1986;36(7):973–87.
10. Hirose T et al. Immunohistochemical demonstration of EMA/Glut1-positive perineurial cells and CD34-positive fibroblastic cells in peripheral nerve sheath tumors. Mod Pathol. 2003;16(4):293–8.
11. Rodriguez FJ et al. Pathology of peripheral nerve sheath tumors: diagnostic overview and update on selected diagnostic problems. Acta Neuropathol. 2012;123(3):295–319.
12. Sofroniew MV, Vinters HV. Astrocytes: biology and pathology. Acta Neuropathol. 2010;119(1):7–35.
13. Wang DD, Bordey A. The astrocyte odyssey. Prog Neurobiol. 2008;86(4):342–67.
14. Kanski R, et al. A star is born: new insights into the mechanism of astrogenesis. Cell Mol Life Sci. 2014;71(30:433–47.
15. Parpura V et al. Glial cells in (patho)physiology. J Neurochem. 2012;121(1):4–27.
16. Shibuya M. Brain angiogenesis in developmental and pathological processes: therapeutic aspects of vascular endothelial growth factor. FEBS J. 2009;276(17): 4636–43.
17. Sokolowski JD et al. Brain-specific angiogenesis inhibitor-1 expression in astrocytes and neurons: implications for its dual function as an apoptotic engulfment receptor. Brain Behav Immun. 2011;25(5): 915–21.
18. Hardee ME, Zagzag D. Mechanisms of glioma-associated neovascularization. Am J Pathol. 2012; 181(4):1126–41.
19. Sin WC, Crespin S, Mesnil M. Opposing roles of connexin43 in glioma progression. Biochim Biophys Acta. 2012;1818(8):2058–67.
20. Theodoric N et al. Role of gap junction protein connexin43 in astrogliosis induced by brain injury. PLoS One. 2012;7(10):e47311.
21. Yu SC et al. Connexin 43 reverses malignant phenotypes of glioma stem cells by modulating E-cadherin. Stem Cells. 2012;30(2):108–20.
22. Perry A, Brat DJ. Chapter 5. Astrocytic and oligodendroglial tumors. In: Practical surgical neuropathology: a diagnostic approach. Philadelphia: Churchill Livingstone/Elsevier; 2010. p. 63–124.
23. Marko NF, Weil RJ. The molecular biology of WHO grade I astrocytomas. Neuro Oncol. 2012;14(12): 1424–31.
24. Rodriguez FJ et al. Pathological and molecular advances in pediatric low-grade astrocytoma. Annu Rev Pathol. 2013;8:361–79.
25. Tascos NA, Parr J, Gonatas NK. Immunocytochemical study of the glial fibrillary acidic protein in human neoplasms of the central nervous system. Hum Pathol. 1982;13(5):454–8.

5 The Genitourinary System

The Kidney

Overview

Normal Renal Histology and Physiology

The normal renal parenchyma is composed of tightly packed tubules and glomeruli which are delimited by a capsule. The tubules are situated on a thin basement membrane which is supported by a complex network of specialized interstitial fibroblasts [1, 2]. The interstitial cells also play important roles in the modulation of hemodynamic tubular reabsorption and erythropoietin production. There are at least two types of cortical interstitial cells and three types of medullary interstitial cells to accommodate the normal function of the organ. Importantly, the type 1 medullary interstitial cells are characterized by their prominent lipid storage capabilities and peroxidase activity.

The normal renal tubules are tasked with the tremendous job of continuous reabsorption excretion, and secretion in keeping an adequate volume of sanitized blood. Accordingly, the cells are fitted with extraordinary metabolic capabilities which are reflected in the characteristic metabolic changes present in the common renal malignancies [1, 3–5]. It has been suggested that kidney cancer is actually a metabolic disease.

Adult Renal Tumor Progression Pathways

In stark contrast to most other organs in which the progression from epithelial dysplasia to carcinoma is well characterized, the concept of renal dysplasia has been only occasionally mentioned in the literature and the pathway of epithelial dysplasia to carcinoma has not been firmly established [6–8]. The premalignant dysplasia probably has slow proliferative rates as the normal tubule cells. When the accumulation of chromosomal defects reaches a threshold, the tumor cells gain the capacity to break the spatial constraints imposed by the tightly packed basement membrane, interstitium, renal capsule and renal pelvis, and calyces at the parenchymal borders. The spatial restraint allows little space for significant premalignant growth.

Papillary carcinoma is thought to derive from papillary adenoma [7]. The fact that some renal stem cells reside in the mesenchyme further supports the notion that renal epithelial malignancy might arise directly from the mesenchyme without going through the conventional tubular dysplasia to carcinoma pathway [9].

Tumor Circumscription and Capsulation: Two Important Features of Renal Malignancy

In this book on well-differentiated malignancies, we focus on the commonly encountered, less aggressive renal epithelial malignancies (clear cell carcinoma, papillary carcinoma, and chromophobe carcinoma). Importantly, instead of having an infiltrative border, these tumors present as well-circumscribed masses and papillary carcinoma is usually encapsulated (counterintuitively,

X. Sun, *Well-Differentiated Malignancies: New Perspectives*, Current Clinical Pathology,
DOI 10.1007/978-1-4939-1692-4_5, © Springer Science+Business Media New York 2015

angiomyolipoma sometimes has an infiltrative appearance). These malignancies exhibit an infiltrative border when a sarcomatous component becomes evident. The presence of a sarcomatous component represents tumor progression to a higher grade and portends a prognosis. Morphologically, it resembles high-grade sarcoma. Importantly, this sarcomatous component should not be confused with benign bone formation associated with clear cell carcinoma, the mucinous tubular ad spindle cell carcinoma, and angiomyolipomas in which the spindle or osteoid tissue is cytologically benign. Counterintuitively, in the business of differentiation of papillary adenoma vs papillary carcinoma and nephrogenic rest (also metanephric adenoma) vs nephroblastomas (not discussed in this book), the presence of a capsule is an important criterion for malignancy.

The Analogy to Epithelial Malignancies in the Hepatobiliary Tract

An overview of all renal epithelial malignancies reveals striking similarity to the carcinoma in the hepatobiliary tract. Corresponding to the spectrum of classical hepatocellular carcinoma, hepatocellular carcinoma variants and cholangiocarcinoma are clear cell carcinoma, papillary carcinoma, and chromophobe carcinoma and collecting duct carcinoma and medullary carcinoma, respectively. At one end of the spectrum are classical hepatocellular carcinoma and clear cell carcinoma. Both of them are characterized by well circumscription, a rich sinusoidal microvessel network, and minimal other stromal components. At the other end are cholangiocarcinoma, collecting duct carcinoma, and medullary carcinoma which are featured by a highly infiltrative border and abundant desmoplasia elicited by tumor cells. In the middle of the spectrum are hepatocellular carcinoma variants, papillary carcinoma and chromophobe carcinoma. These entities have moderate amount of stroma and are moderately vascularized.

Even though hepatic adenoma rarely progresses to hepatocellular carcinoma, an analogy can be drawn between it and renal papillary neoplasm in that the malignant entity is often encapsulated while the benign counterpart lacks a capsule. Thus, rather than being a restrictive force, the tumor capsule here probably plays an important guiding and cheering role in the carcinogenesis akin to that of the stroma in the invasive front of pulmonary non-small cell carcinoma [10, 11]. Disrupting the underlying mechanism(s) might provide therapeutic benefits.

Key Morphologic Features of Low-Grade Clear Cell Carcinoma

- Bland cells with clear and/or eosinophilic cytoplasm in nests, trabeculae
- Enshrouding sinusoidal vessels (Figs. 5.1 and 5.2)

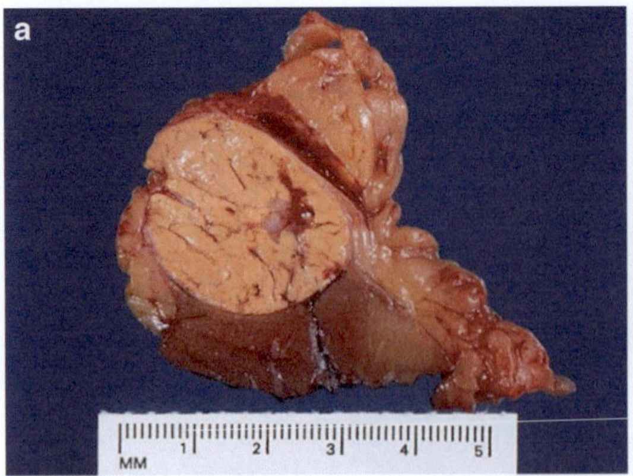

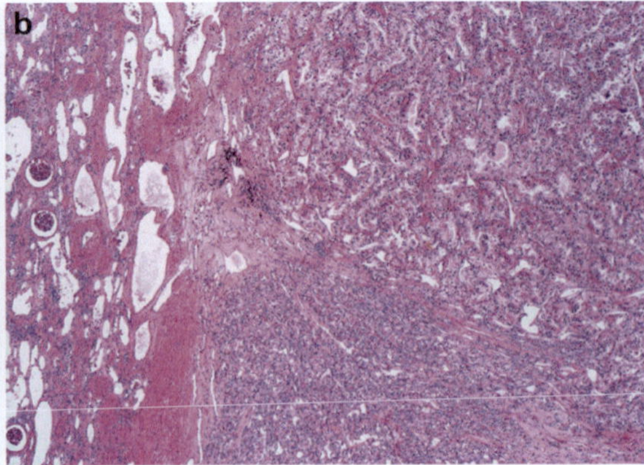

Fig. 5.1 Clear cell carcinoma. Well circumscription

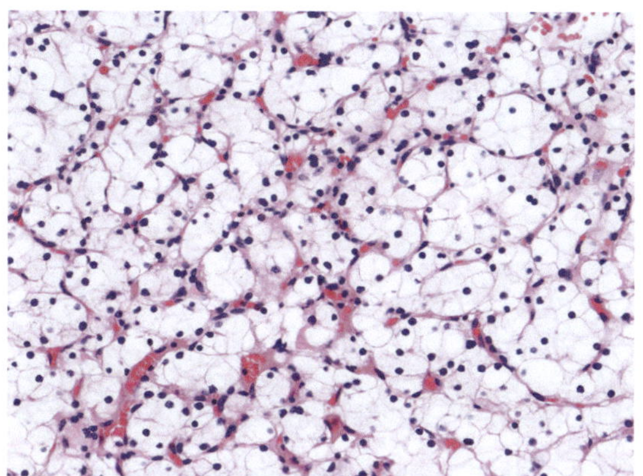

Fig. 5.2 Low-grade clear cell carcinoma. Nests or trabeculae of tumor cells with clear to eosinophilic cytoplasm enshrouded by sinusoidal vessels (Tumors of the Kidney, Bladder and Related Urinary Structures, *Armed Force Institute of Pathology/American Registry of Pathology*, 2004 with permission)

Discussion

Typically, clear cell carcinoma cells form nests and trabeculae; however, occasional tubules, cysts, and even papillary structures can been seen. When malformed mitochondria are abundant, the cytoplasm can even become eosinophilic. The tumor is graded according to the nuclear features (Fuhrman nuclear grading) with the low-grade tumor being characterized as having a nuclear size comparable to that of a red blood cell.

Clear cell carcinoma is a neoplasm in which the pseudohypoxic condition is induced through the loss of VHL tumor suppressor gene (Von–Hippel–Lindau) [3, 4]. The resultant overexpression of hypoxia-inducible factor (HIF) underlies the morphological changes characteristic of the tumor. The classical clear cytoplasm of this entity is due to aerobic glycolysis and accumulation of lipids through genes controlled by HIF. An imbalance between hepatocyte growth factor activator inhibitor (HAI) and hepatic growth factor activator (HGFA) in the tumor favors epithelial growth at the cost of tumor stroma [12]. The tumor nests and trabeculae are surrounded by a rich network of sinusoidal vessels as a result of activation of VEGF, Glut-1, and EPO. Furthermore, the cells express high levels of CA IX in response to increased hydrogen ion production due to aerobic glycolysis [13]. This feature can be used in difficult cases to confirm a diagnosis of clear cell carcinoma.

Even though clear cell carcinoma is highly vascularized, the pseudohypoxic condition forces the cells to rely on aerobic glycolysis and might even resort to drastic means such as autophagy for survival [14–17]. Ultrastructurally, the tumor cells contain few organelles except for malformed mitochondria. Other circumferential supporting evidence for increased autophagy activity in clear cell carcinoma includes tumor cell overexpression of CD68, alpha-1-antitrypsin, and alpha-1-antichymotripsin and lack of parvalbumin or beta-defensin-1 [18, 19].

Differential Diagnosis

Adrenal Cortical Tumors

Adrenal cortical tumor is easily confused with clear cell carcinoma because it also has clear cells arranged in nests and alveoli and surrounded by sinusoidal vessels. The tumor cells are, however, positive for inhibin and Melan A and negative for RCC antigen and cytokeratins.

Xanthogranulomatous Pyelonephritis

The lipid laden macrophages in xanthogranulomatous pyelonephritis might be mistaken for clear cell carcinoma cells. In some cases where abundant fibroblastic proliferation is evident, a more serious diagnosis of clear cell carcinoma with a sarcomatoid component could be rendered. However, the lesion lacks sinusoidal vessels and contains a mixed inflammatory infiltrate which tends to be more prominent in the vicinity of the renal collecting system

Angiomyolipoma

Angiomyolipoma is composed of blood vessels, smooth muscle, and adipose tissue of various portions in a haphazard arrangement. The vessels usually have thick walls, many of which contain dense fibrous tissue. The smooth muscle fibers are typically arranged in a radial fashion and are perpendicular to the vessels. Thus, it usually causes no diagnostic problems even though the muscle cells may contain enlarged and hyperchromatic nuclei and show mitotic activity. However, the tumor may entrap normal renal tubules creating a pseudo-invasive pattern. Moreover, the tumor may coexist with epithelial malignancies, and the benign smooth muscle fibers can be mistaken as a sarcomatous component subjecting the patient to unnecessary overtreatment.

Immunostainings for HMB 45 and Mart-1 can be helpful in making the distinction. Except for the danger for life-threatening hemorrhages and failure associated with the tumor, angiomyolipoma is generally considered a neoplasm with a benign prognosis. On the other hand, the epithelioid angiomyolipoma variant is now considered malignant. The epithelioid smooth muscle cells can have clear to eosinophilic cytoplasm and contain multinucleation, prominent nucleoli, necrosis, and even brisk mitotic figures. In this variant, the characteristic thick-walled vessels sometimes can be inconspicuous or even absent. Important clues include the presence of benign fat tissue and lack of sinusoidal vessels.

Oncocytoma

Oncocytoma contains nests, trabeculae, microcysts, or even tubules. Focal areas of cytoplasmic vacuolization can be noted. Furthermore, focal nuclear atypia, hemorrhage, and even extension into the perirenal fat are present. Nevertheless, the tumor usually has a conspicuous stromal component and lacks shrouding microvessels. It lacks necrosis or brisk mitotic activity.

Papillary Carcinoma

See papillary carcinoma section.

Key Morphological Features of Papillary Carcinoma

- Encapsulated mass composed of papillae, tubule cystic structures
- Abundant foamy cells in the stroma (Figs. 5.3 and 5.4)

Discussion

Typically, papillary carcinoma is composed of one layer of cells arranged in papillae or tubule cystic structures. The cell cytoplasm can be eosinophilic, basophilic, or clear. The same Fuhrman nuclear grading system applies here.

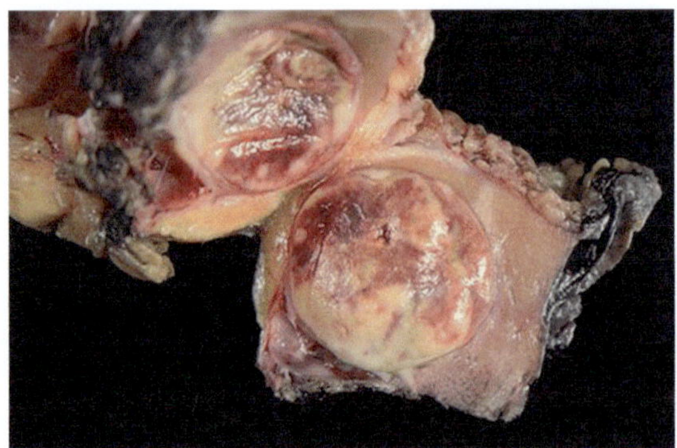

Fig. 5.3 Papillary carcinoma with encapsulation (Tumors of the Kidney, Bladder and Related Urinary Structures, *Armed Force Institute of Pathology/American Registry of Pathology*, 2004 with permission)

Renal papillary carcinoma shows differentiation toward both proximal and distal tubules, and it has a more conspicuous stroma than does clear cell carcinoma. The stroma component presents largely as fibrovascular cores and a tumor capsule. Characteristically, the fibrovascular cores often contain abundant foamy cells which occasionally expand the cores. The foamy cells may well be macrophages in nature. However, since they preferentially present in the fibrovascular core and there is lack of apparent correlation with the degree of tumor hemorrhage or necrosis [17, 19], they might derive from interstitial fibroblast (cortical or outer medullary) as a fuel (lipid) depot to meet the tumor cell metabolic needs. Papillary carcinoma cells express high levels of alpha-methylacyl-CoA racemase (AMACR), an important enzyme for lipid metabolism in mitochondria and peroxisomes [20]. Immunostaining for the enzyme can be used in difficult cases to confirm a diagnosis of papillary carcinoma (Fig. 5.5). As cirumferential evidence for this interstitial lipid depot hypothesis, there exists a little known tumor: mucinous tubular and spindle cell carcinoma. Typically, this rare entity contains elongated tubules in a bubbly myxoid stroma. However, it shares striking immunochemical and cytogenetic features with papillary carcinoma indicating that it might be a variant of the latter [21]. The tumor cells overexpress AMACR, and the commonly present foamy cells also lack correlation with tumor necrosis or hemorrhage.

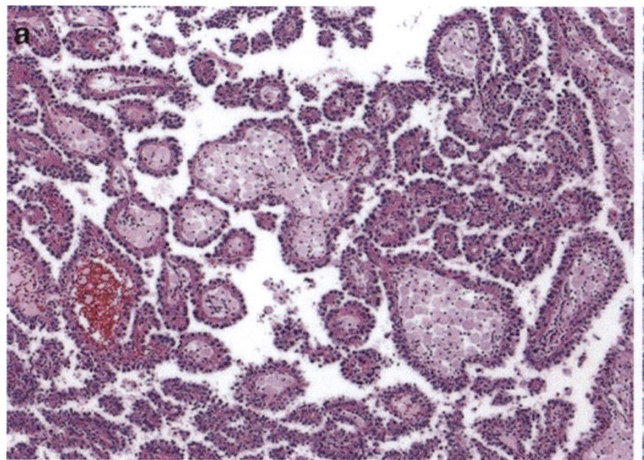

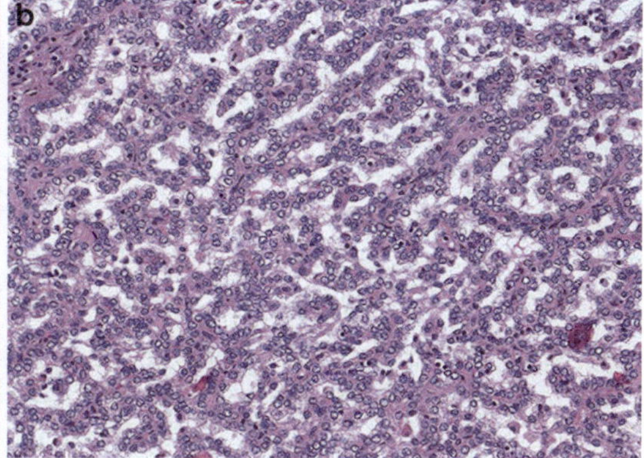

Fig. 5.4 Papillary carcinoma. (**a**) Papillary and tubulocystic growth patterns. (**b**) Note foamy cells in the stroma (Tumors of the Kidney, Bladder and Related Urinary Structures, *Armed Force Institute of Pathology/American Registry of Pathology*, 2004 with permission)

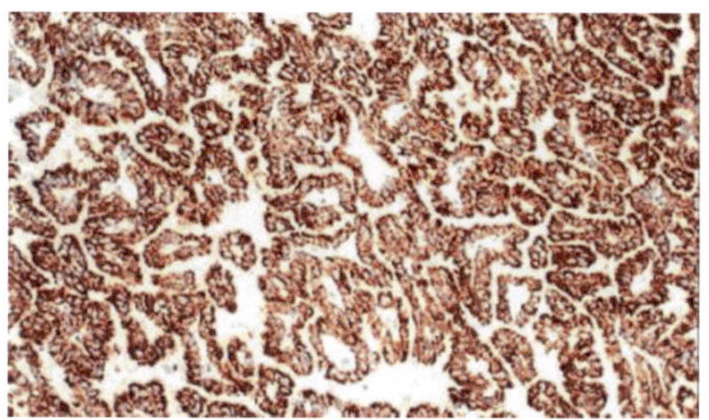

Fig. 5.5 Papillary carcinoma. Tumor cells are diffusely positive for alpha-methylacyl-CoA racemase (American Journal of Roentgenology, *American Roentgen Ray Society*, 2012; American Journal of Surgical Pathology, *Wolters Kluwer/Lippincott Williams & Wilkins*, 2004 with permission)

Papillary carcinoma probably develops as a result of self-perpetuating cellular HGF/MET signaling. The cells are characterized by increased uptake of nutrients (through PI3K pathway) and altered energy- and nutrient-sensing pathways [3]. Paradoxically, papillary carcinoma is not equipped with an accommodating stroma from a conventional point of view in that it is hypovascular compared to most solid tumors and seems to rely heavily on lipid metabolism for energy extraction. The hypovascularity and preference for lipids might be due to the overexpression of onconeural cerebellar degeneration-related antigen (Cdr2) in the tumor cells (Fig. 5.6). Papillary carcinoma expresses high levels of Cdr2 which correlate well with significantly attenuated expressions of the HIF target genes [22, 23].

Differential Diagnosis

Papillary Adenoma

Papillary adenomas is believed to be a precursor lesion for papillary carcinoma. It is small in size (less than 0.5 cm in diameter) and is composed of densely packed papillae which lack foamy cells in the fibrovascular core. Importantly, the tumor lacks a fibrous capsule.

Metanephric Adenoma

Metanephric adenoma is composed of small tubules and papillary components in a paucicellular stroma. In some cases necrosis and hemorrhage can be present. However, it lacks capsule and foamy cells in the fibrovascular core. And mitotic figures are rarely seen. In difficult cases, immunostainings for WT-1, CD57, and Pax2 can be used to light out the tumor cells.

Clear Cell Carcinoma

Clear cell carcinoma can sometimes have papillary structures composed of cells.

Non-clear Cytoplasm

The papillae are usually small and contain no fibrovascular cores. Furthermore, the tumor lacks a capsule and sinusoidal vessels are evident. In unequivocal cases, a panel of five stains (CAIX, CK7, AMACR, c-kit, and CD10) allow differentiation among the four common renal tumors.

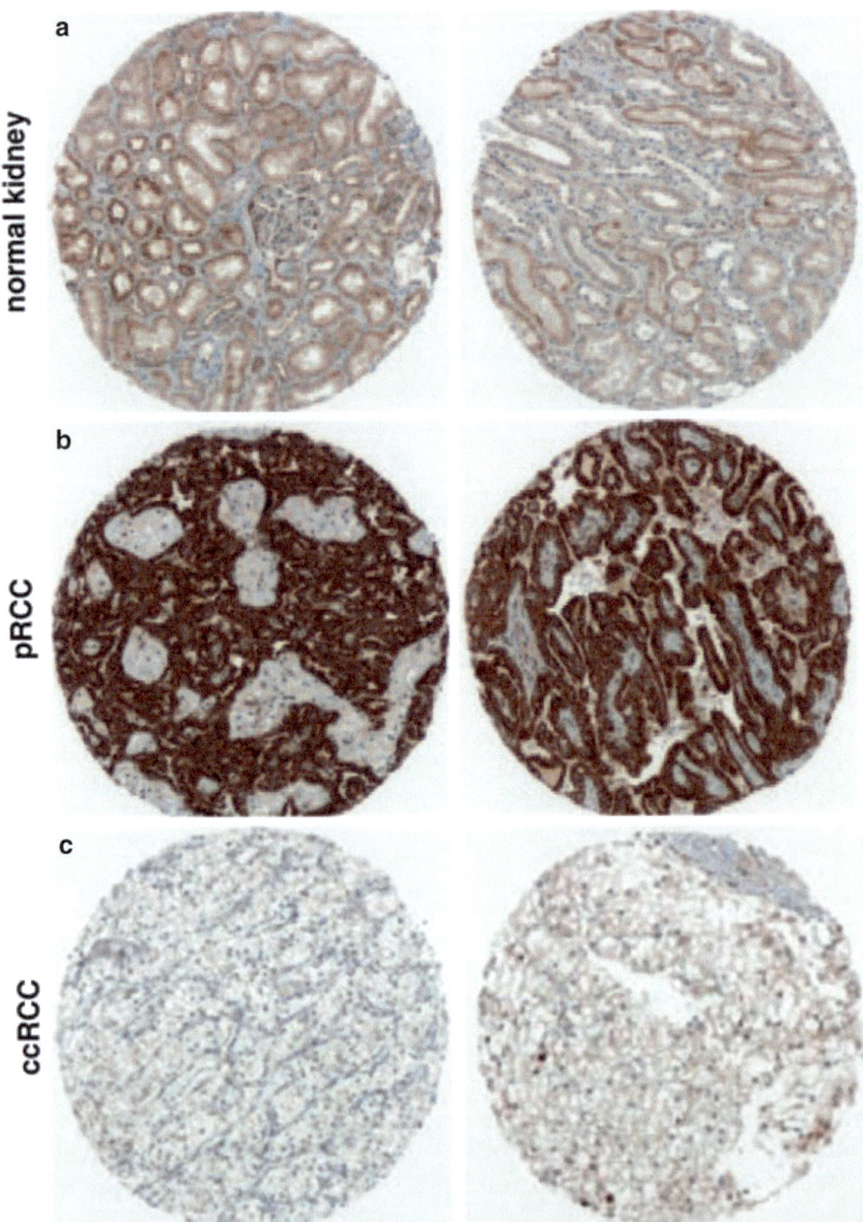

Fig. 5.6 Papillary carcinoma. Tumor cells overexpress onconeuronal cerebellar degeneration-related antigen (Cdr2) (**b**). Normal renal tubule (**a**) and clear cell carcinoma cells (**c**) have very low expression levels. Immunostaining on microarray sections (Oncogene, *Nature Publishing Group*, 2009 with permission)

Collecting Duct Carcinoma

Collecting duct carcinoma can have papillary structures and remaining glomeruli structures. However, the tumor is highly infiltrative with brisk desmoplastic reaction. Although the tubules and papillae are also lined by one layer of epithelial cells, the lining cells are apparently high grade and characteristic hobnailing is evident.

Key Morphological Features of Chromophobe Carcinoma

- Plantlike cells with pale or eosinophilic cytoplasm, perinuclear clearing in nests and trabeculae
- Nuclear polymorphism with raisinoid features (Figs. 5.7, 5.8, and 5.9)

Discussion

Chromophobe carcinoma is a renal malignancy with differentiation toward the intercalated cells in the collecting ducts. The tumor cells have abundant cytoplasmic microvesicles which compress the cytoplasmic organelles to the periphery. This accounts for the pale cytoplasm, plantlike thick cell membrane, and perinuclear clearing. The raisinoid nuclear appearance is probably due to damaged nuclear matrix scaffold which is not replaced in a timely fashion.

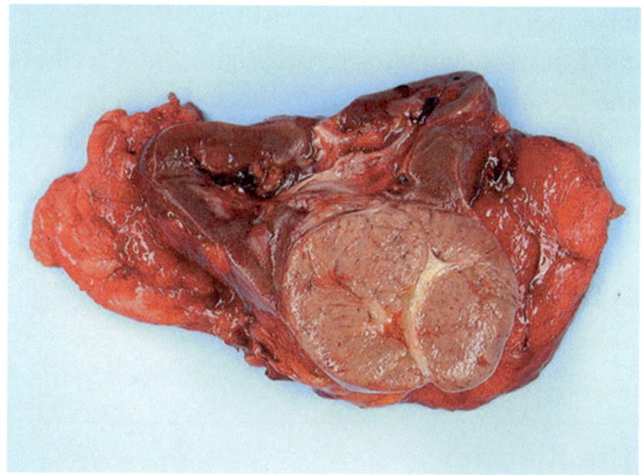

Fig. 5.7 Chromophobe carcinoma with circumscription

Like in clear cell carcinoma, tubule structures can be present but are rarely the predominant structure. The cytoplasm can sometimes be eosinophilic probably due to increased numbers of mitochondria.

The tumor cells of chromophobe carcinoma have abnormal mitochondria with tubulovesicular, circular, and lamellar cristae [24]. The abnormal mitochondria demonstrate high levels of alpha subunit of OXPHOS complex V (ATP5A1) and HSPB1. This leads to increased glycolytic activity, subjecting the cells to free radical stress with subsequent organelle damage. Furthermore, the tumor cell autophagy seems to be faulty. This probably results in the accumulation of double-membrane autophagosomes which fail to fuse with lysosomes or endosomes to form single-membrane autolysosomes. Supporting this autophagy hypothesis is that the tumor cells show diffuse, strong reticular positivity for Hale colloidal iron stain which correlates well with abundant microvesicles at the ultrastructural level [25] (Fig. 5.10). The diffuse positivity for the stain indicates the presence of mucopolysaccharides which might represent damaged cell organelles

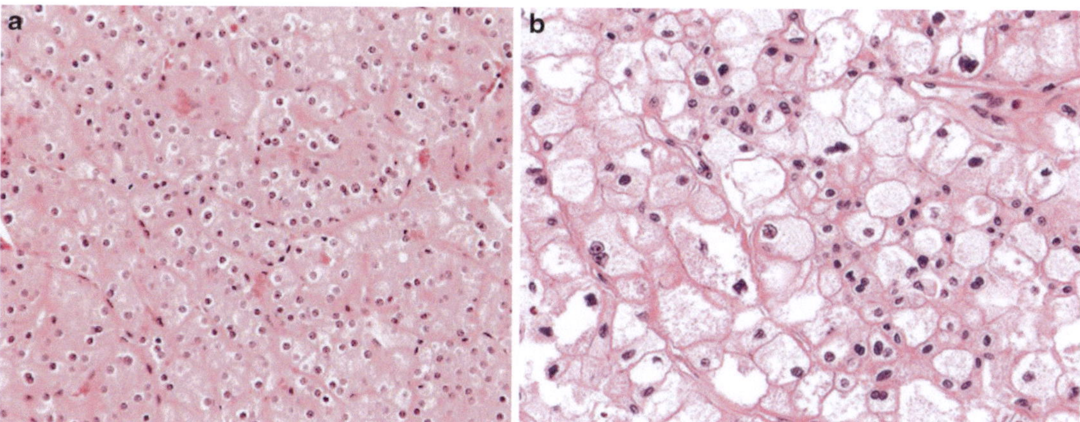

Fig. 5.8 Chromophobe carcinoma. Note plantlike cells with pale to eosinophilic cytoplasm, perinuclear clearing in nests or trabeculae (Tumors of the Kidney, Bladder and Related Urinary Structures, *Armed Force Institute of Pathology/American Registry of Pathology*, 2004 with permission)

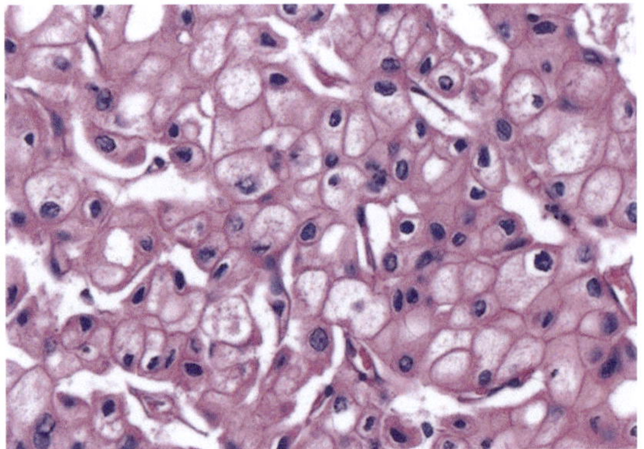

Fig. 5.9 Chromophobe carcinoma. Nuclear polymorphism with rasinoid features (Tumors of the Kidney, Bladder and Related Urinary Structures, *Armed Force Institute of Pathology/American Registry of Pathology*, 2004 with permission)

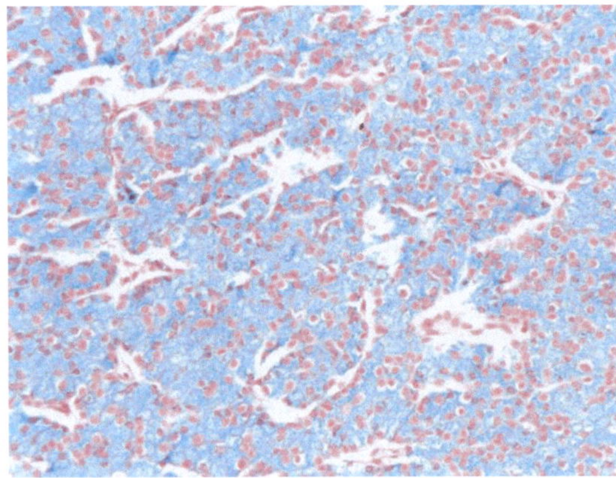

Fig. 5.10 Chromophobe carcinoma. Diffuse positivity with Hale colloidal iron stain (Tumors of the Kidney, Bladder and Related Urinary Structures, *Armed Force Institute of Pathology/American Registry of Pathology*, 2004 with permission)

such as mitochondria and endoplasmic reticulum. Moreover, the tumor cells overexpress aspartic protease, a major lysosomal enzyme [24].

Differential Diagnosis

Oncocytoma

Oncocytoma is arranged nests, trabeculae, and even tubules composed of cells with eosinophilic cytoplasm. The increased number of mitochondria could be the result of compensatory biogenesis since the levels of the complex I chain are decreased. The tumor lacks other important cytological features of chromophobe carcinoma as well as frequent mitotic activity and sheetlike growth pattern. In addition to Hale colloidal iron stain, CK7 is useful in the distinction. Oncocytoma cells lack reactivity for both stains.

Carcinoid

Carcinoid tumor can show nests and trabeculae which are composed of cells with pepper-salt chromatin but lack the cytological features of chromophobe carcinomas.

Clear Cell Carcinoma

Clear cell carcinoma can resemble chromophobe carcinoma in several ways. For instance, both entities can manifest as nests and trabeculae and the tumor cells can have clear and/or eosinophilic cytoplasm. Some clear cell carcinoma cells can have perinuclear clearing. However, clear cell carcinoma has characteristic sinusoidal vessels and lacks the most of the other cytological features of chromophobe carcinoma. In difficult cases, immunostainings for CK7 and c-kit would be helpful. Clear cell carcinoma is negative for both.

Epithelioid Angiolipoma

See clear cell carcinoma section.

The Bladder

Overview

Normal Urothelial Physiology and Histology

The normal urothelium is not just a passive blood–urine barrier. Rather, it plays an essential role in accommodating the bladder filling, emptying, sensing, and modulation of the urine [26, 27]. Even though the normal turnover rate is low (about 3–6 months), the urothelium has the capacity to regenerate the whole epithelium in less than 72 h when damaged. The traditional view holds that the urothelial stem cells reside in the niches at the basal layer and are influenced by the lamina propria stromal cells via paracrine factors such as epithelial growth factor (EGF) and fibroblast growth factor (FGF). The urothelium differentiation seems to follow a similar pathway to that for the squamous epithelium (even though at a much slower rate) in that the cells move from the basal layer (one cell thick) to the intermediate layer (several cells thick) before they become fully differentiated (as a one cell layer of umbrella cells). Recently, new evidence has emerged indicating that there is another pool of stem cells which can give rise to mature umbrella cells without going through the intermediate stage [28, 29].

The Papillary Neoplasm Family

Analogous to mammary neoplasms, there exist two distinct pathways for urothelial epithelial tumors [30–32]. The papillary neoplasm family includes papilloma, noninvasive papillary urothelial carcinoma (grade 1 to 3), and rarely invasive carcinoma. Papilloma is the predominant tumor type. This family is characterized by genetically stable activation mutations of fibroblast growth factor receptor 3 (FGFR3). The mutation gives the cells increased growth potential. The tumor suppressor gene p53 and cell cycle regulators are affected more frequently with increasing tumor grade (from grade 1 to grade 3 carcinoma). The grade 1 carcinoma (2004 WHO classification: papillary urothelial) neoplasm of low malignant potential (PUNLMP) is characterized by increased number of epithelial layers with no cellular atypia and the grade 2 urothelial carcinoma (2004 WHO classification: low-grade urothelial carcinoma) contains slender papillae and cytological atypia. Grade 3 papillary urothelial carcinomas are cytologically high grade and shares molecular changes with the invasive urothelial carcinoma.

The High-Grade Flat Lesion Family

It includes the flat neoplastic lesions and invasive urothelial carcinoma and is featured by loss of function or missense mutations of the *TP*53 tumor suppressor gene. The two pathways are not mutually exclusive as papillary neoplasms can acquire p53 mutations and progress to higher grades and become invasive [30–32]. Alternatively, there are maybe concurrent mutations of both types in one tumor.

Invasive Urothelial Carcinoma

The unsurpassed plasticity of invasive urothelial carcinoma cells is evident in that more than twenty histological variants have been recognized and divergent differentiation is present in one fourth of the cases. Corresponding to this enormous cellular and architectural plasticity of urothelial carcinoma, up to 2,300 coding sequences involving up to 150 genes have been reported in high-grade urothelial carcinoma [33]. In some cases epigenetic modifications are involved since they do not have mutations of the two classical genes. All invasive urothelial carcinomas are considered by many experts as high grade, even though the tumor cells can be cytologically bland. This is particularly true for the variants we discuss in this book. For instance, the micropapillary variant carries a worse prognosis than the usual invasive urothelial carcinoma even though only mild cytological atypia is present. The nested and tubular variants have the same (or even worse) clinical outcomes as does the usual high-grade urothelial carcinoma despite their bland cytological features. In a similar manner to renal carcinomas, sarcomatoid dedifferentiation in urothelial carcinoma portends a dismal prognosis. Therefore, it should not be confused with urothelial carcinomas with pseudosarcomatous stromal proliferation or the variant with osseous and chondroid metaplasia [34].

Currently, the histological grading of invasive urothelial carcinoma is secondary to the tumor staging in clinical correlation. Hopefully, this would change with future tumor classifications which incorporate data from both histological and immunohistochemical evaluation. Recently, three major clinically relevant urothelial carcinoma categories have been proposed based on the information on molecular markers and histopathological features [35]. Promising immunostainings include CK5, p-cadherin, EGFR, and cell cycle activity indicator CCND1.

Two Important Issues in Bladder Surgical Pathology

The two important issues in bladder surgical pathology are the distinction of dysplasia (including carcinoma in situ) from reactive atypia and identifying stroma invasion [36]. A detailed discussion of them is beyond the scope of this book. Briefly, the first issue can usually be tackled with a panel of immunostainings including CK20, CD44, p53, Ki67, and even p16. In normal and reactive urothelium, CK20 positivity is restricted to the superficial layer. CD44, on the other hand, stains the basal and intermediate layers of the normal urothelium with expansion to the superficial layer which shows reactive changes. Benign urothelial cells have low reactivity for p53, Ki67, and p16.

The dysplastic urothelial cells have aberrant expression of CK20 (expansion to all cell layers) and CD44 (loss of reactivity) and increased positivity for Ki67, p53, and p16.

A set of morphological changes have been proposed to represent stromal invasion in the bladder [34, 36]. They include irregularly shaped nests and cysts, tentacular projections, single cells, and some stromal changes such as desmoplasia, pseudosarcomatous stroma proliferation, myxoid stroma and retraction artifact around nests, and even associated inflammation.

However, identification of invasion in small bladder biopsies is frequently complicated by tangential sectioning, obscuring inflammation, thermal effect, and even unusual growth patterns. The phenotypical changes in the tumor stroma offers some promise in identifying invasive carcinoma [37]. The stromal changes are loss of CD34-positive fibroblasts with parallel gain of alpha SMA-positive myofibroblasts and increased expression of SPARC (secreted protein, acidic and rich in cysteine) (Fig. 5.11).

In this book we focus on the invasive urothelial carcinoma variants with bland cytological and/or architectural features. Familiarity with them is essential in avoiding in potentially catastrophic underdiagnosing.

Key Morphological Features of Invasive Urothelial Carcinoma with Bland Cytology Nest Variant

- Random, small cords, and nests of variable size with occasional fusion
- Infiltrative border with random cytological atypia (Fig. 5.12)

Discussion

This variant frequently coexists with the usual urothelial carcinoma, but it can present in pure nested forms [38]. Despite their cellular blandness and seemingly benign nesting patterns, this variant actually carries worse prognosis than does the usual urothelial carcinoma. Histologically, the small, variably sized nests are randomly arranged and infiltrative at the periphery. Occasionally, the nests fuse or become elongated (cord-like). Sometimes, small lumens can be formed giving rise to tubules. The overall cytological feature is bland nuclei; however, an interesting finding is that scattered cytological atypia can be identified in the deeper parts of the tumor, and the cytologi-

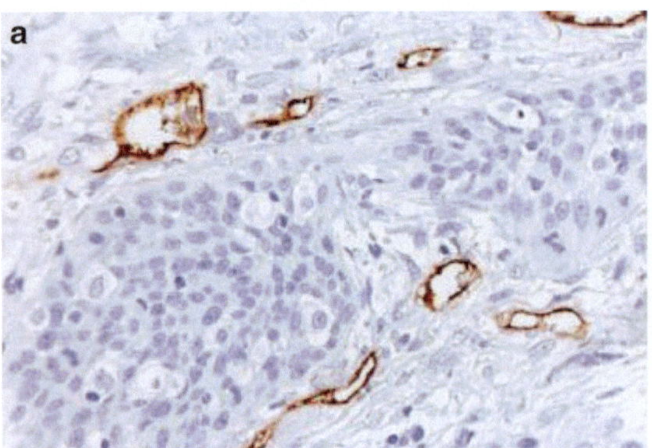

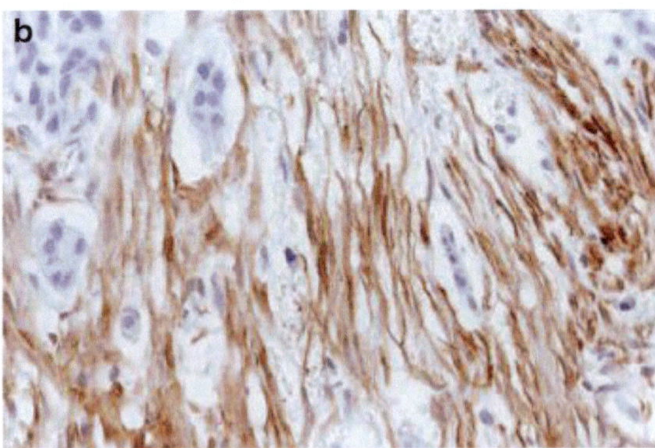

Fig. 5.11 Invasive urothelial carcinoma, nest variant. Tumor stroma contains SMA-positive cells and lacks CD34+fibroblasts

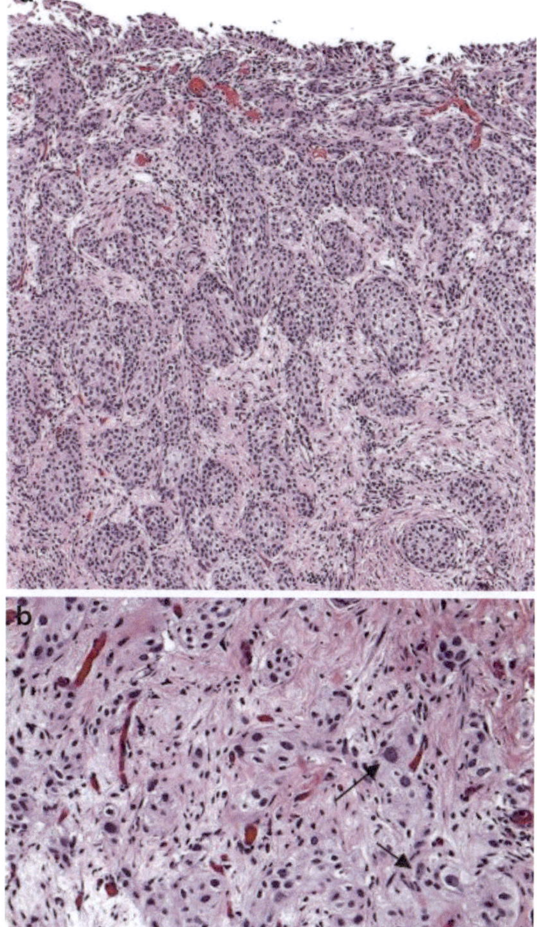

Fig. 5.12 Invasive urothelial carcinoma, nest variant. Random small cords and nests of variable sizes with occasional fusion. Infiltrative border and random cytological atypia are evident (Human Pathology, *Elsevier/Saunders*, 2010; Biopsy Interpretation of the Bladder, *Wolters Kluwer/ Lippincott Williams & Wilkins*, 2004 with permission)

cal atypia seems to increase with the tumor depth with high-grade atypia at the base of the tumor. This variant shares the same immunohistochemical features as the usual urothelial carcinoma.

Differential Diagnosis

Von Brunn's Nests

Von Brunn's nests have been considered a normal variant of bladder mucosa. They present as well-circumscribed nests located immediately beneath the urothelium. When they become florid, they may simulate nested variant of urothelial carcinoma. However, the benign nests are usually larger, more regular in shape and distribution, and lack deep invasion. Even though reactive atypia can be seen, it lacks the characteristic correlation with tumor depth in nested variant carcinoma. In difficult cases, a panel of immunostaining can offer some help. While CK20 might not be very useful, significantly greater staining for Ki67 and p53 favors carcinoma.

Cystitis Cystica and Glandularis

Cystitis cystica and glandularis derive from central cavitation of von Brunn's nests. In the latter, the lining cells have changed from cuboidal to columnar cells. When the lining cells show goblet differentiation with abundant mucin production, it is called cystitis glandularis intestinal type. They enter into the differential diagnosis because nested variant can have variable lumen formation. In general, these benign lesions lack cellular atypia and an infiltrative base. The panel of immunostainings can be used in questionable cases. However, it is important to know that cystitis glandularis intestinal type are positive for CK20.

Nephrogenic Adenoma

Nephrogenic adenoma has a mixed growth pattern including tubular, papillary, and tubulocystic and even solid structures. Cells can be cuboidal, low columnar and sometimes flat, and hobnail-like. The luminal structures usually contain eosinophilic secretions, and prominent basement sheath is present around nests. Nuclear atypia can be present but is reactive or degenerative in nature. Even though it might contain admixed superficial muscle fibers, the tumor is largely confined to the lamina propria and appear well circumscribed. The tumor cell might show focal p53 staining. Positive reactivity for PAX2 is confirmative.

Paraganglionic Tissue, Paraganglioma

Paraganglionic tissue has the characteristic Zellballen pattern with intervening vascular stroma. Sustentacular cells are present and can be lighted up with immunostaining for S100. The tumor cells are positive for chromogranin and synaptophysin.

Key Morphological Features of Microcystic Variant

- Haphazardly arranged cysts of variable sizes

Key Morphological Features of Urothelial Carcinoma with Small Tubules

- Small- to medium-sized tubules with attenuated cells with infiltrative pattern (Fig. 5.13)

Discussion

This rare entity of microcystic variant is characterized by tubulocystic structures which infiltrate the bladder wall. Intracellular lumens are also often seen. This infiltrative feature sets it apart from those benign mimickers. Only in small biopsies where the infiltrative nature is not evident, differentiation may become an issue. The variation in size of the tubulocystic and cytological atypia (mild) should alert the pathologist.

Some authorities consider urothelial carcinoma with small tubules as within the spectrum of nested variant due to their bland cytology and lumen formation. Urothelial carcinoma with small tubules has an exclusive component of small- to medium-sized tubules. The malignant tubules are lined by attenuated cells. Its bland cytological and histological features stand in stark contrast to those of the benign nephrogenic adenoma which is composed of cells with a mixture of morphology. In small biopsies where the infiltrative nature is not evident, it can be easily passed over as a benign lesion.

These two variants should not be confused with adenocarcinoma and urothelial carcinoma with glandular differentiation [34, 36, 39]. A diagnosis of adenocarcinoma in the bladder requires a pure glandular component, and tumor cells are positive for villin and CdX2. Urothelial carcinoma with glandular differentiation is defined as urothelial carcinoma containing true glandular spaces or signet ring cells. The tumor cells are CK7 positive and villin negative.

Differential Diagnosis

Florid Polypoid Cystitis Cystica and Glandularis

See differential diagnosis for the nested variant.

Nephrogenic Adenoma

See differential diagnosis for the nested variant.

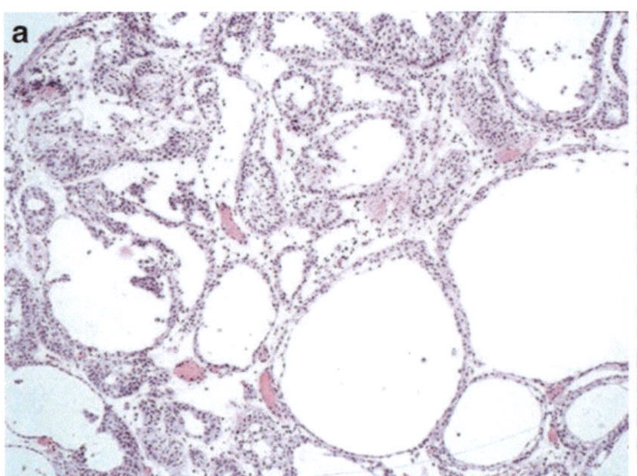

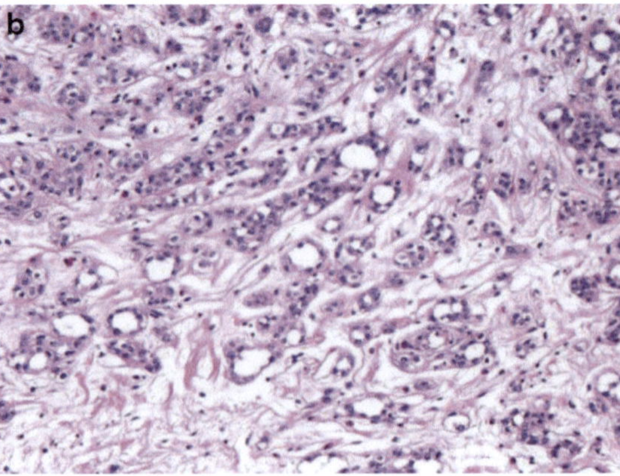

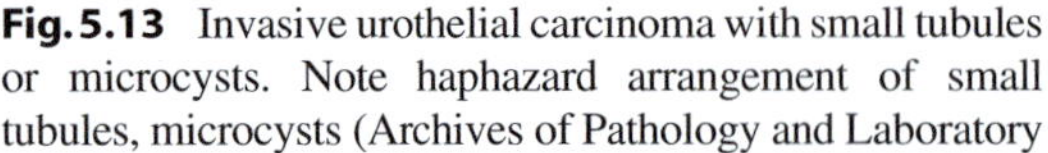

Fig. 5.13 Invasive urothelial carcinoma with small tubules or microcysts. Note haphazard arrangement of small tubules, microcysts (Archives of Pathology and Laboratory Medicine, *American Society of Clinical Pathology*, 2007; Biopsy Interpretation of the Bladder, *Wolters Kluwer/Lippincott Williams & Wilkins*, 2004 with permission)

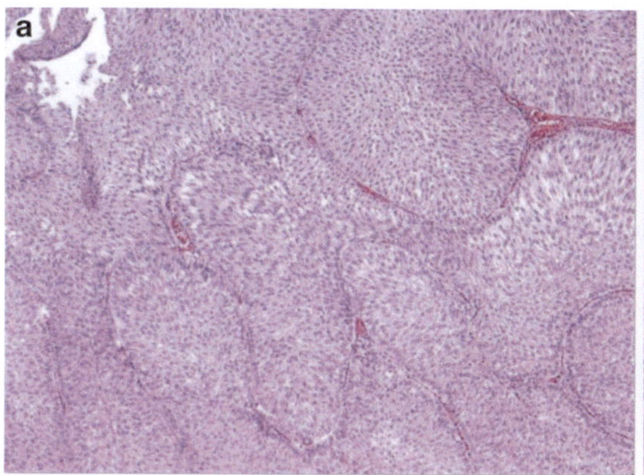

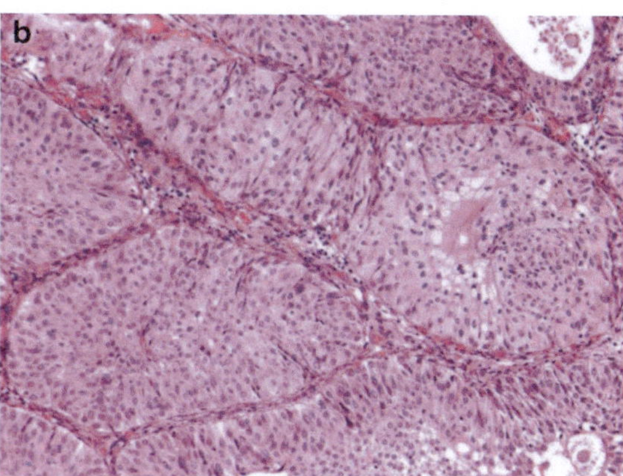

Fig. 5.14 Invasive urothelial carcinoma, inverted variant. Wide trabeculae or papillae of variable thickness with no maturation. Pushing border (Biopsy Interpretation of the Bladder, *Wolters Kluwer/Lippincott Williams & Wilkins*, 2004 with permission)

Key Morphological Features of Inverted Papilloma Pattern

- Wide trabeculae of variable thickness with no maturation
- Or wide ball-like invaginations with broad pushing border (Fig. 5.14)

Discussion

This variant often contains thick trabeculae or wide ball structures without maturation [36]. Nuclear atypia is usually present even though it is sometimes mild and mitotic figures are commonly noted. Furthermore, on the surface a coexisting exophytic papillary component or carcinoma in situ is present and the tumor is frequently associated with stromal inflammation. In difficult cases, a panel of immunostaining can be helpful as the inverted papilloma pattern shares the same cytogenetic and immunochemical features as the usual urothelial carcinoma.

Differential Diagnosis

Inverted Papilloma

Inverted papilloma can present as anastomosing islands and trabeculae and even true papillae. Focal cellular atypia sometimes accompanied by prominent nucleoli can be present. However, the tumor is well circumscribed and the thin nests and trabeculae show central maturation and peripheral palisading. Spindling is also often common. In contrast to urothelial carcinoma, the surface urothelium is usually smooth or dome shaped and lacks an exophytic component. The tumor cells are CK20 negative and have low or negative Ki67 and p53 expressions.

The Prostate

Overview

Normal Prostate Physiology and Histology

The adult prostate gland represents a unique glandular organ in which the histology is designed for the slow production of essential substances for the sperm, storage, and rapid expulsion of its products. In the prostate, the distinction of ducts and acini is blurred with both seeming to function as distensible secretory reservoirs [40]. The distensible secretory reservoirs appear to be cramped into a fibromuscular stroma creating an undulating luminal border. Luminal undulation can still be appreciated in adenosis which manifests as genuine acinic structures. The prostatic epithelium is composed of a luminal layer surrounded by basal cells. The basal layer contains stem cells and transit amplifying cells, and their ratio is tightly controlled by the stem cell niche via androgen and related paracrine factors [41, 42].

Carcinogenesis and Nuclear Changes and Lack of Basal Cell Differentiation

The current predominant view holds that prostatic carcinoma derives from the luminal cells in a chronically inflammatory milieu [41–43]. Through androgen receptor-driven chromatin looping mechanisms, many genes are affected as a result of either gene fusion (*TMPRSS2-ERG*) or direct interaction with target gene promoters [43–47]. Importantly, the *PTEN gene* is a tumor suppressor gene, and its reduction or loss can lead to not only overexpression of lamin A/C via the PI3K/AKT/PTEN pathway but also the activation of *MYC* oncogene. These changes are likely to play important roles in the nuclear changes characteristic of prostatic acinic carcinoma: nuclear enlargement and prominent nucleoli.

This luminal cell view also explains the lack of basal cell differentiation of malignant glands, a feature that has important diagnostic significance. This lack of basal cell differentiation bears remarkable resemblance to the lack of myoepithelial cells in breast cancer. In both organs, epithelial malignancies seem to be closely related to steroid hormone (s), and the precursor lesions are known to have a spectrum of architectural presentations. However, important differences are noteworthy. First, instead of having two seemingly distinct pathways for low- and high-grade breast cancers, low-grade prostatic carcinoma frequently coexists with higher-grade components representing tumor progression. Secondly, tumor stroma in prostatic carcinoma assumes an inconspicuous profile with desmoplasia being a rare occurrence.

Stromal Changes in Prostatic Carcinoma

Through the production of proliferative and antiproliferative factors, the prostatic stroma exerts important influence on the normal epithelial proliferation, maturation [48, 49]. The rapid expulsion of prostatic secretion products is effected by a fibromuscular stroma which negates the need for a myoepithelial layer in the glandular structures.

Whereas being inconspicuous in prostatic carcinoma, progressive decrease of stromal smooth muscle phenotype is noted in the progression from prostatic intraepithelial neoplasia (PIN) to low-grade and high-grade adenocarcinomas [50]. This progressive loss of smooth muscle phenotype corresponds to a spectrum of changes. The loss of one copy is believed to participate in tumor initiation, and the loss of both copies coincides with invasive and metastatic carcinoma.

Therefore, the status of the stromal smooth muscle phenotype might provide both diagnostic and prognostic values in prostatic pathology.

This stromal inconspicuousness in prostatic carcinoma stands in contrast to the dominant role that stroma plays in benign nodular hyperplasia [51]. In nodular hyperplasia, the stroma/epithelium ratio is increased from a normal 2:1 to 5:1. This important feature can be used in the differentiation of hyperplastic glands from the pseudohyperplastic variant of carcinoma.

Key Morphological Features of Gleason 2 and 3 Pattern Carcinoma

- Small rigid glands with enlarged nuclei and prominent nucleoli
- Lack of a basal cell layer (Fig. 5.15)

Discussion

In theory, well-differentiated prostatic adenocarcinomas should only include Gleason 1 and 2 patterns. However, a diagnosis of these two patterns is rarely made in needle biopsies because the tumor edge is unavailable for evaluation and the original Gleason 1 tumor probably represents adenosis.

The Gleason 2 and 3 patterns differ mainly in that the former has well circumscription with probably larger glands than the latter. Gleason 3 pattern infiltrates among benign prostatic acini and represents the most commonly diagnosed pattern in needle biopsies. Thus, it is for this practical purpose that these two patterns are discussed as one entity in this book. The two patterns are characterized as small rigid glands composed of cells with nuclear enlargement and prominent nucleoli and with no basal cell differentiation.

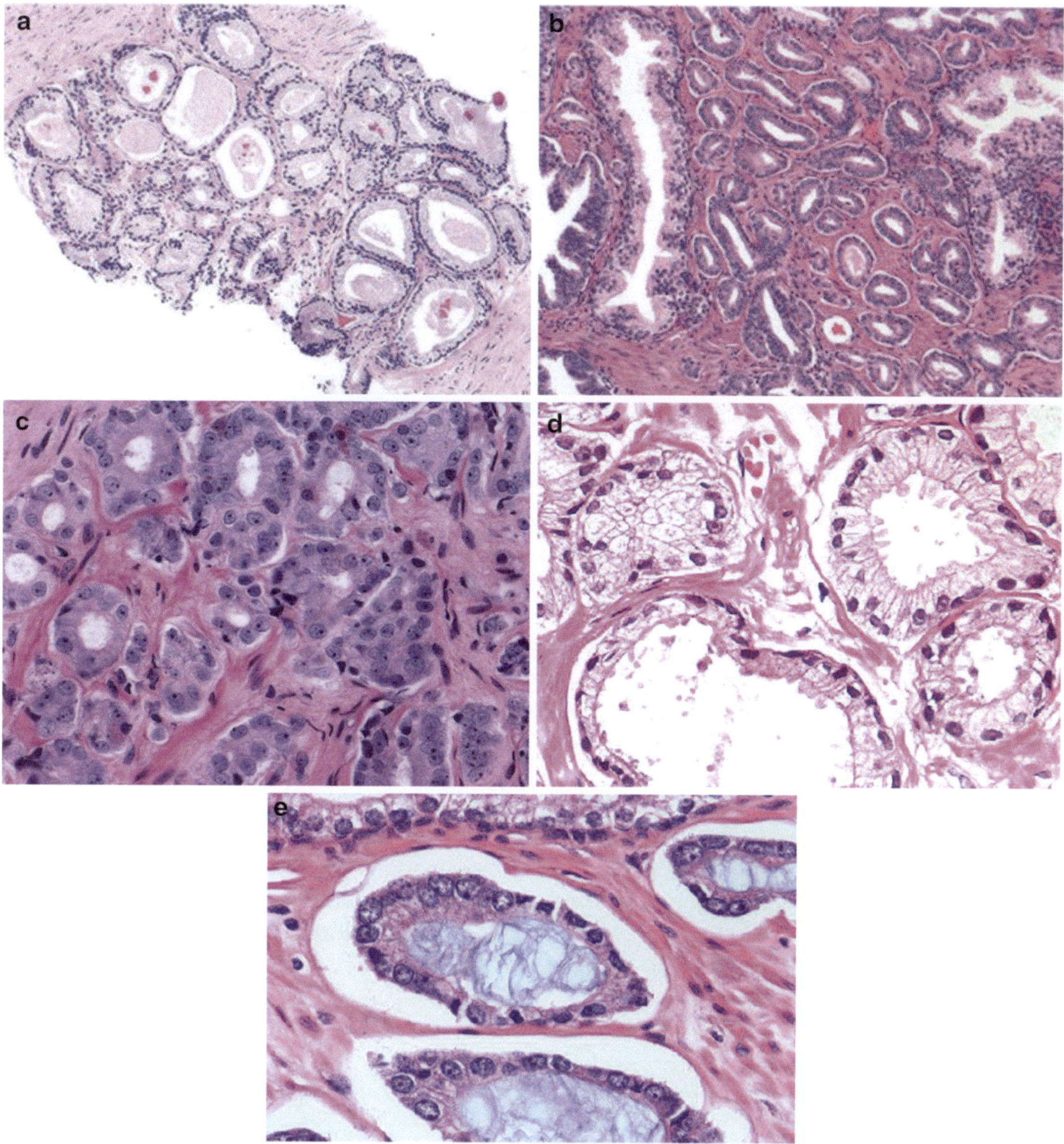

Fig. 5.15 Low-grade prostatic adenocarcinoma. Small rigid glands with nuclear enlargement and prominent nucleoli. Lack of a rim of basal cells around the glands is evident (**a, b, c, d, e**) (Biopsy Interpretation of the Prostate, *Wolters Kluwer/Lippincott Williams & Wilkins*, 2008 with permission)

As discussed in the differential diagnosis, the evaluation of nuclear size and presence of basal cell differentiation requires comparing with the adjacent benign glands because nuclear size is a relative, subjective thing and benign glands sometimes can have enlarged nuclei. Furthermore, if the questionable glands have the same morphological features as the adjacent benign glands, they should be interpreted as benign even though basal cell markers fail to light up. This is to acknowledge that some benign glands can have a focal or an attenuated basal cell layer.

Recently, a p63-positive prostatic carcinoma variant has been reported. The tumor cells are positive for BcL-2 but have negative or focal weak expression of the other basal cell marker (high molecular weight keratins). This variant has been associated with a less aggressive behavior.

Recently, a p63-positive prostatic carcinoma variant has been reported. The tumor cells are positive for BcL-2 but have negative or focal weak expression of the other basal cell marker (high molecular weight keratins). This variant has been associated with a less aggressive behavior [52].

Other important features that have been reported to be helpful in identifying malignant prostatic glands include abundant amphophilic or pale cytoplasm, lack of lipofuscin, presence of crystals, blue-tinged mucinous secretions, and pink amorphous material in the luminal spaces [53]. These changes indicate an increased or altered cellular productive activities in malignant glands. Interestingly, inflammation is rarely associated with prostatic carcinoma even though it has been increasingly recognized to play an important role in carcinogenesis. Oftentimes inflammation is located away from malignant glands. Awareness of this feature avoids overdiagnosing inflammatory atypia.

Important Adenocarcinoma Variants

The above discussed morphological features can even be applied to the important adenocarcinoma variants with some modifications.

Atrophic variant: Even though the atrophic variant resembles atrophy in that there is minimal cytoplasm, the atrophic malignant glands have enlarged nuclei and prominent nucleoli. A basal cell layer is lacking (Fig. 5.16).

Pseudohyperplastic variant: It is easily confused with hyperplastic glands on cursory examination. The nuclear features and absence of basal cells are evident. Furthermore, the pseudohyperplastic malignant glands are back-to-back with minimal intervening stroma (Fig. 5.17).

Foamy gland variant: This variant is more easily missed than the pseudohyperplastic variant because the low nuclear grade pattern is characterized by abundant cytoplasm with small and often pyknotic nuclei with nuclear enlargement and prominent nucleoli present only in high-grade ones [54–56]. The high-grade foamy gland variant can have a prominent stromal reaction. However, lack of basal cell differentiation can still be applied to the foamy gland variant (Figs. 5.18 and 5.19), even though the high-grade ones tend to show increased frequency in aberrant expression of HMMCK and p63. High-grade foamy gland tumors, however, can be picked up by their nuclear and architectural features.

The foamy gland variant contains the same ETS gene aberrations as the conventional prostate carcinoma with which it often coexists. Noteworthy is that one quarter of this variant is negative for AMACR. Ultrastructurally, the foamy cytoplasm is full of intracytoplasmic vesicles which are analogous to those in the cytoplasm of the chromophobe variant of renal cell carcinoma. Thus, this variant might represent an entity with a faulty tumor cell autophagy.

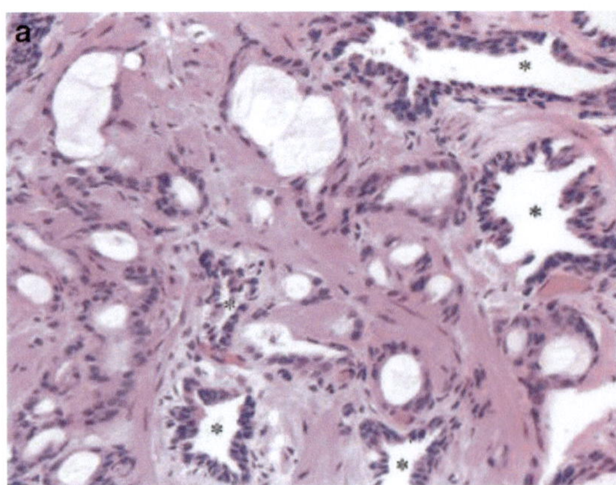

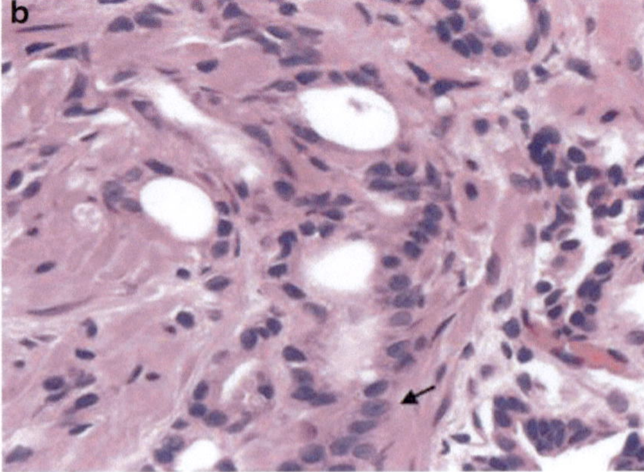

Fig. 5.16 Prostatic adenocarcinoma, atrophic variant. The atrophic glands contain cells with nuclear enlargement and prominent nucleoli. No basal cells are present (Biopsy Interpretation of the Prostate, *Wolters Kluwer/ Lippincott Williams & Wilkins*, 2008 with permission)

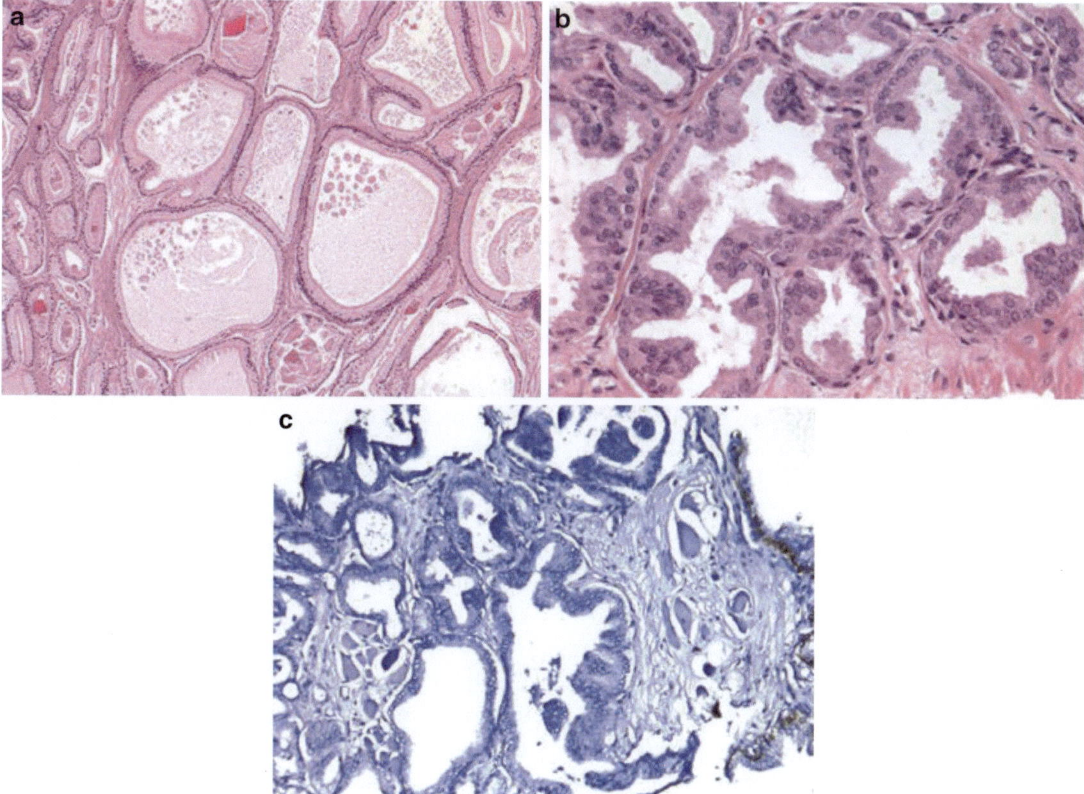

Fig. 5.17 Prostatic adenocarcinoma, pseudohyperplastic variant. The malignant glands are back-to-back (**a, b**). Characteristic nuclear features as well as lack of basal cells (**c**) are evident (Biopsy Interpretation of the Prostate, *Wolters Kluwer/Lippincott Williams & Wilkins*, 2008 with permission)

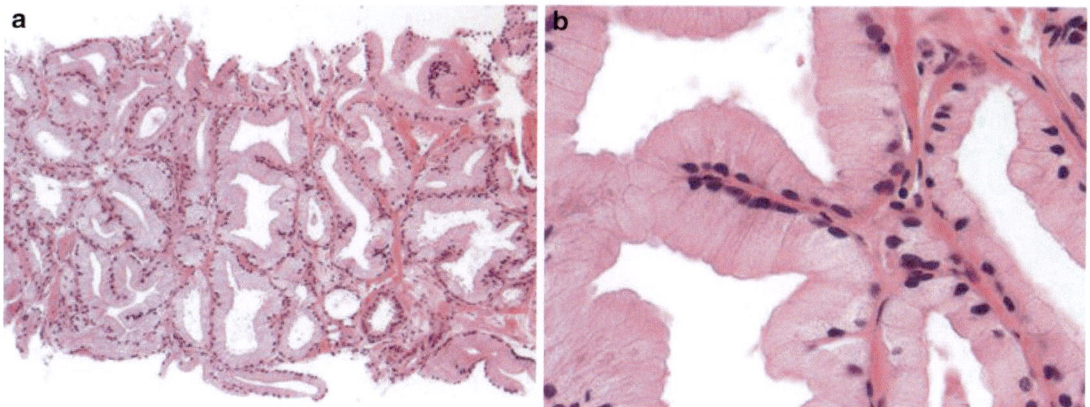

Fig. 5.18 Prostatic adenocarcinoma, foamy gland variant. Note abundant foamy cytoplasm and nuclear pyknosis. There is lack of basal cells (Biopsy Interpretation of the Prostate, *Wolters Kluwer/Lippincott Williams & Wilkins*, 2008 with permission)

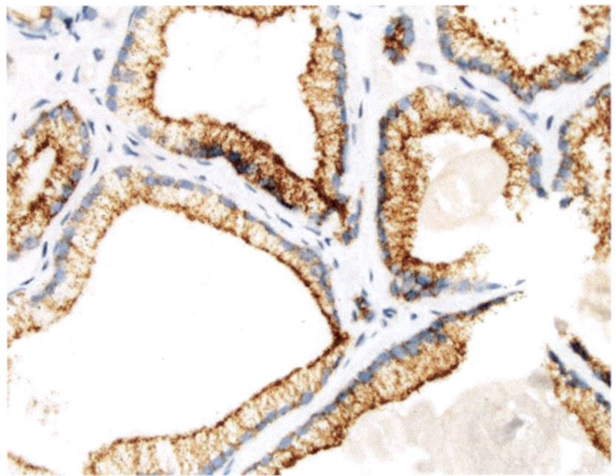

Fig. 5.19 Prostatic adenocarcinoma, foamy gland variant. Tumor cells are positive for AMACR stain (American Journal of Surgical Pathology, *Wolters Kluwer/Lippincott Williams & Wilkins*, 2013 with permission)

Differential Diagnosis

Adenosis (Atypical Adenomatous Hyperplasia)

Typically, adenosis is composed of a lobular proliferation of small glands. However, the lobular growth pattern is not always present, and limited infiltrative border can be seen. Even though nuclear enlargement is not a feature of the lesion, prominent nucleoli can be present in sizable number of lesions. An important clue to this lesion is that the small glands are admixed with larger glands, and they are often seen to bud off them. The two components have similar cytological features. This is in contrast to invasive glands around benign larger glands with benign cytological features. Furthermore, the luminal borders of adenomatous glands lack the rigidity of malignant glands. In difficult cases, PIN-4 immunostaining can offer some help. As a note of caution, AMACR has been reported in up to 18 % of cases, and basal cells may be very focal (10 % of the glands). The notion is that if those questionable glands have similar cytological features to the adjacent benign ones, they should be considered benign [57, 58].

Atrophy

There are three types of atrophy in the prostate gland and they often are admixed [58, 59]. Simple and post atrophic hyperplasia are usually not diagnostically challenging because of their lobular or circumscription feature even though the lack of cytoplasmic maturation might give an erroneous impression of nuclear enlargement or crowding.

Partial atrophy is more likely to be confused with carcinoma. First, a lobular growth pattern sometimes is not evident. Instead, the glands show a diffuse configuration. Second, the decreased cytoplasm can also evoke an impression of high N/C ratio and the nuclei can be slightly enlarged with visible nucleoli. Even though in most of the cases, the glands have an undulating luminal border, some glands can be rigid with a smooth luminal contour. As in adenosis, basal cell presence can be focal and AMACR overexpression can present. Therefore, the same note of caution is applied here. As long as the basal cell marker-negative and/or AMACR-positive glands have similar cytological features as the adjacent benign ones, they should be deemed as such.

Cowper's Glands

Cowper's glands are lobular mucinous glands arranged around a central duct. Their lobular arrangement and the presence of an attenuated basal cell layer set them apart from the foamy gland variant. In difficult cases, PSA, PSAP, and high molecular weight keratin can be used. The glandular cells are negative for PSAP and show variable staining pattern for PSA. The ductal cells and basal cells stain positively for high molecular weight keratin.

Nephrogenic Adenoma, Mesonephric Remnants

Nephrogenic adenoma can present mainly around the prostatic urethra as small tubules composed of cuboidal to columnar cells with eosinophilic cytoplasm. In addition, it can have nuclear enlargement and prominent nucleoli and lacks a basal cell layer. The tubules can even show positivity for AMACR, PSA, and PSAP. These features can lead to an erroneous diagnosis of carcinoma by the unwary. However, in most cases, other histological patterns are evident (including papillae, signet ring-like, and vascular-like). The tubules are often surrounded by a thick hyaline sheath and contain thyroid-like material. The nuclear atypia is usually local and is associated with degeneration (smudged chromatin). Even though no basal layer is present, the tumor cells can be positive for high molecular weight keratin in many cases. Moreover, oftentimes there is always associated inflammation which is rarely seen in carcinoma. In difficult cases, immunostaining for PAX2 or PAX 8 makes the distinction.

Mesonephric remnants are lined by a layer of cuboidal cells with dense secretion. They lack the cytological features of malignancy. In questionable cases, immunostainings for PSA and PSAP can be used due to their negative reactivity.

Verumontanum Mucosal Gland Hyperplasia

Verumontanum mucosal gland hyperplasia contains well-circumscribed, compact, small glands which might be confused with Gleason patterns 2 and 3 carcinomas. However, the glands lack the cytological features of carcinoma and compose a basal cell layer. Their location underneath the urothelium and eosinophilic secretions are important clues.

Seminal Vesicles and Radiation Atypia in Benign Glands

Seminal vesicle is characterized by small glands clustered around a dilated lumina. Scattered cells might show prominent nuclear atypia which exceeds the severity for even high-grade prostatic adenocarcinoma. Similar to radiation atypia, the nuclear atypia is degenerative in nature. The gland contains a basal layer and lipofuscin pigment can readily be identified.

The radiation atypia is characterized by fewer glands with atrophy and nuclear atypia in a fibrotic stroma which might also show nuclear atypia and significant vascular damage. However, the glands are non-infiltrative. Basal cells are present and oftentimes demonstrate concomitant nuclear atypia. The glands are negative for AMACR.

References

1. Brenner BM. Chapter 2. Anatomy of the kidney. In: Brenner & Rector's the kidney, vol. 1. 8th ed. Philadelphia: Saunders/Elsevier; 2011. p. 25–85.
2. Kaissling B, Le Hir M. The renal cortical interstitium: morphological and functional aspects. Histochem Cell Biol. 2008;130(2):247–62.
3. Pinthus JH, et al. Metabolic features of clear-cell renal cell carcinoma: mechanisms and clinical implications. Can Urol Assoc J. 2011;5(4):274–82.
4. Linehan WM, Srinivasan R, Schmidt LS. The genetic basis of kidney cancer: a metabolic disease. Nat Rev Urol. 2010;7(5):277–85.
5. Murphy WM, Grignon DJ, Perlman EJ. Chapter 1. Kidney tumors in children. In: Tumors of the kidney, bladder, and related urinary structures. Washington, DC: American Registry of Pathology; 2004. p. 1–101.
6. Kirkali Z, Yorukoglu K. Premalignant lesions in the kidney. Sci World J. 2001;1:855–67.
7. Wang KL, et al. Renal papillary adenoma–a putative precursor of papillary renal cell carcinoma. Hum Pathol. 2007;38(2):239–46.
8. Van Poppel H, et al. Precancerous lesions in the kidney. Scand J Urol Nephrol Suppl. 2000;205:136–65.
9. Reule S, Gupta S. Kidney regeneration and resident stem cells. Organogenesis. 2011;7(2):135–9.
10. Ponnusamy M, Ma L, Zhuang S. Necrotic renal epithelial cell inhibits renal interstitial fibroblast activation: role of protein tyrosine phosphatase 1B. Am J Physiol Renal Physiol. 2013;304(6):F698–709.
11. Maruyama E, et al. Involvement of angiopoietins in cancer progression in association with cancer cell–fibroblast interaction. Anticancer Res. 2005;25(1A): 171–7.
12. Yamauchi M, et al. Hepatocyte growth factor activator inhibitor types 1 and 2 are expressed by tubular epithelium in kidney and down-regulated in renal cell carcinoma. J Urol. 2004;171(2 Pt 1):890–6.
13. Tostain J, et al. Carbonic anhydrase 9 in clear cell renal cell carcinoma: a marker for diagnosis, prognosis and treatment. Eur J Cancer. 2010;46(18):3141–8.
14. Banerjee P, et al. Heme oxygenase-1 promotes survival of renal cancer cells through modulation of apoptosis- and autophagy-regulating molecules. J Biol Chem. 2012;287(38):32113–23.
15. Bastola P, et al. Folliculin contributes to VHL tumor suppressing activity in renal cancer through regulation of autophagy. PLoS One. 2013;8(7):e70030.
16. Wang Z, Choi ME. Autophagy in kidney health and disease. Antioxid Redox Signal. 2014;20(3):59–37.
17. Maclennan GT, Cheng L. Chapter 2. Neoplasms of the kidney. In: Bostwick DG, Cheng L, editors. Urologic surgical pathology. 2nd ed. London: Mosby/Elsevier; 2008. p. 77–172.
18. Kim MK, Kim S. Immunohistochemical profile of common epithelial neoplasms arising in the kidney. Appl Immunohistochem Mol Morpholo. 2002;10: 332–8.
19. Murphy WM, Grignon DJ, Perlman EJ. In: Silverberg SG, editor. Tumors of the kidney, bladder, and related urinary structures, AFIP atlas of tumor pathology series 4. Washington, DC: American Registry of Pathology; 2004. Chapter 2: Kidney tumors in Adults.
20. Tretiakova MS, et al. Expression of alpha-methylacyl-CoA racemase in papillary renal cell carcinoma. Am J Surg Pathol. 2004;28(1):69–76.

21. Shen SS, et al. Mucinous tubular and spindle cell carcinoma of kidney is probably a variant of papillary renal cell carcinoma with spindle cell features. Ann Diagn Pathol. 2007;11(1):13–21.
22. Balamurugan K, et al. Onconeuronal cerebellar degeneration-related antigen, Cdr2, is strongly expressed in papillary renal cell carcinoma and leads to attenuated hypoxic response. Oncogene. 2009;28(37):3274–85.
23. O'Donovan KJ, et al. The onconeural antigen cdr2 is a novel APC/C target that acts in mitosis to regulate c-myc target genes in mammalian tumor cells. PLoS One. 2010;5(4):e10045.
24. Yusenko MV, Ruppert T, Kovacs G. Analysis of differentially expressed mitochondrial proteins in chromophobe renal cell carcinomas and renal oncocytomas by 2-D gel electrophoresis. Int J Biol Sci. 2010;6(3):213–24.
25. Kuroda N, et al. Review of chromophobe renal cell carcinoma with focus on clinical and pathobiological aspects. Histol Histopathol. 2003;18(1):165–71.
26. Khandelwal P, Abraham SN, Apodaca G. Cell biology and physiology of the uroepithelium. Am J Physiol Renal Physiol. 2009;297(6):F1477–501.
27. Kreft ME, et al. Formation and maintenance of blood-urine barrier in urothelium. Protoplasma. 2010;246(1–4):3–14.
28. Ho PL, Kurtova A, Chan KS. Normal and neoplastic urothelial stem cells: getting to the root of the problem. Nat Rev Urol. 2012;9(10):583–94.
29. Hatina J, Schulz WA. Stem cells in the biology of normal urothelium and urothelial carcinoma. Neoplasma. 2012;59(6):728–36.
30. Cheng L, et al. Bladder cancer: translating molecular genetic insights into clinical practice. Hum Pathol. 2011;42(4):455–81.
31. Castillo-Martin M, et al. Molecular pathways of urothelial development and bladder tumorigenesis. Urol Oncol. 2011;28(4):401–8.
32. DeGraff DJ, et al. When urothelial differentiation pathways go wrong: implications for bladder cancer development and progression. Urol Oncol. 2011; 31(6):802–11.
33. Di Pierro GB, et al. Bladder cancer: a simple model becomes complex. Curr Genomics. 2012;13(5):395–415.
34. Epstein JI, Amin MB, Reuter VE. In: Epstein JI, editor. Bladder biopsy interpretation, Biopsy interpretation series. Philadelphia: Lippincott Williams & Wilkins; 2004. p. 55–99. Chapter 5: Invasive Urothelial Carcinoma.
35. Sjodahl G, et al. Toward a molecular pathologic classification of urothelial carcinoma. Am J Pathol. 2013;183(3):681–91.
36. Cheng L, Lopez-Beltran A, Bostwick DG. Chapter 17. Bladder tumors with inverted growth. In: Lopez-Beltran A, Cheng L, Bostwick DG, editors. Bladder pathology. Hoboken: Wiley-Blackwell/Wiley; 2012. p. 383–98.
37. Nimphius W, et al. CD34+ fibrocytes in chronic cystitis and noninvasive and invasive urothelial carcinomas of the urinary bladder. Virchows Arch. 2007;450(2): 179–85.
38. Wasco MJ, et al. Nested variant of urothelial carcinoma: a clinicopathologic and immunohistochemical study of 30 pure and mixed cases. Hum Pathol. 2010;41(2):163–71.
39. Cheng L, Lopez-Beltran A, Bostwick DG. Bladder pathology. Hoboken: Wiley-Blackwell; 2012. Chapter 12: Histological variants of urothelial carcinoma.
40. Bostwick DG, Cheng L. Chapter 8. Nonneoplastic diseases of the kidney. In: Urologic surgical pathology. London: Mosby/Elsevier; 2008. p. 381–442.
41. Miki J. Investigations of prostate epithelial stem cells and prostate cancer stem cells. Int J Urol. 2010;17(2):139–47.
42. Wang ZA, et al. Lineage analysis of basal epithelial cells reveals their unexpected plasticity and supports a cell-of-origin model for prostate cancer heterogeneity. Nat Cell Biol. 2013;15(3):274–83.
43. Lai KP, et al. Loss of stromal androgen receptor leads to suppressed prostate tumourigenesis via modulation of pro-inflammatory cytokines/chemokines. EMBO Mol Med. 2012;4(8):791–807.
44. Wu D, et al. Androgen receptor-driven chromatin looping in prostate cancer. Trends Endocrinol Metab. 2011;22(12):474–80.
45. Kong L, et al. Lamin A/C protein is overexpressed in tissue-invading prostate cancer and promotes prostate cancer cell growth, migration and invasion through the PI3K/AKT/PTEN pathway. Carcinogenesis. 2012;33(4):751–9.
46. Koh CM, et al. Alterations in nucleolar structure and gene expression programs in prostatic neoplasia are driven by the MYC oncogene. Am J Pathol. 2011;178(4):1824–34.
47. Han B, et al. Characterization of ETS gene aberrations in select histologic variants of prostate carcinoma. Mod Pathol. 2009;22(9):1176–85.
48. Thomson AA. Mesenchymal mechanisms in prostate organogenesis. Differentiation. 2008;76(6): 587–98.
49. Yu S, et al. Altered prostate epithelial development in mice lacking the androgen receptor in stromal fibroblasts. Prostate. 2012;72(4):437–49.
50. Knudsen BS, Vasioukhin V. Mechanisms of prostate cancer initiation and progression. Adv Cancer Res. 2010;109:1–50.
51. Schauer IG, Rowley DR. The functional role of reactive stroma in benign prostatic hyperplasia. Differentiation. 2011;82(4–5):200–10.
52. Giannico GA, et al. Aberrant expression of p63 in adenocarcinoma of the prostate: a radical prostatectomy study. Am J Surg Pathol. 2013;37(9):1401–6.
53. Epstein JI, Netto GJ. Chapter 7. Mimickers of adenocarcinoma of the prostate. In: Biopsy interpretation of the prostate. Philadelphia: Lippincott Williams & Wilkins/Wolters Kluwer Business; 2008. p. 105–56.
54. Zhao J, Epstein JI. High-grade foamy gland prostatic adenocarcinoma on biopsy or transurethral resection: a morphologic study of 55 cases. Am J Surg Pathol. 2009;33(4):583–90.

55. Hudson J, et al. Foamy gland adenocarcinoma of the prostate: incidence, Gleason grade, and early clinical outcome. Hum Pathol. 2011;43(7):974–9.
56. Tran TT, Sengupta E, Yang XJ. Prostatic foamy gland carcinoma with aggressive behavior: clinicopathologic, immunohistochemical, and ultrastructural analysis. Am J Surg Pathol. 2001;25(5):618–23.
57. Humphrey PA. Histological variants of prostatic carcinoma and their significance. Histopathology. 2012;60(1):59–74.
58. Montironi R, et al. The spectrum of morphology in non-neoplastic prostate including cancer mimics. Histopathology. 2012;60(1):41–58.
59. Epstein JI, Netto GJ. In: Epstein JI, editor. Biopsy interpretation of the prostate, Biopsy interpretation series. 4th ed. Philadelphia: Wolters Kluwer/ Lippincott Williams & Wilkins; 2008. Chapter 7: Mimickers of Adenocarcinoma of the Prostate.

6 Female Reproductive System

Cervix

Review of Pertinent Histology, Physiology

The ectocervix of the adult female is lined by a nonkeratizing squamous epithelium which shows cyclical changes in response to local steroid hormonal levels [1]. ER and PR are present in the epithelium and stromal fibroblasts. The endocervix is covered by a mucinous columnar epithelium which also invaginates to line the cleft-like structures in the stroma (endocervical glands). The glandular clefts are arranged in a collateral tunnellike pattern and usually penetrate less than 5 mm from the surface (but can be as deep as 1 cm). In contrast to the marked cyclic morphological changes in the ectocervical squamous cells, the columnar cells manifest minimal cytological changes. Instead, it shows dramatic variations in the production of secretion during the menstrual cycle. Importantly, mitotic activity is extremely rare in benign nongravid columnar epithelium. The subepithelial microvessel network of the endocervix is better developed than that of the ectocervix and the glandular structures largely shun from larger vessels and nerve bundles [2]. Furthermore, the endocervical stroma has twice as many stromal cells as does the ectocervical counterpart. The stromal cell from the two regions has different immunohistochemical features with the former showing reactivity for SMA and the latter for desmin. Moreover, the normal stroma also contains a dense network of CD34+ fibrocytes which are more predominantly located in the subepithelial and perivascular areas. In deep locations of the stroma, smooth muscle fibers are present and they are usually surrounded by CD34+ stromal cells [3].

The cervix plays important roles in the reproductive function. Not only is it involved in providing a port of entry for the sperm and a chemical barrier to infectious microorganism; the cervix also contributes to the creation of a safe haven for the implanting embryo and subsequently the growing fetus and a passageway for the ripe product of conception. The dramatic changes in the process of remodeling and ripening are effected through steroid hormones and complex epithelial–stromal interactions. It is only during the late phase of pregnancy that the endocervical glands are fully developed and manifest as lobules of tightly packed glands [4–6]. The destruction and rearrangement of collage fibers and other changes in the extracellular matrix apparently provide space for this remarkable glandular expansion. During the subsequent postpartum months, the hyperplastic glands involute gradually reverting to the baseline collateral clefts. Defective involution of some of the hyperplastic glands might result in diffuse laminar glandular hyperplasia.

X. Sun, *Well-Differentiated Malignancies: New Perspectives*, Current Clinical Pathology,
DOI 10.1007/978-1-4939-1692-4_6, © Springer Science+Business Media New York 2015

Key Morphological Feature of Well-Differentiated Squamous Cell Carcinoma

- Irregular narrow-based squamous nests with no surface connection
- Desmoplasia (haphazard SMA myofibroblasts) and loss of CD34+ fibrocytes (Figs. 6.1 and 6.2)

Discussion

Squamous cell carcinoma of the cervix develops from cervical intraepithelial dysplasia with clear HPV involvement. Well-differentiated squamous cell carcinoma is characterized by abundant keratin pearls and individual cell keratinization and a chronically inflamed stroma. Four common criteria used in the evaluation of invasion are (1) desmoplasia, (2) paradoxical maturation (excessive

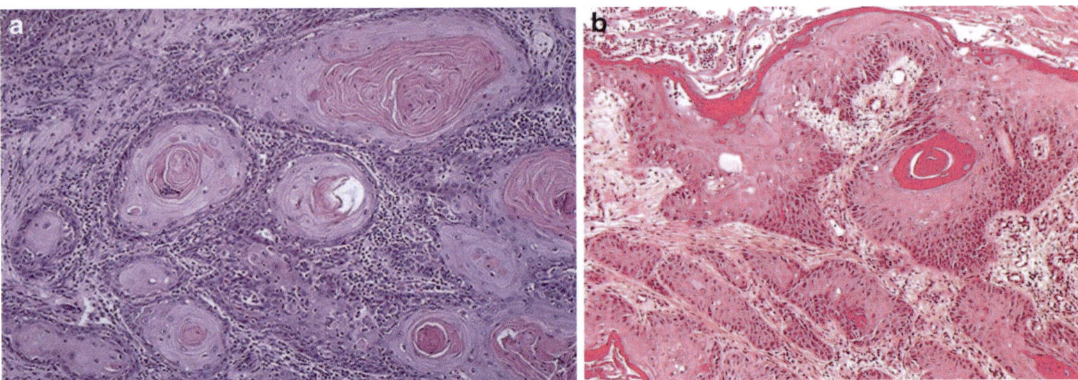

Fig. 6.1 Well-differentiated cervical squamous cell carcinoma. Irregular, narrowly based, or detached squamous nests. Cellular atypia at epithelial–stromal interface

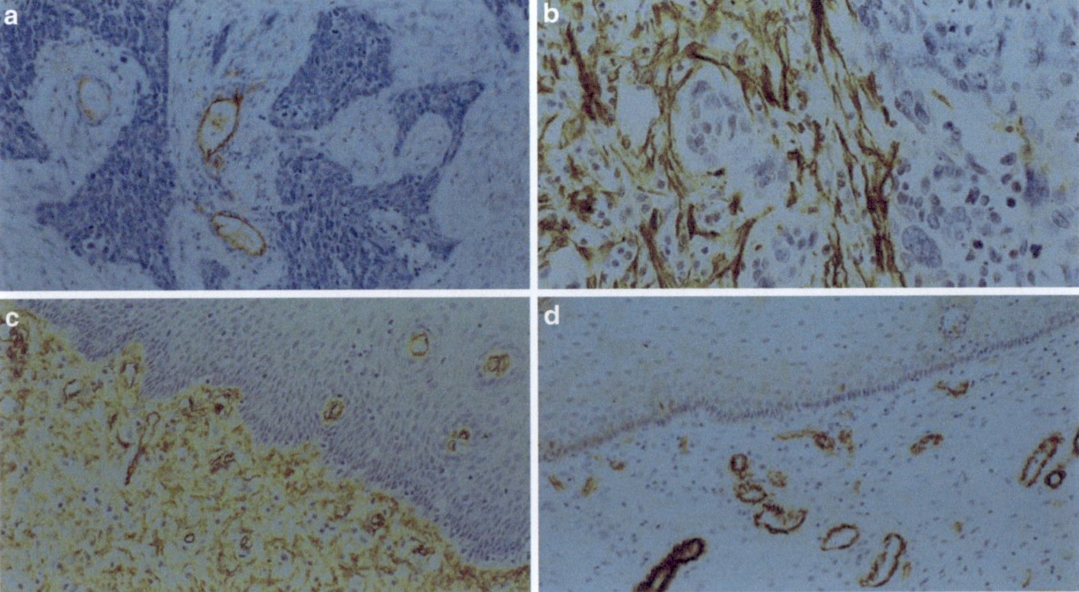

Fig. 6.2 Stroma of cervical squamous cell carcinoma. Note lack of CD34+ fibroblasts (**a**) in tumor stroma and presence of SMA+ fibroblasts (**b**). Normal cervical stroma contains plenty of CD34+ fibroblasts (**c**) and no SMA+ fibroblast (**d**)

cytoplasmic keratinization with conspicuous nucleoli), (3) loss of cell polarity at the basal layer, and (4) and the blurring of the epithelial–stromal interface.

However, the evaluation of stromal invasion is frequently compromised by tangential sectioning, cautery effect, obscuring inflammation at the tumor border and other inflammatory process, and even glandular involvement by metaplasia or dysplasia. In order to avoid overcalling metaplasia or dysplasia involving the glandular clefts, attention should be directed to the smooth contour of the tumor nests, their cytological features in comparison to those of the surface dysplastic epithelium, and polarity of tumor cells. In difficult cases, immunostainings for CD34 and SMA hold the promise for making the distinction [7, 8]. The stromal cells of invasive squamous carcinoma lack reactivity for CD34. SMA stain lights up haphazardly arranged myofibroblasts (desmoplasia). To differentiate pseudoepitheliomatous hyperplasia from well-differentiated squamous cell carcinoma would require the appreciation of the underlying inflammatory process and shape of the invasive components and their connection to the surface and shape (jagged pointed tips and a broad base connected to the surface). In addition to the panel of p53, MMP-1, and Ki67 which is used in other squamous locations, p16 can be used [9, 10].

Important Squamous Cell Carcinoma Variants

Awareness of the presence of variants would avoid passing them off as benign mimics.

Verrucous carcinoma lacks a central fibrovascular core and koilocytosis. Instead of having an infiltrative growth pattern, the tumor has a characteristic pushing border.

Condylomatous (warty) carcinoma has marked condylomatous changes. It has basal atypia and an infiltrative component at the base.

Papillary squamous (transitional) carcinoma has prominent papillary structures lined by cells with squamous and/or transitional cell differentiation. Interestingly, the transitional cells still maintain their cellular polarity. The invasive component manifests as well-circumscribed nests which are composed of squamous cells which are basal cell-like and resemble high-grade dysplasia.

Differential Diagnosis

Condyloma Acuminatum

Condyloma acuminatum shows squamous papillomatous growth with acanthosis, parakeratosis, and hyperkeratosis. Koilocytotic atypia, multinucleation, and individual cell keratinization are evident. The lack of stromal invasion sets it apart from condylomatous carcinoma.

Immature Squamous Metaplasia, Dysplasia Involving Glands

Squamous metaplasia and dysplasia frequently extend downward to the endocervical glands, and they show cellular atypia and mitotic activities. They however remain connected to the surface and keep the smooth glandular contours.

Placental Site Nodule and Epithelioid Trophoblastic Tumor, Decidual Changes

Placental site nodules are well-circumscribed nests composed of intermediate trophoblasts surrounded by hyaline material. Epithelioid trophoblastic tumor also shows preference for nest formation. The tumor often contains geographic necrosis. In difficult cases, immunostainings for CK18, inhibin, and p16 can help make the distinction since the trophoblast is positive for inhibin and CK18 and negative for p16 [11]. The reverse is true for squamous cell carcinoma cells.

Decidual changes can be confused with well-differentiated squamous cell carcinoma because of the abundant pink cytoplasm and well-defined cellular contours. However, the cells are degenerative in nature and a history of recent pregnancy is evident.

Reparative Changes with Chronic Granulomatous Inflammation and Pseudoepitheliomatous Hyperplasia

Reparative changes and pseudoepitheliomatous hyperplasia associated with chronic inflammatory diseases can be mistaken for invasive squamous carcinoma. The presence of extensive chronic inflammatory infiltrate alerts the pathologist to a possible infectious etiology. The hyperplastic squamous projections are usually connected to the surface with a broad base and have a jagged contour with pointed tips. Special stains for microorganisms and p16 can help confirm a diagnosis.

Key Morphological Features of Cervical Well-Differentiated Adenocarcinoma

- Nonlobular, irregular glandular, or villoglandular proliferation
- Deep location (Figs. 6.3, 6.4, and 6.5)

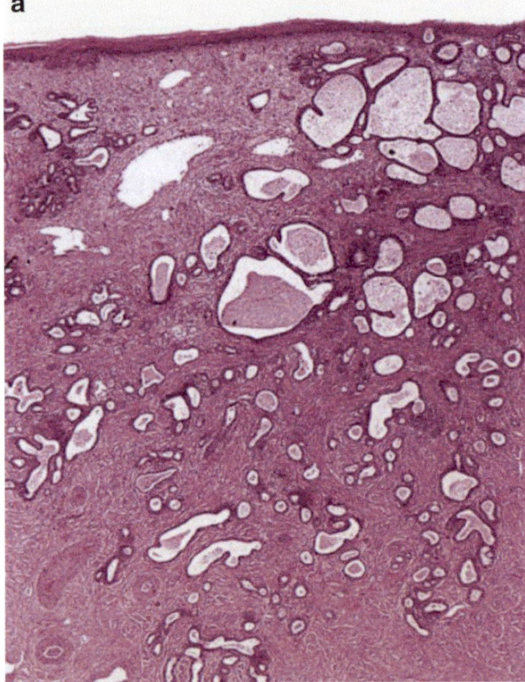

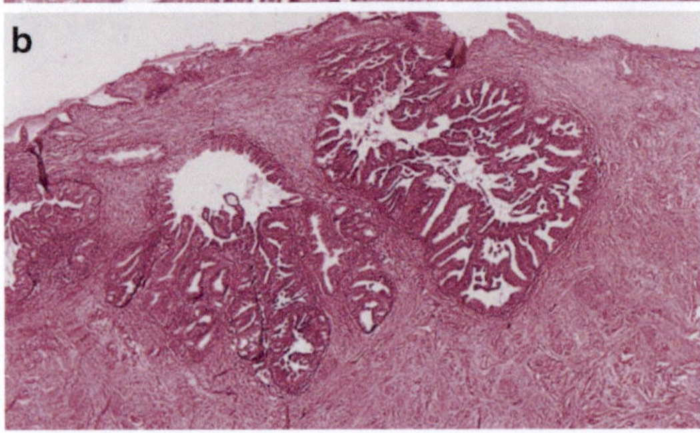

Fig. 6.3 Well-differentiated adenocarcinoma. Nonlobular, irregular glands (**a**). Expansive growth pattern (**b**) (Diagnostic Gynecologic and Obstetric Pathology, *Elsevier/Saunders*, 2011 with permission)

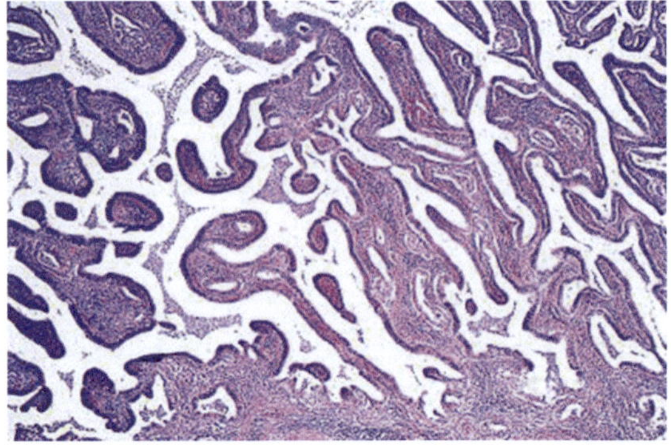

Fig. 6.4 Adenocarcinoma. Villoglandular growth pattern (Diagnostic Gynecologic and Obstetric Pathology, *Elsevier/Saunders*, 2011 with permission)

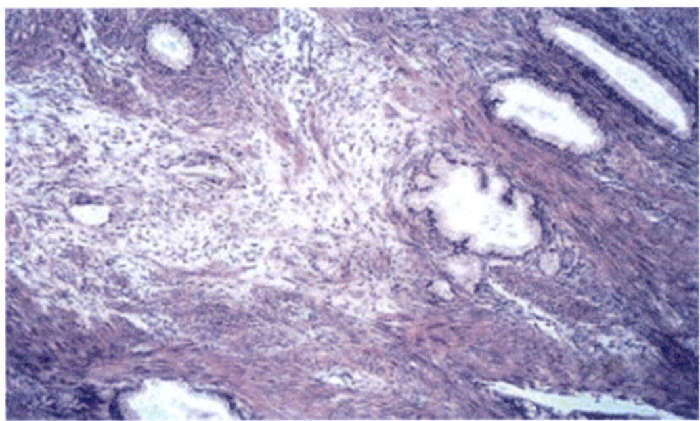

Fig. 6.5 Adenoma malignum. Note bland-looking glands with deep penetration (Diagnostic Gynecologic and Obstetric Pathology, *Elsevier/Saunders*, 2011 with permission)

Discussion

It has been increasingly realized that there are two pathways for cervical glandular carcinogenesis. The vast majority of endocervical adenocarcinomas are HPV related and progress through the dysplasia to carcinoma in situ progression pathway. The second pathway is independent of HPV infection and follows the pathway from lobular endocervical glandular hyperplasia to minimal deviation adenocarcinoma and mucinous adenocarcinoma [12, 13].

It is generally known that invasion should be suspected if there are nonlobular exuberant glandular growth in the form of extensive budding, confluency, cribriform, and exophytic papillary projections. However, the adenocarcinoma in

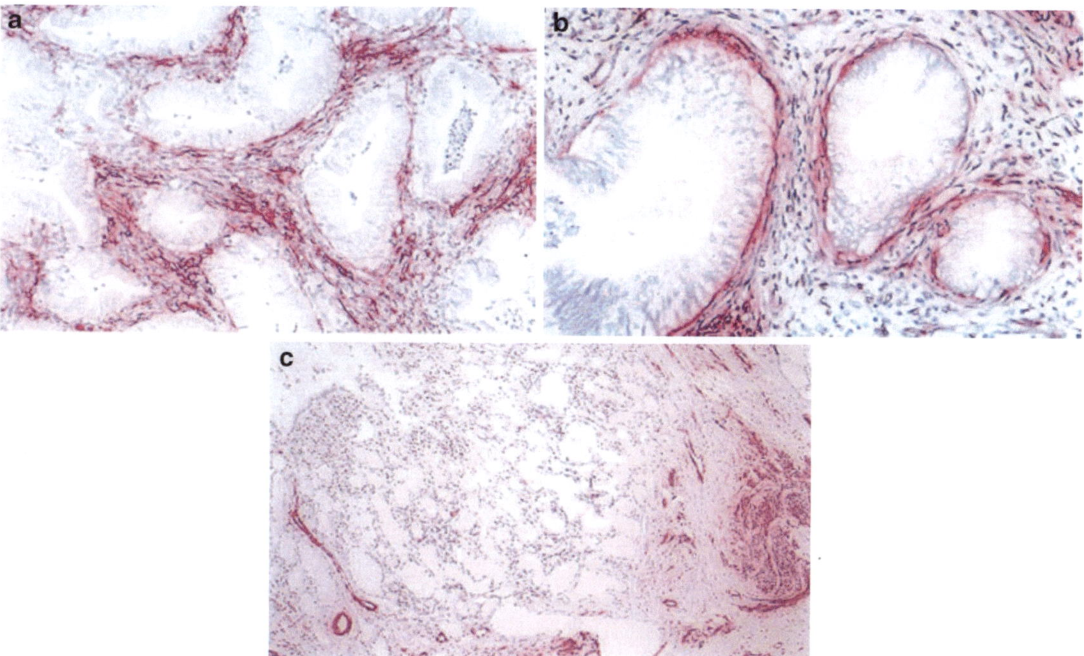

Fig. 6.6 Stroma of adenocarcinoma. Note presence of SMA+ myofibroblasts in stroma (**a**). A rim of SMA+ myofibroblasts around minimal deviation adenocarcinoma (**b**). Benign glands between preexisting smooth muscle bundles (**c**) (Histopathology, *John Wiley&Sons, Inc*, 2005 with permission)

situ can have complex papillary formation and even cribriform formation, and some benign glandular lesions are not lobular. Deep location, inflammatory, and desmoplasia of the stroma and presence adjacent to large vessels and nerve fibers are some important features of stromal invasion. Nevertheless, they are not always present. For instance, endocervical adenocarcinoma can also invade in expansile pattern without eliciting salient desmoplastic reaction. Some other promising indicators of stromal invasion include increased periglandular expression of SMA-positive myofibroblasts and stromal expression of CD44 and tenascin [14, 15] (Fig. 6.6).

The depth of glands is a very important index for the minimal deviation adenocarcinoma because it lacks exuberant epithelial growth and contains only focal cytological atypia. Most of the benign glands are confined to the inner 1/3 of the cervical wall. If the questionable glands extend more than 1 mm deeper than the adjacent benign ones, they are considered deep enough. This "deep concept" is not to be confused with those benign lesions usually located in the outer layer of the cervical wall. As discussed in the differential diagnosis section, some benign lesions can also be deep and even transmural.

To differentiate from those benign mimics of adenocarcinoma, a panel of immunostaining can be very helpful. The panel includes CEA, Ki67, and p16. Benign lesions usually show low mitotic activity and are negative for CEA and p16 [16, 17].

Another common dilemma in gynecological pathology is to distinguish a primary cervical adenocarcinoma from uterine extensions since several variants (such as villoglandular, endometrioid, and even mucinous) can be seen in both locations. Clues to a cervical origin include the presence of cervical dysplasia and lack of benign squamous morules and stromal foamy cells. Endocervical adenocarcinoma cells are positive of CEA and negative for ER, PR, and vimentin (the cells at the invasive front can be vimentin positive due to epithelial– mesenchymal transition)

[16, 17]. Apparently, the HPV infection messes up the epithelial–stromal coupling through the steroid hormones with the resultant loss of ER and PR expressions [18–20]. Endometrial carcinoma is ER, PR, and vimentin positive and negative for CEA.

Differential diagnosis

Nabothian Cysts and Deep Glands

The lining epithelium of Nabothian cysts is attenuated and sometimes shows squamous metaplasia. When cysts rupture, the spilled mucin can induce reactive changes in both the stroma and the epithelium. However, the cysts lack significant nuclear atypia and an infiltrative pattern even though they might be deep in location.

Deep tubo-endometrioid metaplasia can be mistaken for adenocarcinoma of endometrioid variant. The irregular and crowded glands are composed of columnar cells with high N/C ratios with occasional mitotic figures and are sometimes surrounded by a myxoid to edematous stroma. The presence of cilia and apical snouts are important clues.

Microglandular Hyperplasia

Microglandular hyperplasia consists of tightly packed glands in various sizes and shapes and may involve both the surface and deeper endocervical clefts. In general, the cells are bland with only occasional nuclear atypia. The lesion can be diagnosed by its lobular arrangement, presence of reserve cell hyperplasia and squamous metaplasia, low mitotic activities, and associated inflammation in the stroma.

Problem arises when the lesion becomes florid and contains more cytological atypia and even signet ring cells. The hyperplastic glands are arranged in reticular or solid patterns mimicking stromal invasion. Compounding the situation even further is when microglandular hyperplasia is involved by glandular dysplasia. In both situations, the presence of typical areas provides an important clue. Immunostainings for CEA, p16, and ki67 offer additional help in its distinction from adenocarcinoma. To differentiate from microglandular variant of endometrial carcinoma involving the cervix, ER, PR, and vimentin stains can be applied. The hyperplastic epithelial cells are positive for ER but negative for PR and vimentin [21].

Tunnel Clusters

Two frequently admixed types of tunnel clusters exist in the cervix. Type A tunnel cluster contains close-packed glands lined by columnar cells which might exhibit nuclear enlargement and pleomorphism. However, their superficial location and well circumscription differentiate them from invasive carcinoma.

Type B tunnel clusters are grossly mucin-containing cysts which are lined by an attenuated epithelium. They share the superficial location and demarcation features of type A tunnel clusters. Nevertheless, these two types probably should be separated further since type A has been shown to be related to lobular endocervical glandular hyperplasia, a likely precursor to cervical adenocarcinoma [22].

Lobular Endocervical Glandular Hyperplasia

Lobular endocervical glandular hyperplasia represents a metaplastic process which is a precursor lesion to cervical adenocarcinoma independent of human papilloma virus infection [23, 24]. It is characterized by a lobular proliferation of mucinous glands with pyloric gland phenotype. The glands are centered around larger glands (ducts) and are confined to the inner half of the endocervix. Typically, there is no significant cytological atypia. A diagnosis of atypical LEGH is made nuclear by the presence of atypia, mitotic figures, or apoptotic body or loss of cell polarity.

LEGH NOS has been used to describe endocervical lesion which shows neither a lobular nor laminated appearance. Most of them are incidental findings.

Diffuse Laminar Endocervical Gland Hyperplasia

Rather than being a mass lesion, diffuse Laminar endocervical gland hyperplasia presents as an incidental finding [25]. This lesion is characterized by a laminar proliferation of small- or medium-sized glands limited to the inner 1/3 of the cervical wall. When affected by inflammation, nuclear atypia can be present. The fact that the glandular proliferation is circumferential and appears to stop at the same level in a straight line at the base suggests that it might result from incomplete involution of pregnancy-related glandular hyperplasia.

Mesonephric Remnants and Hyperplasia

Mesonephric remnants are small tubules in clusters and contain thyroid-like material. They are commonly located deep in the lateral wall. A transmural lesion can result when the remnants become hyperplastic. The lobular type of hyperplasia sometimes has a central ductal structure. The diffuse type has evenly distributed pattern without stromal reaction, even though mild atypia and even mitotic figures can be seen. The tubular epithelium is positive for PAX2 and negative for CEA [26].

Endocervicosis, Endometriosis, and Endosalpingiosis

Endocervicosis in the cervix presents in the outer wall as variably shaped and sized mucinous glands which can become cystic. The extravasation of mucin can induce reactive changes. Thus, lesion is differentiated from adenocarcinoma by the presence of normal uninvolved stroma between the lesion of the surface and superficial normal glands.

Endosalpingiosis has the same anatomical location as endocervicosis, and the same criterion can be used in its distinction from invasive carcinoma.

Endometriosis of the cervix should not be confused with tubo-endometrioid metaplasia (discussed earlier). It is confined to the superficial one third of the cervical wall and contains both endometrial glands and stroma resembling proliferative endometrium.

The Uterus

Review of Pertinent Histology and Physiology

The uterus is an important organ in the reproductive system in that it is the actual site where a new life is formed and develops to term. In order to accommodate the inception, growth, and subsequent expulsion of the new life, the three major structural components of the uterus are brought under the coordinated influence of steroid hormones [27].

The Uterine Mucosa

The mucosa of the uterine body can be divided into three functional/histological layers. During reproductive years, the epithelial and stromal cells in the spongiosa undergo dramatic, cyclic changes in the repetitive business of preparing fresh receptive soil in anticipation of a possible implantation. In the process, the uterine epithelium and stroma form a structural and functional unit mediated through steroid hormone and paracrine factors. It is now known that endometrial epithelial and stromal cells probably share a common stem cell pool which gives rise to a mucosa composed of roughly equal amount of each component at the end of the proliferative phase [27–29]. The normal proliferative glands are straight and nonbranching.

The Uterine Stromal Cells

In the functional and structural units, the stromal cells not only provide structural support but also exert important dual effects on the epithelium. In providing structural scaffold for the cyclic endometrium, the stromal cells produce an elaborate network of reticulin fibers for each of them and develop a close relationship with small arterioles which might even derive from the same stem cells as the stromal cells.

On the one hand, the uterine stromal cells secrete growth factors via estrogen receptor pathways to facilitate the epithelial growth. On the other hand, in response to progesterone, they inhibit exuberant epithelial proliferation in response to progesterone [27]. Lack of or defect in this inhibitory effect leads to endometrial hyperplasia and carcinoma with resultant glandular crowding, branching, and even confluent growth.

Regional Mucosal Variance and Plasticity

The uterine endometrium is known for its regional variations and epithelial plasticity. The basalis and the compact (surface) show little change in morphology during the menstrual cycle (caveat; the surface get shed and the basalis remain throughout the menstruum). The lower uterine segment has a thinner and sluggish mucosa and often contains hybrid endocervical/endometrial components. The epithelial plasticity manifests in the form of metaplastic changes which are frequently present in endometrial specimens [30].

The Myometrium

The uterine myometrium is different from the smooth muscle tissues in other organs in two major aspects. First, uterine smooth muscle cells are responsive to steroid hormones. As a result, cyclic changes do occur even though they are not dramatic as those of the endometrium. During pregnancy, the myometrium undergoes extraordinary increase in mass through hyperplasia and hypertrophy. Concurrently, the uterine vasculature proliferates and remodels resultant from concerted effect of high levels of steroids and trophoblasts [31–33]. Secondly, the uterine smooth muscle fibers also have the capability to produce extracellular matrix material such as collage and elastin. Some smooth muscle cells at the endometrium/myometrium junction can have a hybrid stromal/smooth muscle phenotype.

Key Morphological Feature of Well-Differentiated Endometrial Adenocarcinoma

- Confluent growth pattern or complex papillary and villous glands
- Minimal intervening or altered stroma (fibrosis) (Figs. 6.7 and 6.8)

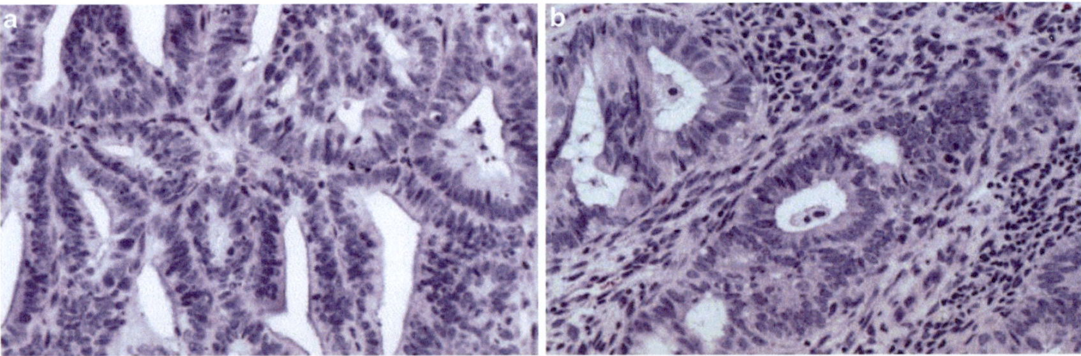

Fig. 6.7 Well-differentiated endometrial adenocarcinoma. Confluent growth pattern (**a**) and back-to-back glands (**b**) (Annals of Diagnostic Pathology, *Elsevier/Churchill Livingstone*, 2005 with permission)

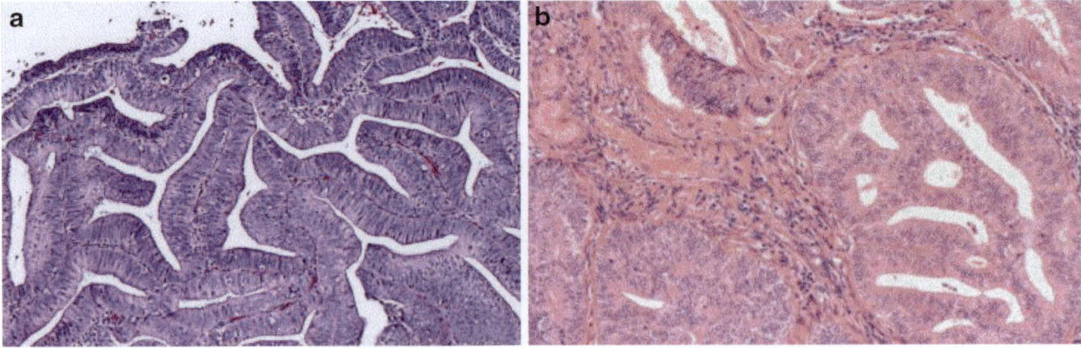

Fig. 6.8 Endometrial carcinoma. Villoglandular growth pattern (**a**) and altered stroma (**b**)

Discussion

Endometrial carcinoma develops from endometrial hyperplasia with PTEN mutation and PAX2 downregulation. The tipping point is reached when stromal invasion is evident. In this specialized organ where the epithelial and stromal components are derived from the same stem cells, stromal invasion manifests in three different forms [34]. They are (1) confluent glandular growth (or back-to-back glands) with no evident intervening stroma, (2) complex papillary or villoglandular structures, and (3) altered stroma.

Confluent glandular growth pattern manifests as complex branching or cribriform formations so that individual glands are surrounded by minimal or nil uterine stromal component. Complex papillary and villous glands are defined as branching papillary or villous structures with a fibrovascular core. Those intraglandular papillation and delicate papillae which are commonly present in metaplastic and hyperplastic processes should be excluded. To avoid overcalls, it is essential that the integrity of the specimen be not compromised.

In the evaluation of stromal alteration as evidence for stromal invasion, the shape and arrangement of the collagen-producing stromal cells are important features. They are more elongated, wavy, and eosinophilic than the normal stromal cells and are arranged in parallel fascicles compressed by collagen fibers. Caution should be exercised so that this stromal alteration is not confused with the fibrous stroma of endometrial polyps and tissue from the lower uterine segment. Endometrial polyps seem to be monoclonal stromal proliferation with secondary epithelial growth which is usually mild and seems undisturbed by stromal component. The stromal proliferation is frequently hyalinized and contains thick-walled blood vessels. The lower uterine segment stroma, particularly that of the inferior portion, is very fibrous. However, glandular proliferation in the form of glandular crowding and branching is lacking.

The grading of endometrial carcinoma employs a different set of criteria from those of most other adenocarcinomas. Well-differentiated carcinoma is defined as a tumor which contains less 5 % solid areas and lacks high-grade nuclei. In a case where the nuclei are markedly enlarged, hyperchromatic with prominent nucleoli, a higher grade is rendered (moderately differentiated, grade 2). Moderately differentiated carcinoma typically contains solid growth involving between 5 and 50 % of the tumor. Presence of marked nuclear atypia upgrades the tumor to grade 3 (poorly differentiated). Therefore, tumor necrosis and mitotic rate are left out of the grading system. In the evaluation of solid masses, it is very important that the squamous nests and sheets be excluded.

Similar to the nonneoplastic endometrial epithelium, the transformed epithelial cells can also manifest remarkable plasticity and the tumor shows frequent squamous, mucinous, ciliated, and even secretory and sex cord differentiation. Awareness of this important phenomenon avoids mistaking the differentiated components as benign tissue or confusing them as high carcinomas (such as clear cell carcinoma and serous cell carcinoma).

Finally, endometrial carcinoma, particularly in the well differentiated, can undergo dedifferentiation [35, 36]. Together with those entities showing sex cord differentiation (with spindle cells and hyalinized stroma) or containing benign chondroid and osteoid stroma, it needs to be differentiated from malignant mesodermal mixed tumor (MMMT). Malignant mesodermal mixed tumor (MMMT) contains separable high-grade epithelial and mesenchymal components.

Differential Diagnosis

Glandular Crowding Due to Stromal Breakdown or Artifact, Exaggerated Papillary Hyperplasia

Glandular crowding due to stromal breakdown or artificial displacement represents a common pitfall of overdiagnosis. In endometrial breakdown commonly seen in menstruation or anovulatory cycles, the epithelial structures lose the stromal support and become piled up with altered cellular polarity and even chromatin texture. Important clues to menstrual endometrium include secretory changes, predecidual changes in the stroma, nuclear dusts, and abundant neutrophils. In both menstruating and non-menstruating endometrium, endometrial tissue can be seen in the vessels. This should be interpreted as a sign of malignancy.

For small biopsies, crowding due to artifact can be recognized when the tissue adjacent to the displaced glands show signs of artificial shearing. Sometimes atrophic surface epithelium can aggregate and causes confusion with adenocarcinoma. It lacks true glandular crowding, epithelial stratification, or nuclear atypia.

Papillary hyperplasia is commonly seen on the surface of an endometrial polyp. Occasionally intracystic growth pattern is seen. The lining cells can undergo mucionous, eosinophilic, and ciliated metaplasia. The papillae can show branching and tufting. When present without a polyp, it can be misdiagnosed as endometrioid carcinoma or even papillary carcinoma. The nuclei are bland looking. No epithelial stratification nor real glandular crowding is evident.

Polyp, Mid- to Late Secretory Endometrium

Endometrial polyps can have irregular glands with focal glandular crowding. The crowding usually does not reach a level at which differentiation from carcinoma needs to be made. However, if involved by papillary hyperplasia, a differentiation is necessary.

Mid- to late secretory endometrium can have significant crowding. Since the cells show nuclear polymorphism and enlargement as well as loss of cell polarity when not accompanied by predecidual stroma, it can be mistaken as carcinoma in small biopsies when a predecidual stroma is evident.

Endometrial Hyperplasia

Compared to the proliferative endometrium, endometrial hyperplasia has an increased gland/stroma ratio with or without cytological atypia. With complex hyperplasia, the glandular structures can show significant branching and crowding. There is lack of the three criteria of endometrial carcinoma.

Atypical Polypoid Adenomyoma

The atypical polypoid adenomyoma typically presents in the lower uterine segment as a polypoid lesion. It contains irregular and haphazardly arranged endometrial glands in a fibromuscular stroma, simulating myometrium invasive endometrial carcinoma. The glands can show pseudostratification with mild to moderate cytological atypia. Abundant squamous morules are an important component, and they are frequently involved by necrosis. Important clues to this lesion are the polypoid presentation, short interlacing fibromuscular fascicles, and lack of endometrial stromal rimming.

Adenomyosis and Adenomyoma

Adenomyosis is defined as an endometrial tissue in myometrium. When a mass is formed, it is called adenomyoma. Typically the lesion contains both epithelial and stromal components even though either component can become inconspicuous. The important features of the lesion are its lobular appearance and hypertrophy of the surrounding muscle fibers. It lacks squamous morules as well as stromal desmoplasia.

Microglandular Hyperplasia and Endocervical Adenocarcinoma

Microglandular hyperplasia is a benign cervical lesion in young females. The morphology of the lesion can be mimicked by endometrial carcinoma with microcystic structures, focal squamous metaplasia, and inflammatory infiltrate. The malignant glands have, however, more glandular complexity and cytological atypia (Fig. 6.9).

Occasionally, a distinction of endometrial carcinoma from endocervical adenocarcinoma is needed in biopsy or curettings specimens. The distinction can be made easier by employing a panel of immunostainings (ER, PR, p16, and vimentin). Endometrial adenocarcinoma is diffusely positive for ER, PR, and vimentin and focally positive for p16. As the vast majority of endocervical adenocarcinomas are HPV related, they are usually negative for ER, PR, and vimentin. Instead, the tumor cells manifest diffuse reactivity to p16 antibody.

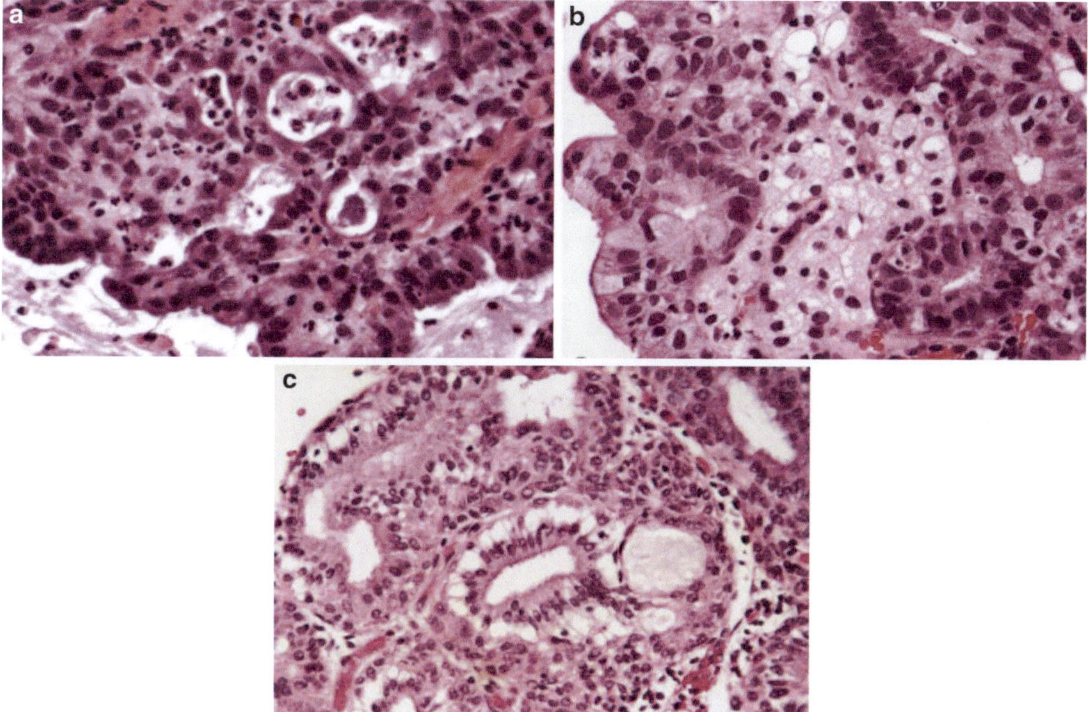

Fig. 6.9 Adenocarcinoma, microglandular variant (**a**, **b**). Note mitotic figures and foamy cells (**b**). Microglandular hyperplasia (**c**) (Diagnostic Gynecologic and Obstetric Pathology, *Elsevier/Saunders*, 2011 with permission)

Key Morphological Feature of Low-Grade Uterine Stromal Sarcoma

- Myometrial or vascular invasion (Fig. 6.10)

Discussion

Uterine stromal sarcomatous cells overexpress Bcl-2 probably as a result of chromosomal rearrangement, and they typically show low mitotic activity and negligible tumor cell necrosis and/or apoptosis. In contrast to the parameters used in the evaluation of uterine leiomyomatous lesions, muscle or vascular invasion becomes the yardstick in the differentiation between a benign stromal nodule and stromal sarcoma. Typically, myometrial invasion is in the form of tentacles, but may also present as an intramyometrial nodule or rarely diffuse myometrial thickening with no evident tumor mass formation. While uterine stromal cells develop a close functional/histological relationship with arterioles, sarcomatous cells tend to invade lymphatics and veins.

Uterine stromal lesions frequently show divergent differentiations, and unfamiliarity with this important feature could lead to erroneous diagnoses. For instance, frequent sex cord elements, glandular structures, and heterologous elements can be seen. Stromal hyalinization and smooth muscle differentiation can also be present resulting in a diagnosis of mixed stromal–smooth muscle tumor.

Adenosarcoma and adenofibroma can also show sex cord differentiation and heterologous elements. They can, however, be differentiated from low-grade endometrial stromal sarcoma with glandular differentiation by the presence of their leaflike growth pattern. Adenosarcoma differs from adenofibroma in that it has periglandular condensation of stromal cells which have increased cellularity, mitotic activity, and cytological atypia [37]. This is in stark contrast to mammary phyllodes tumors in which periglandular stromal cell

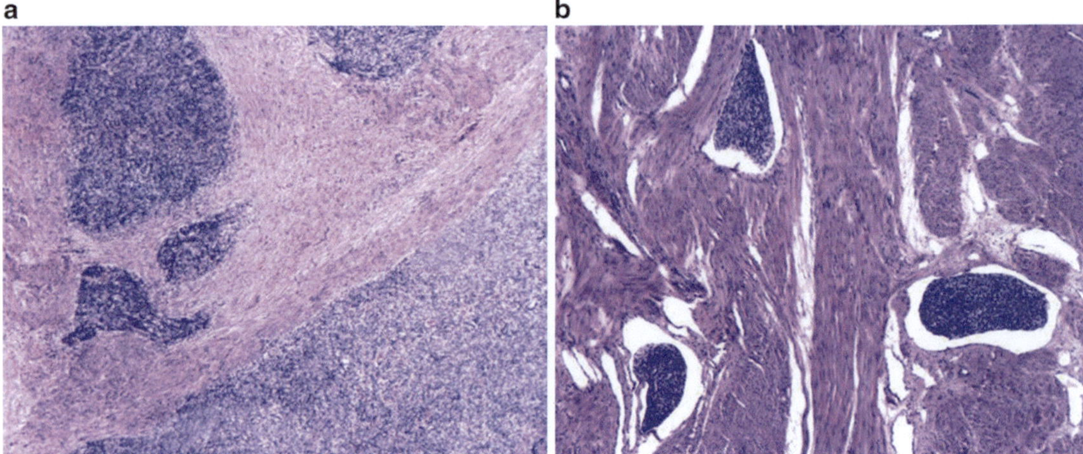

Fig. 6.10 Low-grade uterine stromal sarcoma. Myometrial (**a**) and vascular invasion (**b**) (Diagnostic Gynecologic and Obstetric Pathology, *Elsevier/Saunders*, 2011 with permission)

condensation is not a sign of malignancy. Instead, malignant phyllodes tumor is characterized by marked stromal overgrowth. Only a small fraction of adenosarcomas share this feature.

Differential Diagnosis

Endometrial Stromal Nodule

An endometrial stromal nodule is composed of uniform, small cells with scant to moderate cytoplasm and poor cellular borders. Glandular and sex cord-like elements can be present. The lesion, however, lacks invasion into the endometrium, myometrium, or vessels. Importantly, an extension or protrusion of less than 3 mm into the adjacent tissue is not considered invasion. As this stromal lesion can frequently show smooth muscle and fibrous differentiation, it is also important that the intermingling metaplastic smooth muscle fibers and stromal cells are not interpreted as evidence of myoinvasion.

Cellular Leiomyoma and Intravenous Leiomyomatosis

Highly cellular leiomyoma can be confused with uterine stromal sarcoma in small biopsy/curettage specimens because the tumor border cannot be evaluated. Cellular leiomyoma is composed of larger spindle-shaped smooth muscle fibers. Important clues include large thick vessels in the lesion.

Intravenous leiomyomatosis (IVL) can mimic uterine stromal sarcoma in that it invades vessels and dissects into adjacent myometrium. The tumor cells, however, are larger and tend to show a predominant intravascular component. Immunostaining for SMA, desmin, caldesmon, and CD10 and even reticulin stain can help make the distinction.

Adenomyosis and Adenomyoma

Two variants of adenomyosis are particularly prone to be confused for stromal sarcoma. In one variant, the endometrial tissue has a propensity to protrude into the myometrial vessels. However, this is not a true vascular invasion. Immunostainings for endothelial cells would reveal a complete layer of endothelium covering the endometrial tissue.

The other variant has an inconspicuous glandular component, and its stromal component maintains a lobular appearance with hypertrophy of adjacent smooth muscle fibers. Typical adenomyosis areas can be found in other location.

Adenomyoma is a well-circumscribed mass composed of endometrial stroma, glands, and smooth muscle fibers.

Key Morphological Feature of Well-Differentiated Uterine Leiomyosarcoma

- Tumor cell necrosis and mitotic figures >10/10HPF
- Or tumor cell necrosis with significant nuclear atypia (Figs. 6.11 and 6.12)

Discussion

The uterine smooth muscle tissue (myometrium) is programmed to respond to steroid hormones in order to provide a muscular conglomerate for labor. During pregnancy, the uterine smooth muscle tissue undergoes tremendous increase in mass through cellular hyperplasia and hypertrophy. Understandably, there should be multiple protective mechanisms to keep this extraordinary growth potential in check in nongravid conditions. Commonly encountered uterine leiomyomas are characterized by a variety of

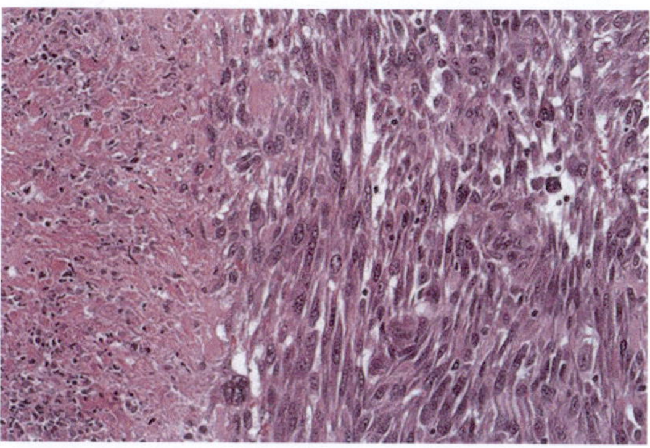

Fig. 6.11 Leiomyosarcoma with tumor necrosis (Journal of Clinical Pathology, *American Society of Clinical Pathology*, 2007; Best Practice & Research in Clinical Obstetrics and Gynecology, *Elsevier/Churchill Livingstone*, 2011 with permission)

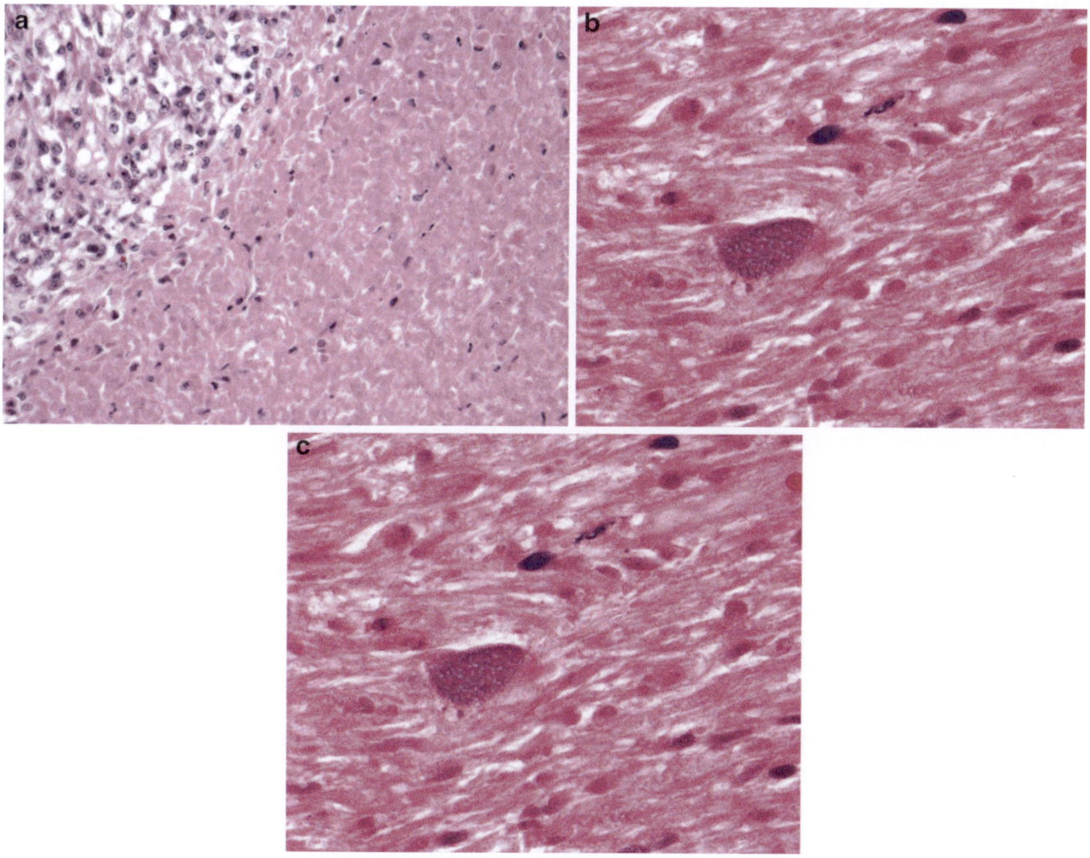

Fig. 6.12 Tumor necrosis. Note abrupt and sharp interface between necrotic and viable tissue. Ghost cells present (Diagnostic Gynecologic and Obstetric Pathology, *Elsevier/Saunders*, 2011 with permission)

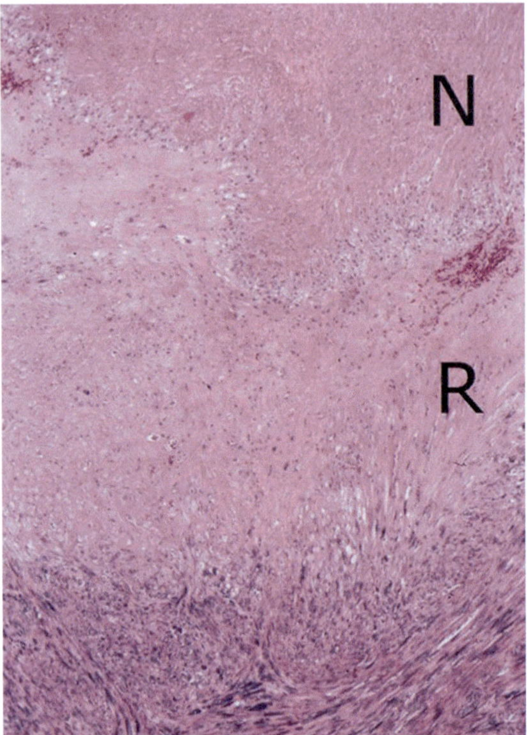

Fig. 6.13 Bland (coagulative) necrosis. Distinctive zonation with necrosis, hyalinized collagen, and viable tissue (Diagnostic Gynecologic and Obstetric Pathology, Elsevier/Saunders, 2011 with permission)

simple genetic changes involving multiple pathways (mechanisms) [38]. The multiple involved pathways might account for the many variants of uterine leiomyoma. Some of them show concerning features and they include mitotically active, cellular, atypical (with bizarre nuclei), dissecting, vascular invasion and even metastasizing variants.

The predominant view holds that most leiomyosarcomas arise de novo and they contain far more complex cytogenetic changes than leiomyomas. These complex chromosomal abnormalities lead to genomic instability and knockdown of the protective mechanisms, allowing aggressive growth, recurrence, and frequent metastasis.

In the evaluation of uterine leiomyomatous lesions, many of the common malignant parameters such as infiltrative border, hemorrhage, cellularity, vascular invasion, and even metastasis are left out of the picture (Fig. 6.13). Tumor cell differentiation is also largely clinically irrelevant (except for the fact that a lower mitotic threshold has been proposed for epithelioid tumors). Instead, the evaluation should focus on three indices: tumor cell necrosis, mitotic count, and cytological atypia.

Tumor cell necrosis needs to be differentiated from hyaline necrosis (infarction) which is a common occurrence in uterine leiomyoma (Fig. 6.14). Apparently resultant from compromised blood supply probably due to defective anticoagulation/fibrinolytic function in the tumor vessels, hyaline necrosis has distinctive zonation in that the central necrotic region is surrounded by a layer of granulation tissue which is separated from the viable tissue by hyalinized collagen [39, 40].

Tumor cell necrosis is typically geographic (multifocal and irregular in shape), and its interface with the viable tissue is sharp and abrupt and lacks fibroblastic proliferation. At a low power, viable cells can be seen in the periphery of small vessels. However, acute ischemic necrosis is difficult to differentiate from tumor cell necrosis since both lack a zonal pattern with abruption transition from viable dead and viable cells. Important clues favoring tumor cell necrosis include ghost cells with persevered hyperchromatic and pleomorphic nuclei and lack of associated inflammation. Acute infarction is usually associated with acute inflammation and other regions at various stages of infarction.

Mitotic counting should be conducted in the most active areas which are free of erosion and/or attenuated mucosa. It is important not to confuse lymphocytes, pyknotic, nuclei and even mast cells as mitotic figure. In difficult cases, the stain for Ki67 can be used. Atypical mitotic figure is placed under the significant cytological atypia category.

Significant atypia includes moderate to severe atypia which can be diffuse or focal. Typically, it presents as nuclear hyperchromasia and pleomorphism at low power magnification. Less commonly, atypia manifests as uniform nuclear enlargement and hyperchromasia.

The above discussed criteria need to be modified in the diagnosis of myxoid leiomyosarcoma which has low mitotic counts. A mitotic count

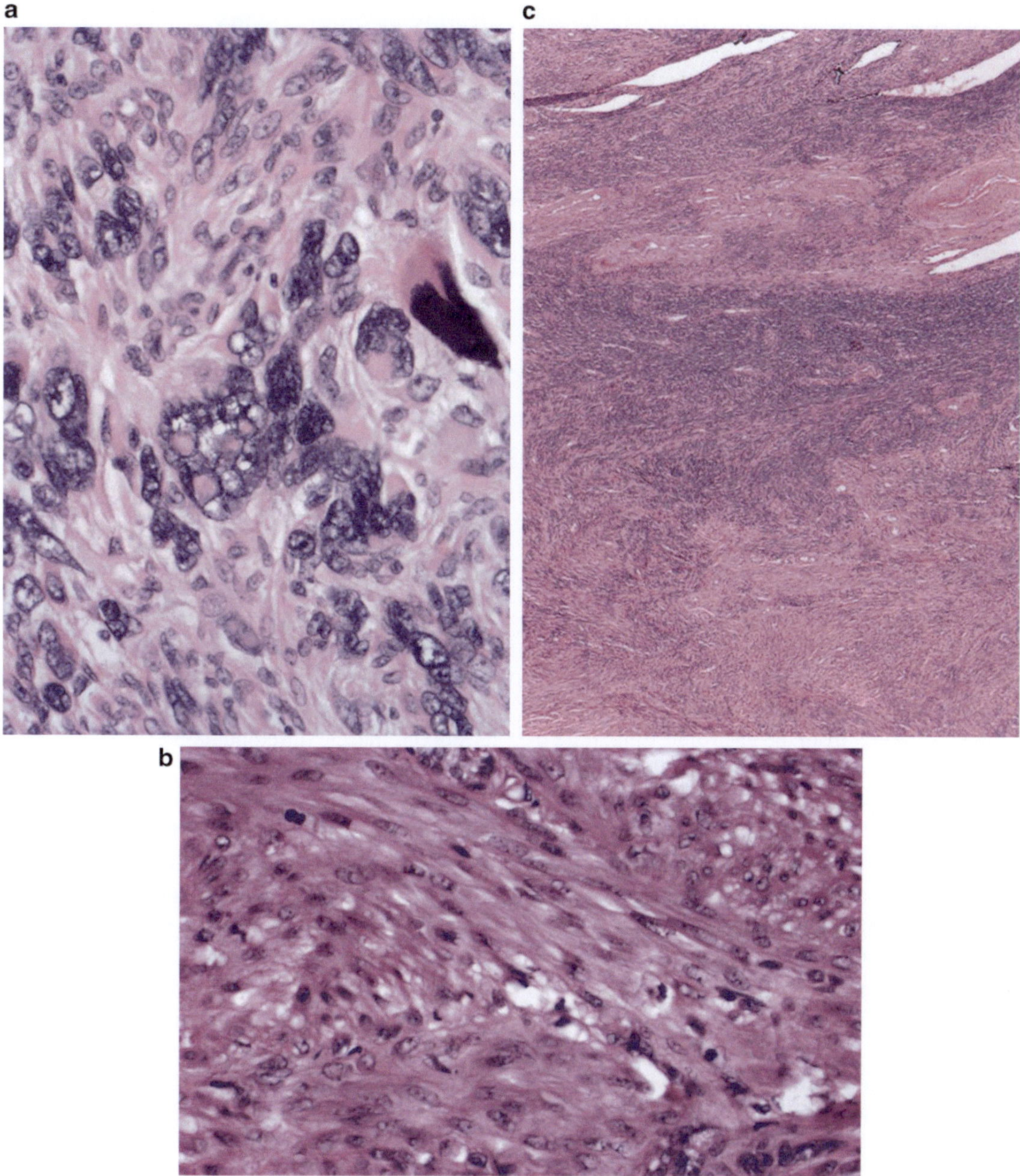

Fig. 6.14 Leiomyoma variant. With cellular atypia (**a**), increased mitotic figures (**b**), and hypercellularity (**c**) (Diagnostic Gynecologic and Obstetric Pathology, *Elsevier/Saunders*, 2011 with permission)

greater than 2/10 HPF has been proposed. Some experts make a malignant diagnosis in the presence of any of three criteria or a destructive pattern.

The diagnosis of epithelioid leiomyosarcoma also requires a lower mitotic count (greater than 5 MF/10hpf). Its frequent reactivity for pan cytokeratin and decreased reactivity for SMA might lead to an erroneous diagnosis of epithelial lesion.

Differential Diagnosis

Leiomyoma Variants

Mitotically active leiomyoma can have up to 10–20 MF/10 HPF. It occurs mainly in premenopausal women and lacks significant cellular atypia including atypical mitosis and tumor cell necrosis.

Atypical leiomyoma (leiomyoma with bizarre nuclei) refers to a variant with moderate to severe nuclear atypia. Typically the nuclei are enlarged and hyperchromatic with frequent multinucleation and smudgy chromatin texture. It lacks tumor necrosis and the mitotic count is less than 10/10HPF.

Leiomyoma with vascular invasion defines a rare variant with prominent intravenous growth. This pattern can also be seen in leiomyosarcoma. However, this growth pattern does not represent true vascular invasion since the tumor clusters are lined with a layer of endothelium. This variant lacks all the three signs of malignancy (tumor necrosis, high mitotic activity, and moderate to severe cytological atypia).

Other rare uterine leiomyoma variants with concerning features for other tissues include dissecting leiomyoma, benign metastasizing leiomyoma, parasitic leiomyoma, and disseminated peritoneal leiomyomatosis. Parasitic leiomyoma is believed to be detached from subserosal uterine leiomyoma and should not be confused with leiomyosarcoma from the gastrointestinal tract or the retroperitoneum. Disseminated peritoneal leiomyomatosis needs to be distinguished from metastatic uterine leiomyosarcoma. Importantly, the tumor nodules are small and are composed of bland spindle cells with smooth muscle, myofibroblast, and fibroblast differentiations which show low mitotic activity and lack of tumor cell necrosis. The tumor is frequently associated with pregnancy and decidual cells can be seen.

Smooth Muscle Tumor of Unknown Malignant Potential (STUMP)

By definition, STUMP defines a group of leiomyomatous tumors with features exceeding those for leiomyoma variants but falling short of those for leiomyosarcoma. Three subcategories can be recognized. Subcategory one encompasses tumors with tumor cell necrosis, but less than 10MF/10 HPF or only mild cytological atypia. Included in subcategory two are tumors with diffuse significant cytological atypia and a mitotic count of 5 to 9/HPF, but no tumor necrosis. Tumors with focal significant atypia with mitotic count greater than 5/HPF but no necrosis fall into subcategory three.

Uterine Stromal Lesions

Uterine stromal lesions have relatively uniform cells with round to ovoid nuclei. Characteristically, they contain abundant small arterioles and frequent hyaline plaques. The tumor cells are not arranged in fascicles. Instead, the individual cell or small nests are surrounded by reticulin fibers. However, fibroblastic or myofibroblastic differentiation is common. In difficult cases, CD10 and smooth muscle markers are useful. Because stromal cells can undergo myofibroblastic differentiation and uterine smooth muscle fibers can show CD10 reactivity, it is recommended that a diffuse stain pattern for each stain be required in the arbitration. It seems that h-caldesmon is more specific for smooth muscle fibers than the other markers.

Nevertheless, stromal lesions can also contain epithelioid abundant cytoplasm and myxoid stroma. Epithelioid leiomyosarcoma is known to have decreased expression of usual smooth muscle markers including h-caldesmon. Histone deacetylase 8 (HADAC-8) might be helpful in confirming its smooth muscle differentiation [38, 41].

PEComa

PEComa is composed of spindle or epithelioid cells with flocculent eosinophilic cytoplasm. It simulates uterine stromal cell lesions more than smooth muscle tumors in its growth patterns. Immunostainings for Melanin A and microphthalmia transcription factors and CD1a are better markers for PEComa since a significant portion of uterine leiomyosarcomas are positive for the stain [38, 42]. Malignant PEComa is characterized by high cellularity, significant atypia and mitosis (>1/10HPF), necrosis, and an infiltrative growth pattern.

The Ovary

Overview

Review of Pertinent Histology and Physiology

The ovary is charged with two important functions of producing oocytes and coordinating physiological and histological changes in the others parts of the female reproductive system (including the mammary glands) via the production of steroid hormones.

The cortical stroma of the ovaries in a woman of the reproductive ages is irregularly strewn with primordial follicles. Along with granulosa cells, they form functionally and architecturally independent units in support of follicular development and steroid production. Except for a small fraction of primordial follicles which are scheduled to embark on the monthly developmental odyssey, the vast majority of follicles and their associated interstitial cells are kept in a dormant state. Out of around twenty of selected primordial follicles, only a few become dominant and move to the next stage. The primary follicles contain a rim of granulosa cells accompanied by the differentiation of the interstitial cells into theca interna cells. Further developments produce secondary follicle(s) and subsequently a tertiary follicle (appearance of a theca externa). The story goes on even after the ovulation with both granulosa and theca cells being transformed into hormone-producing cells (corpus luteum) and end up with the formation of corpus albicans.

The developmental odyssey is orchestrated by the complex interactions among the oocyte, granulosa cells, and ovarian stromal cells with the oocyte being the probable dominant figure [43, 44]. Derived from the embryonal surface epithelium, the granulosa cells are positive for calretinin, CD99, Melanin A, cytokeratin, and vimentin [45]. They connect each other through adherence junctions, gap junctions, and desmosomes, and they seem to lack the capability to attract blood vessels. The desmin- and actin-positive interstitial cells are supported by a rich reticulin network. Along with the associated follicular development, stromal cells evolve into theca inner and theca outer layers. The theca inner cells are positive for inhibin, calretinin, and melan-A, whereas the theca outer cells show smooth muscle differentiation. After ovulation, they become an important component of the corpus luteum.

The ovary is covered by a layer of simple epithelium which shares the same embryonal origin as the epithelium lining the upper part of the vagina, cervix, uterus, and the fallopian tube. The epithelial cells are positive for ER, PR, follicle-stimulating hormone receptor, and EGRF. By no means a passive barrier, the ovarian surface epithelium participates in many aspects of the ovarian physiology such as follicular rupture, oocyte release, and subsequent repair[46, 47]. As a result, cortical and even medullary inclusion cysts are very common in postmenopausal women.

Ovarian Epithelial Tumors, Epithelial–Stromal Interaction, and Stroma Invasion

The epithelial inclusion cysts are believed to be the site of origin of ovarian epithelial neoplasms [47, 48]. The lining cells keep the potential to differentiate along the mullerian line, and their proliferative activity seems to be largely kept in check by an inherently inhibitory stroma which is programmed to support only highly focal and short-lived follicular and epithelial proliferation probably through a p53-related mechanism [49, 50]. This inhibitory mechanism makes the stroma less permissive for tumor growth than the peritoneal stroma and account for the phenomenon of invasive peritoneal implants in ovarian borderline serous and even borderline endocervical mucinous tumors. It may even underlie the fact that primary ovarian carcinomas more often than not manifest an expansile invasion pattern.

Analogous to the situation in hair follicular and sweat gland tumors, benign and borderline epithelial tumors can be seen distributed in cortical or fibrous stroma. Simply being surrounded by the stroma does not signify invasion. Two types of stromal invasion patterns have been recognized in the ovary. Expansive invasion manifests as confluent epithelial growth with little intervening stroma. This important feature also helps differentiate primary ovarian tumor from metastatic malignances which are more likely to be infiltrative or nodular and bilateral with surface and hilar involvement. Infiltrative invasion is characterized by haphazard arrangement of epithelial structures or single cells in an often desmoplastic stroma.

It seems that the epithelial differentiation not only determines the arrangement of the tumor epithelial cells but also affects the tumor stromal composition [50]. For instance, clear cell carcinoma stroma tends to be densely hyalinized with a low fibroblast cell component. The low cellular stroma is also shared by high-grade serous cell carcinoma. Mucinous and low-grade serous carcinomatous stroma instead contains a high proportion of stromal cell contribution. Endometrioid carcinoma has a low to moderate cellular stroma. As in other organs, the cancer-associated stromal cells might have multiple sources including tissue-resident fibroblasts, senescent fibroblasts, recruitment of hematopoietic precursors, and even stromal stem cells. The use of specific molecular markers for cancer-associated stromal cells might have important diagnostic significance in the differentiation between borderline tumors and invasive carcinomas since the former can manifest complex epithelial proliferation. FAP-1 alpha and FSP-1 alpha are some promising markers [51]. Moreover, recent data implicate the involvement of stromal cell p53 attenuation in the epithelial tumorigenic progression. Future studies on stromal p53 in different types of ovarian carcinomas might shed new light on the tumorigenesis [49, 50].

In this book of well-differentiated (low-grade) malignancies, we will also discuss borderline epithelial tumors since they carry a small risk of recurrence and even death. The differentiation between them and invasive carcinomas lies in the presence of stromal invasion in the latter. High-grade serous carcinoma and clear cell carcinoma are largely left out of the discussion.

Ovarian Granulosa Cell and Sertoli Cell Tumors

Recent evidence indicates that the ovarian sex cord components evolve from the embryonal surface epithelium [45]. In the process of organogenesis, a high degree of intimacy develops between them and the stromal interstitial cells in that the stromal cells proliferate, invade, and separate the sex cord components into primordial follicular structures. Such an intimate relationship blurs the interface between them, particularly in sex cord–stromal tumors. As a result, the two components are so closely intertwined that a diagnosis of infiltrative tumor might be rendered if taken out of the context. Furthermore, because the ovary lacks a tunica albuginea-like structure but possesses inherent properties to erupt and repair, the clinically relevant sign of invasion takes on a less conventional form (analogous to neuroendocrine and lymphoproliferative neoplasms): extension beyond the organ boundary. Therefore, clinical staging is required for both granulosa and Sertoli cell tumors and extraovarian extension becomes the most reliable indication for malignancy.

Granulosa cell tumor is generally considered a tumor of low-grade malignancy. Interestingly, the tumor cell differentiation and some of the common malignancy indices such as necrosis and hemorrhage do not correlate with the tumor behavior. In this book, we do not intend to grade granulosa tumors based on histological pattern or differentiation. Instead, we focus on those morphological features which are proved to be associated with an adverse clinical outcome.

On the other hand, tumor differentiation seems to correlate well with clinical outcomes for Sertoli cell tumors. Well-differentiated Sertoli cell tumors behave like benign neoplasms. The majority of poorly differentiated and a fraction of well-differentiated tumors are clinically malignant. We call attention to the histological features of this small fraction of well-differentiated tumors.

Key Morphological Features of Low-Grade Serous Malignancy

- Hierarchical branching papillae with epithelial stratification or micropapillae (borderline) (Fig. 6.15)
- Multiple papillae projecting into clear spaces or infiltrative glands and small nests and papillae in a hyaline of desmoplastic stroma (greater than 0.5 mm, invasive) (Fig. 6.16)

Discussion

The serous borderline tumor displays extensive epithelial proliferation in the form of hierarchical papillary structures with cell stratification, tufting, and detachment. Even though the cells are more atypical than those of the benign serous tumor, the basally located nuclei are ovoid with fine chromatin features. Nucleoli and mitotic figures are much less commonly identified than in serous carcinoma in situ and high-grade serous carcinomas. Because micropapillary/cribriform formations are associated with a higher risk for peritoneal implants, some authorities adopt a term of noninvasive micropapillary serous carcinoma (or low-grade serous intraepithelial carcinoma) for those tumors in which cribriform (fused micropapillae) formation measures greater than 5 mm but lacks stromal invasion [52].

An important feature of borderline serous tumor is the presence of peritoneal implants. As invasive implants are associated with an adverse clinical outcome, accepted criteria require the presence of both desmoplasia and an infiltrative border [52, 53]. Micropapillary structures have been proposed as an additional criterion for invasive implantation. Moreover, borderline serous tumor has also been associated with lymph node involvement. Nodular presentation, desmoplasia, and micropapillary architectures in the involved lymph node portend an unfavorable clinical outcome.

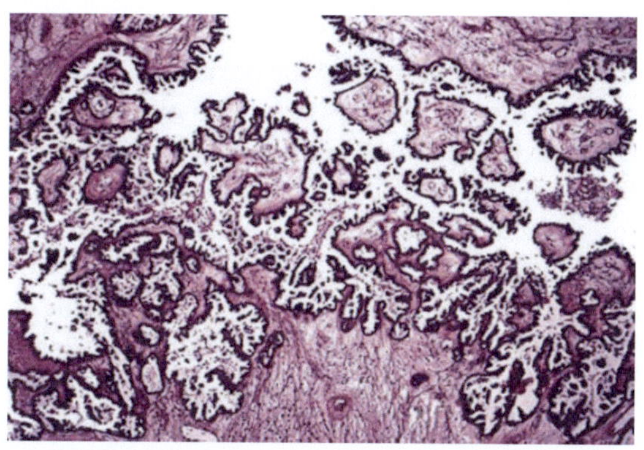

Fig. 6.15 Borderline serous neoplasm. Hierarchical branching papillae with stratification (Diagnostic Gynecologic and Obstetric Pathology, *Elsevier/Saunders*, 2011 with permission)

The ovarian low-grade serous carcinoma evolves from the serous borderline tumor, and they are both genetically (KRAS and BRAF mutations vs p53 mutations) and morphologically different from the high-grade serous carcinoma and carcinoma in situ [53]. The tumor is arranged in well-differentiated papillary structures composed of cells with uniform low-grade nuclei and focal or patchy p53 reactivity. The tumor stroma is typically highly cellular. Stromal invasion usually manifests as irregular infiltration of small glands, nests, and papillae in a desmoplastic or hyaline stroma. Oftentimes, the invasive papillae are separated from the stroma by a clear space. When the invasive growth pattern occupies an area greater than 5 mm across, a diagnosis of invasive carcinoma should be rendered. Microinvasion is used for lesions falling short of the size criteria. Importantly, tangentially cut stromal invagination of complex papillae should not be interpreted as stromal invasion. Psammoma carcinoma refers to a rare form of low-grade serous carcinoma which contains psammoma bodies in more than 75 % of papillae. It behaves like a borderline tumor.

In contrast, high-grade ovarian serous carcinoma is believed to derive from carcinoma in situ in the fallopian tube epithelium and is characterized

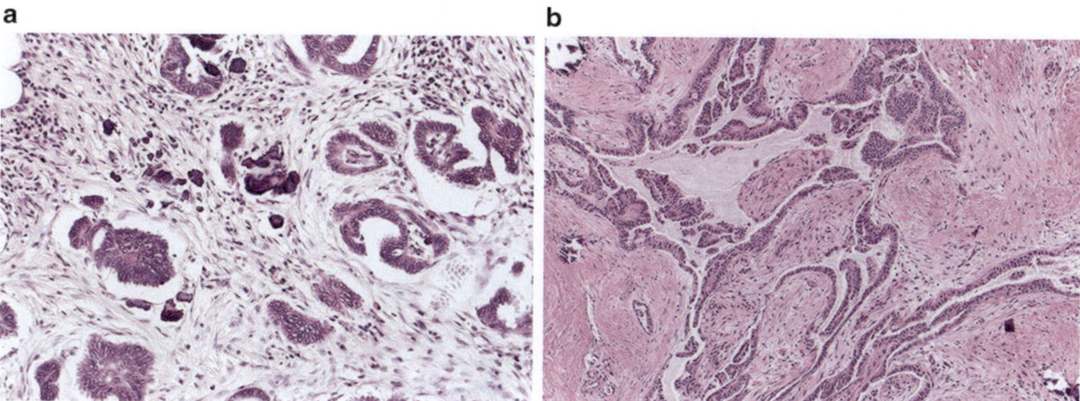

Fig. 6.16 Low-grade serous carcinoma with clefting and desmoplasia (Diagnostic Gynecologic and Obstetric Pathology, *Elsevier/Saunders*, 2011 with permission)

by complex papillary and solid patterns and marked cytological atypia. Lace and labyrinthine growth patterns are frequently seen and the tumor stroma is hypocellular.

Differential Diagnosis

Endosalpingiosis

The lesion consists of simple columnar epithelium with tubular differentiation with mild cytological atypia and simple palpation.

Serous Cystadenoma and Adenofibroma

Benign serous tumors lack the hierarchical branching of papillae, epithelial stratification, tufting, and detachment of small papillae. Cystadenoma with focal atypia has been used for cases with focal areas showing the typical borderline features.

Retiform Variant of Sertoli–Leydig Cell Tumor

Characterized by a network of irregular branching tubules, cysts, and papillae, this variant of Sertoli cell tumor can mimic serous borderline and invasive carcinoma. However, the patient's young age and the presence of other features of Sertoli–Leydig cell tumor are important clues.

Other Types of Ovarian Epithelial Carcinoma

See the description for the other types.

Key Morphological Features of Borderline Clear Cell Tumor

- Cysts and tubules lined by one or two layers of clear cells with nuclear enlargement and hyperchromasia in a fibromatous stroma (Fig. 6.17)

Discussion

The borderline clear cell tumor presents as tubular glands line by one to two layers of clear cells distributed in a compact fibrocollagenous stroma. It is differentiated from the rare benign cell tumor by the presence of significant nuclear atypia and increased mitotic activity. In general, significant epithelial stratification and complex architectural structures are incompatible with borderline clear cell tumor even though slight stratification, budding, and papillation may be present.

Clear cell carcinoma is a high-grade tumor and characteristically manifests as papillary, tubulocystic, and solid structures. Other important features include hyalinized papillary cores and hyaline bodies as well as presence of a variety of cell types including hobnail cells. To facilitate its distinction from the borderline tumor, a single focus of confluent growth greater than 10 mm has been proposed as the yardstick. Although many ovarian malignancies can contain clear cells, they lack the characteristic cytological and architectural features of clear cell carcinoma. As clear cell carcinoma clearly belongs to the high-grade cate-

a

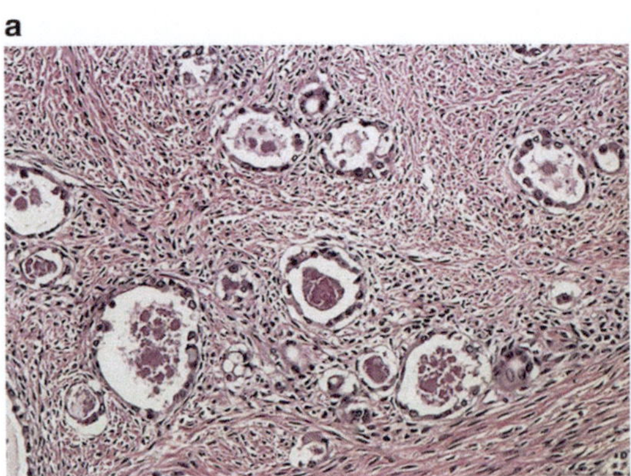

b

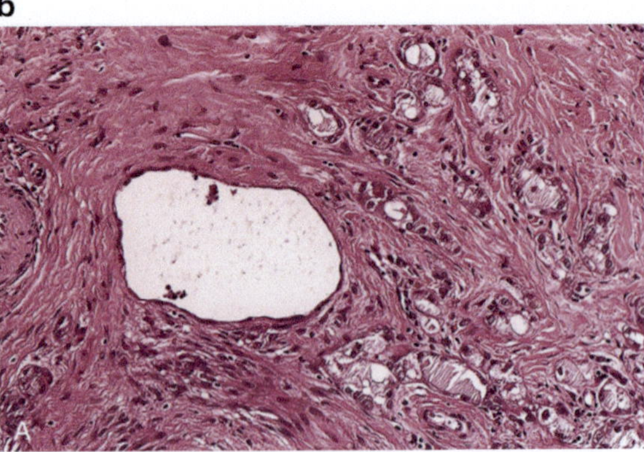

Fig. 6.17 Borderline clear cell neoplasm. Cysts and tubules lined by atypical clear cells (**a**). Focus of invasive clear cell carcinoma arising from borderline neoplasm (**b**) (Diagnostic Gynecologic and Obstetric Pathology, *Elsevier/Saunders*, 2011 with permission)

gory, a more detailed discussion of its differential diagnosis is beyond the scope of this book.

Differential Diagnosis

Clear Cell Adenofibroma and Cystadenofibroma

Benign clear cell adenofibroma is very rare and characterized by tubular glands composed of one or two layers of bland hobnailing or flat cells distributed in a fibroblastic stroma. The cells lack marked cytological atypia and salient mitotic activities.

Key Morphological Features of Low-Grade Mucinous Malignancy (Intestinal Type)

- Multilocular cystic structure lined by stratified mucinous cells with variable cytological atypia or papillary structures (borderline) (Fig. 6.18)
- Confluent growth or infiltrative component greater than 5 mm (invasive carcinoma) (Fig. 6.19)

Discussion

The intestinal borderline mucinous tumor is characterized by a multilocular cystic formation, significant epithelial crowding, stratification, and papillation, but no stromal invasion. A diagnostically important cytological feature is the

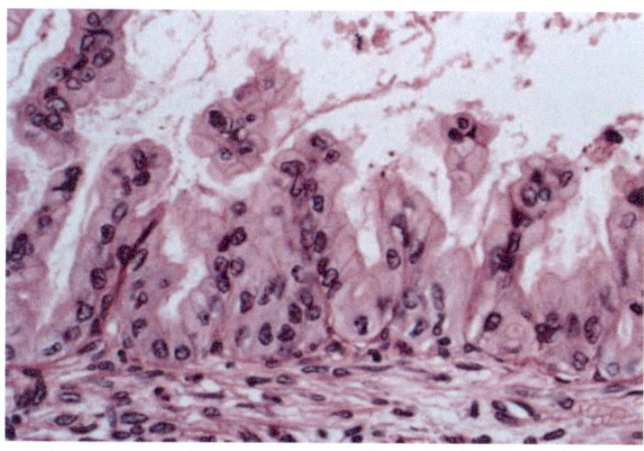

Fig. 6.18 Borderline mucinous neoplasm (Diagnostic Gynecologic and Obstetric Pathology, *Elsevier/Saunders*, 2011 with permission)

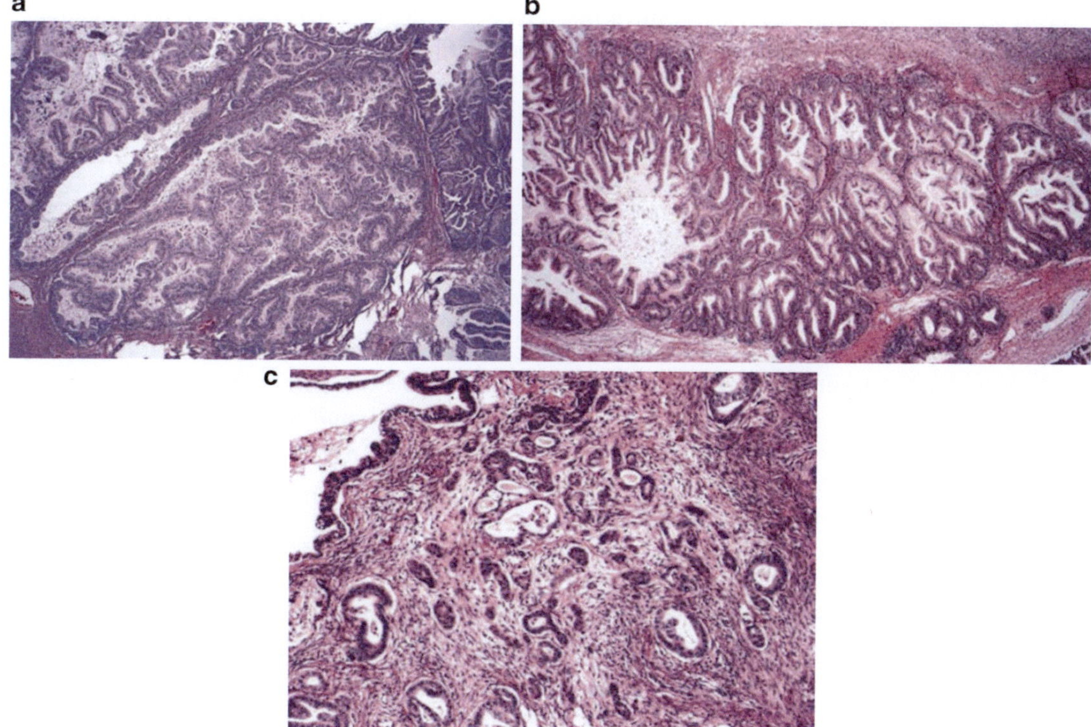

Fig. 6.19 Low-grade mucinous carcinoma. Confluent (**a**), expansive (**b**), and infiltrative growth patterns (**c**) (Diagnostic Gynecologic and Obstetric Pathology, *Elsevier/Saunders*, 2011 with permission)

presence of variable cytological atypia which is usually evident in one individual case.

Most ovarian mucinous carcinomas are well differentiated, and stromal invasion is more commonly in the expansile pattern. The invasive component is composed of ramifying or back-to-back glands or cystic spaces lined by complex papillary structures. Less commonly, infiltrative invasion presents as glands, single cells, and cell clusters distributed in an often desmoplastic stroma. This latter form of invasive pattern is more compatible with metastatic mucinous carcinoma (see differential diagnosis for more clues favoring metastatic over primary carcinoma).

Important Caveat: The much less common endocervical-type mucinous tumor resembles the serous counterpart [52, 53]. Rather than presenting in a multilocular cystic appearance as seen in the intestinal counterpart, the endocervical borderline mucinous tumor has broad bulbous papillae with epithelial stratification and tufting. The cellular atypia is usually mild. Moreover, a small percentage of it is also associated with peritoneal implants. Other mullerian epithelial elements are frequently discernible in both borderline and invasive lesions. The tumor cells are positive for CK7, ER, and PR, but negative for CK20. This is in contrast to the intestinal type cells which show diffuse CK7 and CK20 (less diffuse than CK7) reactivity.

Differential Diagnosis

Benign Mucinous Cystadenoma, Cystadenofibroma, and Adenofibroma (Both Intestinal and Endocervical Variants)

The benign mucinous tumors are lined by a single layer of bland mucinous cells. Even though small papillae can be seen projecting in cystic cavities, no epithelial stratification or tufting should be present. In cases showing focal proliferation (10 %), a diagnosis of mucinous tumor with focal proliferation is adequate. Necrosis can be seen in cases with mucin extravasation.

Mucinous Tumor Arising from Multicystic Mature Teratoma

Even though it has similar histological and immunohistochemical features as ovarian mucinous epithelial tumor, it should be considered of germ cell origin. The presence of typical mature cystic teratoma components is an important clue.

Sertoli–Leydig Cell Tumor with Heterologous Elements

A fraction of Sertoli–Leydig cell tumors show endodermal differentiation. Familiarity of this feature avoids misdiagnosing them as invasive mucinous carcinoma. The patient's younger age and the presence of typical Sertoli–Leydig tumor components are important clues. The Sertoli cells are positive for calretinin and inhibin and negative for EMA, ER, and PR. They show focal reactivity for CD99, AE1/AE3, and CAM 5.2.

Metastatic Mucinous Carcinomas

Features which are more compatible with metastatic mucinous carcinomas include surface and hilar involvement, nodular and infiltrative growth pattern, different growth patterns in different areas, and vascular invasion [54, 55]. Furthermore, metastatic tumors lack benign and borderline lesions in the adjacent regions. Immunostainings offer additional help in difficult cases

Key Morphologic Features of Low-Grade Endometrioid Malignancy

- Hyperplastic endometrioid glands resemble simple or complex endometrial hyperplasia (borderline tumor) (Fig. 6.20)
- Confluent or infiltrative invasion (greater than 5 mm across, carcinoma) (Fig. 6.21)

Discussion

The morphological presentation of borderline endometrioid tumor runs the gamut of simple to complex endometrial hyperplasia in that it encompasses epithelial changes from mild atypia, mild glandular crowding, and stratification to marked atypia and back-to-back or confluent glandular growth (less than 5 mm across). Necrosis is frequently seen inside glandular lumens. Included in this category is an atypical endometriotic cyst which is lined by markedly atypical cells.

Rather than having a stroma composed of uterine stromal cells, the borderline tumor contains a fibrotic ovarian stroma. Occasionally, periglandular condensation of the stromal cells can be perceived. The lack of stromal cell atypia and mitotic figures sets it apart from adenosarcoma.

Invasive endometrioid carcinoma is predominantly well differentiated and more commonly invades in an expansive pattern (back-to-back glands). Infiltrative invasion manifests as variably spaced glands in a fibrous stroma. As an additional sign of its resemblance to endometrial carcinoma, secretory, ciliated, and squamous differentiations are frequently encountered.

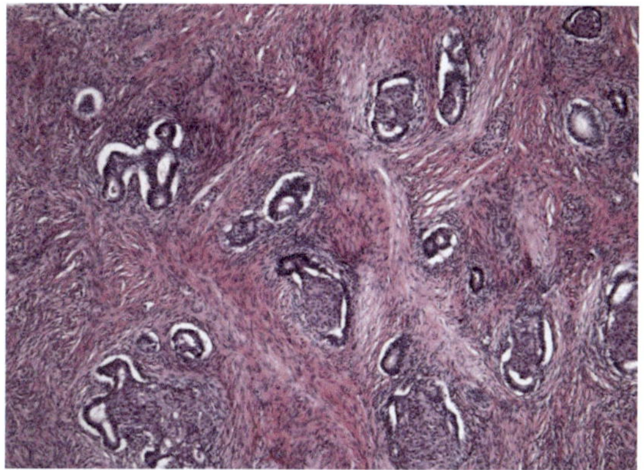

Fig. 6.20 Endometrioid borderline neoplasm. Note the resemblance to simple or complex endometrial hyperplasia (Diagnostic Gynecologic and Obstetric Pathology, *Elsevier/Saunders*, 2011 with permission)

Differential Diagnosis

Endometrioid Adenofibroma and Cystadenofibroma

Benign endometrioid tumor shows branching tubular glands and cysts uniformly distributed in a dense fibrotic or ovarian stroma and bears resemblance to mildly hyperplastic endometrium. There can be epithelial stratification, ciliation, and squamous metaplasia. However, the cells lack cytological atypia, significant stratification, or glandular crowding.

Endometriosis

Ovarian endometriosis is a common neoplastic process. Epithelial proliferation in ovarian endometriosis is differentiated from the endometrioid tumors discussed in this section by the presence of endometrial stroma and lack of mass. The same criteria for endometrial proliferations used in the endometrium apply here. The term "atypical endometriosis" is given to an endometrioid cyst which contains atypical clear cells.

Metastatic Adenocarcinoma

Features which are more compatible with metastatic endometrial carcinoma include high tumor

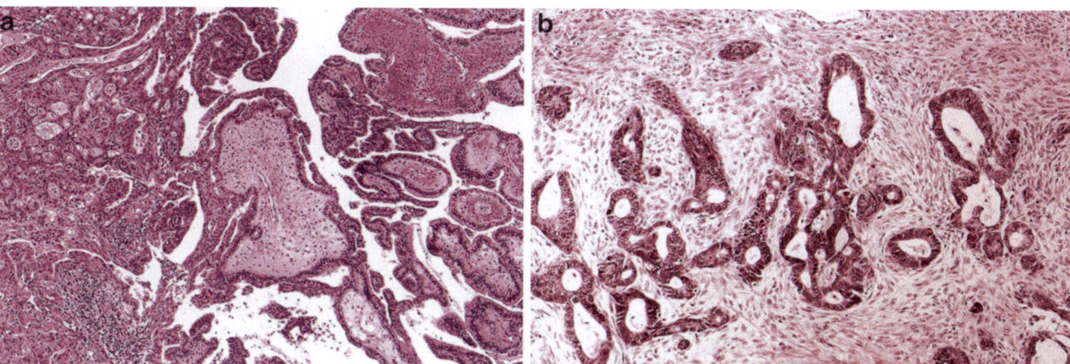

Fig. 6.21 Endometrioid carcinoma. Note confluent, papillary growth (**a**) and infiltrative pattern (**b**) (Diagnostic Gynecologic and Obstetric Pathology, *Elsevier/Saunders*, 2011 with permission)

grade, bilateral involvement, nodular growth pattern, and involvement of the surface, hilar, and blood vessels.

Metastatic colonic carcinoma can be confused with primary endometrioid carcinoma since both can have dirty necrosis and a cribriform pattern. However, the nuclear grade of colonic carcinoma is usually higher. The presence of borderline components and the lack of squamous metaplasia are two important clues. Endometrioid carcinoma cells are diffusely CK7 positive and CK20 negative. The reverse is true for metastatic colonic cells.

Sex Cord–Stromal Tumor

Endometrial carcinoma can have Sertoli cell tumor features. The hallmark of Call–Exner bodies of granulosa cell tumor can be mimicked by endometrioid carcinoma. Furthermore, endometrial carcinoma can also show trabecule and solid growth pattern, and the nuclei can contain grooves. However, sex cord tumor involves a much younger patient population, and it lacks associated benign and borderline lesions, squamous morules, and typical endometrioid areas. In difficult cases, immunostainings for inhibin, calretinin, ER, and PR can be useful.

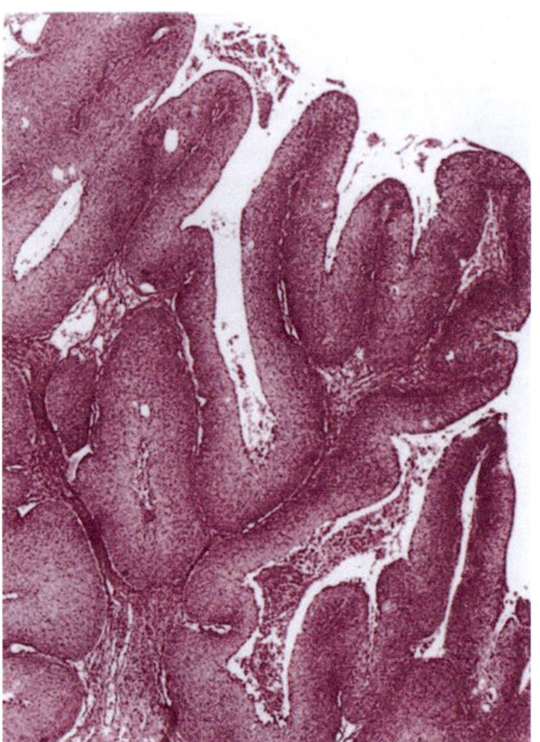

Fig. 6.22 Borderline Brenner tumor. Note the resemblance to noninvasive papillary neoplasm (Diagnostic Gynecologic and Obstetric Pathology, *Elsevier/Saunders*, 2011 with permission)

Key Morphological Features of Low-Grade Transitional Malignancy

- Papillary structures with epithelial stratification protruding into a cystic space or urothelial nests with cytological atypia (borderline tumor) (Fig. 6.22).

  Thick blunt papillae into a cystic wall or solid epithelial proliferation at the bases of papillae or random distribution of angulated nests in a desmoplastic stroma (malignant Brenner tumor) (Fig.6.23).

Discussion

The borderline Brenner tumor presents as either papillary structures with stratified epithelial lining protruding into cystic spaces or usual type of Brenner tumor with cytological atypia which could sometimes be mild. The two criteria for borderline Brenner tumor (papillae and cellular atypia) are analogous to those for urinary noninvasive papillary neoplasm and dysplasia, respectively. Despite the morphological resemblance, different molecular mechanisms are involved. The borderline tumor seems to involve the dysregulation of the cell cycle G1 to S transition (with increased expression of p21 and cyclin D1) as opposed to FGER3 and p53 mutations.

Stromal invasion is most commonly present at the bases of papilla as infiltrative epithelial nests or solid areas into the cyst wall. Slit-like structures and desmoplasia are occasionally present. The tumor is often admixed with other mullerian epithelial components with serous carcinoma being the most common. Glandular formation and squamous differentiation are also common. When no benign or borderline Brenner component is identifiable, a designation of transitional cell carcinoma

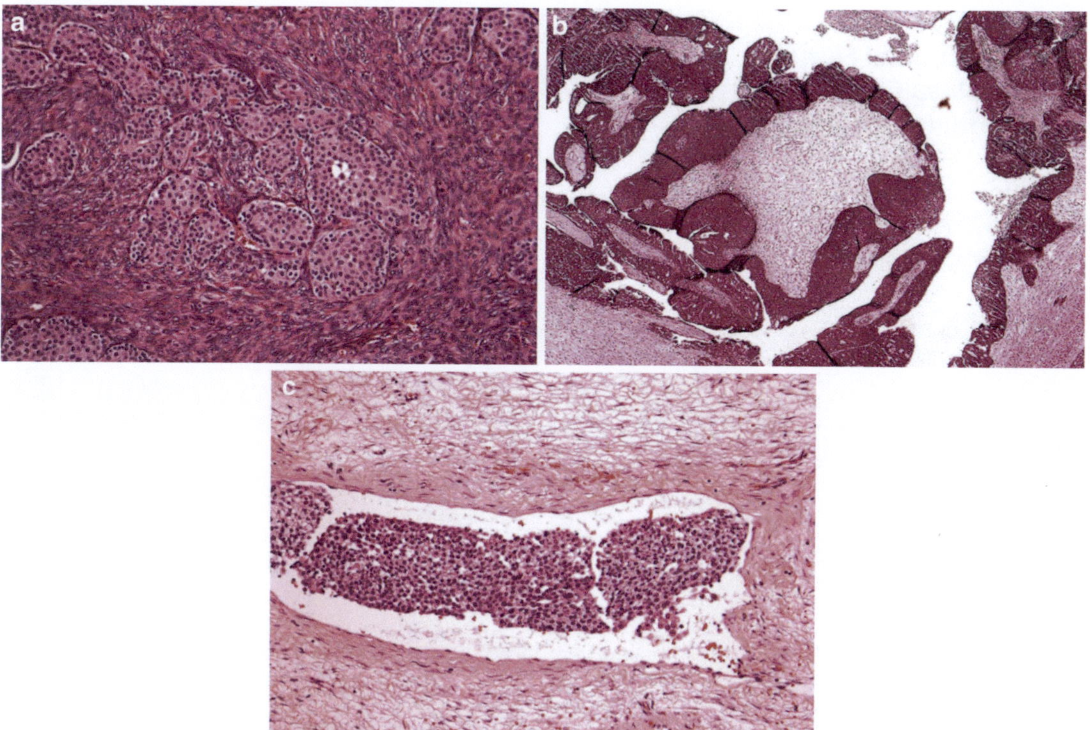

Fig. 6.23 Malignant Brenner tumor. Infiltrative (**a**), broad papillary growth pattern (**b**), and vascular invasion (**c**) (Diagnostic Gynecologic and Obstetric Pathology, *Elsevier/Saunders*, 2011 with permission)

is used. However, there is more to it than meets the eye. It seems that the G1 to S transition control is not altered (preservation of p16 and pRB) in ovarian transitional carcinoma. Instead, the tumor cells overexpress p53 [56, 57]. These molecular and histological differences are reminiscent of those between the ovarian low-grade serous carcinoma and high-grade serous carcinoma. High-grade serous carcinoma lacks a benign or borderline component. Both malignant Brenner tumor and transitional carcinoma cells are, however, positive for CK7 and WT-1 and negative for CK20 in contrast to urinary transitional carcinoma [58, 59].

Differential Diagnosis

Brenner Tumor

The tumor manifests as uniformly distributed small islands or nests in a fibrous stroma which is frequently hyalinized and contains speculated calcifications. The tumor cells are bland transitional cells with frequent mucinous, ciliated, or nondescript differentiation. Cyst formation is common and, when predominant, can obscure the nature of the tumor. It lacks either the epithelial proliferation into papillary structures, cytological atypia, or desmoplasia or haphazard arrangement of nests evident in borderline and malignant Brenner tumors, respectively.

Serous Carcinoma and Endometrial Carcinoma

Invasive transitional cell carcinoma might resemble serous cell carcinoma in that slit-like and papillary structures can be seen in both situations. However, the papillae in serous cell carcinoma are more hierarchical, and the cells are not transitional cell-like.

When transitional cell carcinoma shows glandular differentiation with microspaces, it might resemble endometrioid carcinoma. Endometrioid carcinoma, however, does not have a prominent undulating papillary formation and is more often associated with squamous morules and endometriosis.

Key Histological Features of Granulosa Cell Tumor with Unfavorable Prognosis

- Tumor size greater than 5 cm
- Mitotic activity greater than 3/10 HPF or nuclear atypia (grade II) (Fig. 6.24)

Discussion

Granulosa cell tumor can manifest a wide variety of histological patterns.

Some authorities grade the tumor according to their resemblance to mature follicles with the well differentiated being composed of micro- and macrofollicular, nest, or insular patterns.

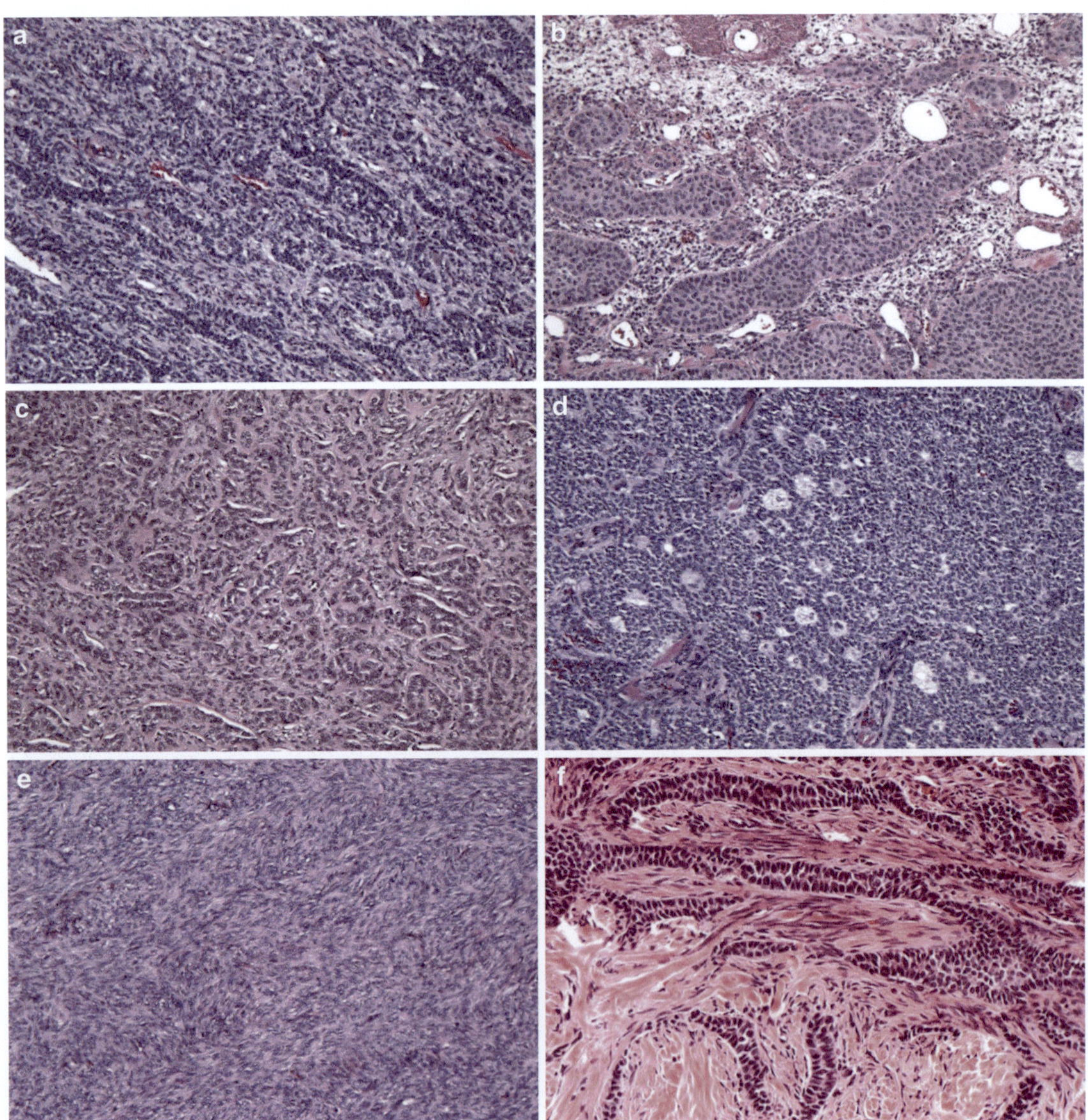

Fig. 6.24 Granulosa cell tumor. Note different growth patterns which do not carry prognostic significance (Diagnostic Gynecologic and Obstetric Pathology, *Elsevier/Saunders*, 2011 with permission)

Probably due to the inherent clumsiness of granulosa cells in handling vessel proliferation, hemorrhage and necrosis are common findings. From a clinical outcome point of view, tumor cell differentiation and necrosis and hemorrhage has no diagnostic significance (Fig.6.25).

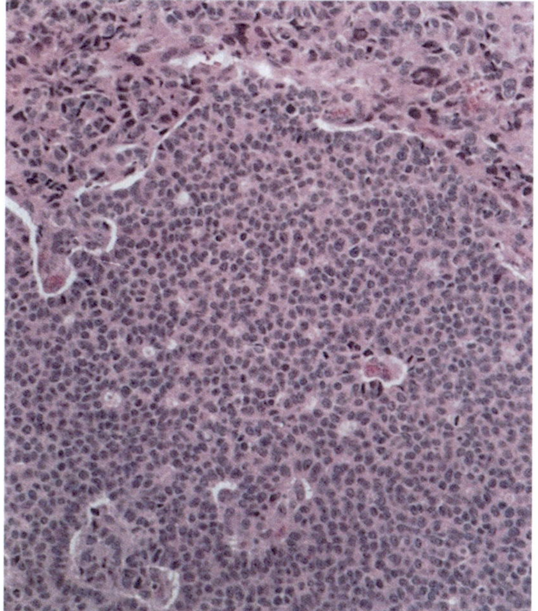

Fig. 6.25 Granulosa cell tumor with cellular atypia (Diagnostic Gynecologic and Obstetric Pathology, *Elsevier/Saunders*, 2011 with permission)

Granulosa cell tumor is considered to have malignancy potential and should be staged. So far the most reliable prognostic indicator for granulosa cell tumor is tumor stage. Relevant morphological parameters include tumor size, mitotic activity, and nuclear grade. However, caution is advised in the evaluation and interpretation of the latter two parameters. For instance, in juvenile granulosa cell tumor which is less differentiated than the adult granulosa cell tumor, a strong correlation of nuclear atypia and mitotic activity with clinical outcome independent of tumor stage is lacking (Fig. 6.26). Nuclear atypia is a subjective index, and interobserver variations are inevitable. As they are likely to be degenerative in nature, the large, multinucleated, bizzare nuclei which are sometimes present in both granulosa cell and Sertoli–Leydig cell tumors should be left out in the evaluation.

Differential Diagnosis for Granulosa Tumor

Cellular Fibroma and Thecoma

Cellular fibroma consists of densely populated spindle cells with frequent storiform or herringbone growth pattern. Thecoma cells are fusiform with vesicular nuclei and likely cytoplasmic differentiation toward granulosa cells. Moreover, granulosa cells tumor can have conspicuous com-

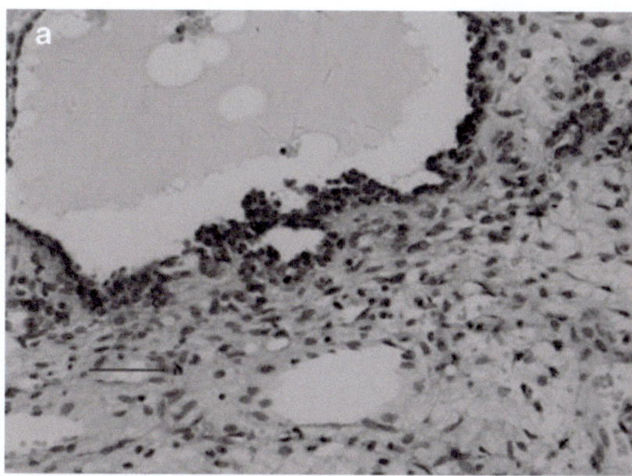

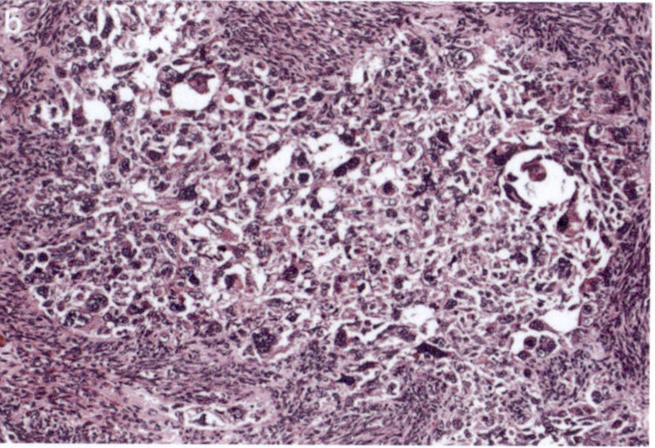

Fig. 6.26 Juvenile granulosa cell tumor. Hyperchromatic nuclei and mitotic figure (Diagnostic Gynecologic and Obstetric Pathology, *Elsevier/Saunders*, 2011; Journal of Pediatric Hematology/Oncology, *Wolters Kluwer/Lippincott Williams & Wilkins*, 2011 with permission)

ponent of fibroblasts and theca cells in the stroma. Therefore, distinction of them from a diffuse pattern of granulosa tumor is needed. Fibroma and thecoma cells lack groove nuclei and other granulosa cell tumor patterns. In difficult cases, reticulin stain may be helpful as fibroma and thecoma cells are surrounded by abundant intercellular reticulin fibers.

Endometrioid Carcinoma and Endometrial Stroma Sarcoma

Both low- and high-grade endometrioid carcinomas can be confused as adult granulosa cell tumor. The presence of squamous morules and higher nuclear grade helps establish the correct diagnosis. Also, endometrial carcinoma lacks the other characteristic growth patterns in one individual tumor. If necessary, immunostainings can be used (inhibin, EMA, and calretinin).

Endometrial stroma sarcoma has characteristic small arterioles and rich reticulin and lacks the other growth patterns.

Poorly Differentiated Carcinoma and Metastatic Malignancy

Poorly differentiated carcinomas in the ovary can be easily misdiagnosed as diffuse granulosa cell tumor, particularly when the latter contains focal atypia and multinucleated and bizzare nuclei. However, poorly differentiated carcinomas contain a much high nuclear grade (nuclear polymorphism, hyperchromasia, high mitotic activity, and abnormal mitosis).

Lobular breast cancer can present as cord-like structures composed of bland cells. Metastatic melanoma may manifest as solid pattern. The presence of pigments, high nuclear grade, and spindle cells should alert the pathologist. All of them lack nuclear grooves and other patterns characteristic of granulosa cell tumor. Immunostainings can be confirmatory in difficult cases.

Carcinoid Tumor

The insular, acini, solid, and trabecular patterns can mimic granulosa cell tumor. However, carcinoid cells have characteristic salt–pepper chromatin and lack nuclear grooves. The tumor cells are negative for sex cord markers.

Key Morphological Features of Moderately Differentiated Sertoli–Leydig Cell Tumor with Unfavorable Clinical Outcome

- Retiform growth pattern (Fig. 6.27)
- Heterologous differentiation, tumor rupture (Fig. 6.28)

Discussion

As with the granulosa cell tumor, extraovarian extension remains the most reliable indicator of

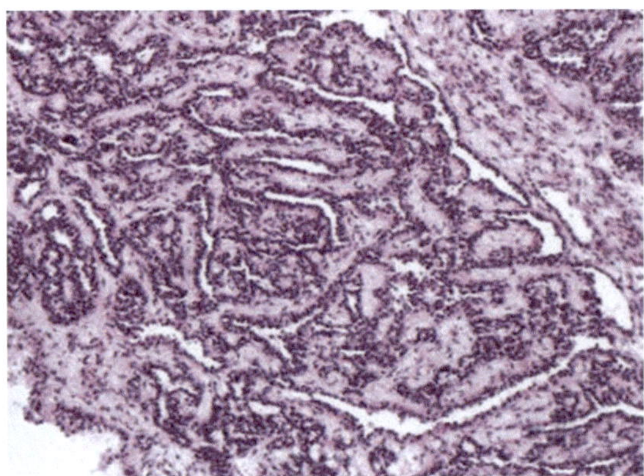

Fig. 6.27 Retiform Sertoli cell tumor (Diagnostic Gynecologic and Obstetric Pathology, *Elsevier/Saunders*, 2011 with permission)

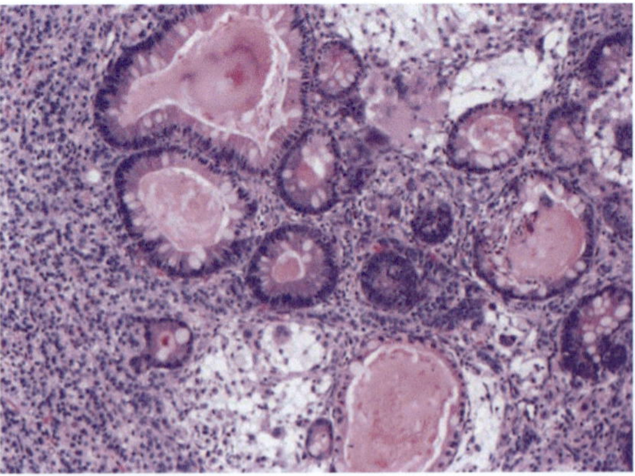

Fig. 6.28 Sertoli cell tumor with heterologous differentiation (Diagnostic Gynecologic and Obstetric Pathology, *Elsevier/Saunders*, 2011 with permission)

clinical malignancy for Sertoli–Leydig cell tumors. Despite earlier reports indicating a lack of correlation between the tumor differentiation and clinical outcome, tumor differentiation has some bearing on the tumor behavior [60]. The well-differentiated Sertoli cell tumor can be considered as a benign neoplasm with a favorable outcome. The majority of poorly differentiated and a small fraction of moderately differentiated tumors have an untoward clinical outcome. Other morphological features associated with clinical malignancy include a retiform growth, heterologous elements, and tumor rupture. Mitotic activity, necrosis, and hemorrhage are left out of the consideration.

Retiform pattern resemble the rete testis and presents as poorly formed tubules and slit-like glandular spaces made up by primitive cells. Cystic and papillary structures can be frequently present, but they lack prominent epithelial proliferation and ciliation. The heterologous elements can be either endodermal or stromal in nature. However, well-differentiated tumor is predominantly associated with mucinous endodermal components [61, 62]. Heterologous stromal elements are often seen in poorly differentiated Sertoli–Leydig cell tumor. In this highly specialized organ of ovary in which the business of producing and releasing well-prepared oocytes is executed via a strong coupling between the sex cord and stromal components, tumor rupture probably is an indicator of soured relationship predisposing to extraovarian extension.

Differential Diagnosis

Yolk Sac Tumor

Similar to granulosa cell tumors, the yolk sac tumor has wide histological presentation patterns which can be present in the same tumor. Even though cystic, glandular, and papillary structures can also be seen in both lesions, yolk sac tumor cells have higher nuclear grade. The hallmark of the tumor is the Schiller–Duval bodies and hyaline globules.

Carcinosarcoma

Carcinosarcoma of the ovary might mimic Sertoli–Leydig cell tumor with heterologous stromal elements. However, both the epithelial and mesenchymal components are usually with a higher nuclear grade. It lacks Leydig cells.

Granulosa Cell Tumor

The microfollicular and trabecular growth patterns of granulosa cell tumor can resemble moderately differentiated Sertoli–Leydig tumor. The presence of characteristic nuclear grooves, a fibrothecomatous stroma, and other growth patterns is usually suffice for the distinction. Retiform pattern and heterologous elements are rare in granulosa cell tumor.

Occasional cases in which the morphological distinction between these two entities is blurry fall into the category of sex cord–stromal tumors unclassified.

Endometrioid Tumor

The endometrioid tumor may closely mimic the Sertoli–Leydig tumor in several aspects. It may present as small tubule and cords, and the stromal cell may even become luteinized. Moreover, the tumor may contain spindle-shaped immature squamous morules and a prominent adenofibromatous component mimicking Sertoli–Leydig tumor with spindle differentiation. Finally, mucinous differentiation might be confused as an epithelial heterologous element.

Nevertheless, the presence of typical squamous morules, older age, and adenofibromatous component are important clues.

Serous Cell Carcinoma and Borderline Tumor

The serous tumor contains papillary structures and slit-like structures which might be mistaken for retiform variant. Important clues include patient's young age, association with virilization, and other patterns. The retiform pattern lacks ciliation, epithelial stratification, and ramification.

Mucinous Neoplasm

The mucinous neoplasms are composed of cells with differentiation toward GI or endocervical epithelium. They are differentiated from the Sertoli–Leydig cell tumor with heterologous epithelial elements by their lack of other areas typical of the latter. Also the latter lacks a multilocular cystic or complex papillary growth pattern.

Teratoma

Teratomatous lesions can be confused with Sertoli–Leydig cell tumors with heterologous elements. The lesions, however, contain various tissues from three germ layers in an organoid pattern.

References

1. Hendrickson MR, Atkins KA, Kempson RL. Chapter 41. Uterus and fallopian tubes. In: Mills SE, editor. Histology for pathologist. 3rd ed. Philadelphia: Lippincott Williams & Wilkins/Wolters Kluwer Business; 2007. p. 1011–62.
2. Wheeler DT, Kurman RJ. The relationship of glands to thick-wall blood vessels as a marker of invasion in endocervical adenocarcinoma. Int J Gynecol Pathol. 2005;24(2):125–30.
3. Kling E, et al. The 2 stromal compartments of the normal cervix with distinct immunophenotypic and histomorphologic features. Ann Diagn Pathol. 2012; 16(5):315–22.
4. Andersson S, et al. Estrogen and progesterone metabolism in the cervix during pregnancy and parturition. J Clin Endocrinol Metab. 2008;93(6):2366–74.
5. Timmons BC, et al. Dynamic changes in the cervical epithelial tight junction complex and differentiation occur during cervical ripening and parturition. Endocrinology. 2007;148(3):1278–87.
6. Timmons B, Akins M, Mahendroo M. Cervical remodeling during pregnancy and parturition. Trends Endocrinol Metab. 2010;21(6):353–61.
7. Barth PJ, Ramaswamy A, Moll R. CD34 (+) fibrocytes in normal cervical stroma, cervical intraepithelial neoplasia III, and invasive squamous cell carcinoma of the cervix uteri. Virchows Arch. 2002;441(6):564–8.
8. Li Q, Huang W, Zhou X. Expression of CD34, alpha-smooth muscle actin and transforming growth factor-beta1 in squamous intraepithelial lesions and squamous cell carcinoma of the cervix. J Int Med Res. 2009;37(2):446–54.
9. Zayour M, Lazova R. Pseudoepitheliomatous hyperplasia: a review. Am J Dermatopathol. 2011;33(2): 112–22; quiz 123–6.
10. El-Khoury J, Kibbi AG, Abbas O. Mucocutaneous pseudoepitheliomatous hyperplasia: a review. Am J Dermatopathol. 2012;34(2):165–75.
11. Kindelberger DW, Krane JF, Lee KR. Chapter 14. Glandular neoplasia of the cervix. In: Crum CP, Nucci MR, Lee KR, editors. Diagnostic gynecologic and obstetric pathology. Philadelphia: Saunders/Elsevier; 2011. p. 328–78.
12. Nara M, et al. Lobular endocervical glandular hyperplasia as a presumed precursor of cervical adenocarcinoma independent of human papillomavirus infection. Gynecol Oncol. 2007;106(2):289–98.
13. Kawauchi S, et al. Is lobular endocervical glandular hyperplasia a cancerous precursor of minimal deviation adenocarcinoma? A comparative molecular-genetic and immunohistochemical study. Am J Surg Pathol. 2008;32(12):1807–15.
14. Danilova NV, et al. Markers of stromal invasion during background and precancerous changes of the glandular epithelium and in adenocarcinoma of the cervix uteri. Arkh Patol. 2012;74(4):28–33.
15. Jordan SM, et al. Desmoplastic stromal response as defined by positive alpha-smooth muscle actin staining is predictive of invasion in adenocarcinoma of the uterine cervix. Int J Gynecol Pathol. 2012;31(4):369–76.
16. McCluggage WG. New developments in endocervical glandular lesions. Histopathology. 2013;62(1):138–60.
17. McCluggage WG. Endocervical glandular lesions: controversial aspects and ancillary techniques. J Clin Pathol. 2003;56(3):164–73.
18. Kwasniewska A, et al. Estrogen and progesterone receptor expression in HPV-positive and HPV-negative cervical carcinomas. Oncol Rep. 2011;26(1):153–60.
19. Nonogaki H, et al. Estrogen receptor localization in normal and neoplastic epithelium of the uterine cervix. Cancer. 1990;66(12):2620–7.
20. Bekkers RL, et al. Down regulation of estrogen receptor expression is an early event in human papillomavirus infected cervical dysplasia. Eur J Gynaecol Oncol. 2005;26(4):376–82.
21. Zamecnik M. Hormone receptors in microglandular hyperplasia of the uterine cervix. Int J Gynecol Pathol. 2002;21(4):424–5.
22. Kondo T, et al. Gastric mucin is expressed in a subset of endocervical tunnel clusters: type A tunnel clusters of gastric phenotype. Histopathology. 2007;50(7): 843–50.
23. Tsuji T, et al. Uterine cervical carcinomas associated with lobular endocervical glandular hyperplasia. Histopathology. 2011;59(1):55–62.
24. Mikami Y, et al. Lobular endocervical glandular hyperplasia is a metaplastic process with a pyloric gland phenotype. Histopathology. 2001;39(4):364–72.
25. Dainty LA, et al. Diffuse laminar endocervical glandular hyperplasia: a case report. Int J Gynecol Cancer. 2009;19(6):1091–3.
26. Rabban JT, et al. PAX2 distinguishes benign mesonephric and mullerian glandular lesions of the cervix from endocervical adenocarcinoma, including mini-

mal deviation adenocarcinoma. Am J Surg Pathol. 2010;34(2):137–46.
27. Bigsby RM. Control of growth and differentiation of the endometrium: the role of tissue interactions. Ann N Y Acad Sci. 2002;955:110–7; discussion 118, 396–406.
28. Morelli SS, Yi P, Goldsmith LT. Endometrial stem cells and reproduction. Obstet Gynecol Int. 2012;2012: 851367.
29. Gargett CE, Masuda H. Adult stem cells in the endometrium. Mol Hum Reprod. 2010;16(11):818–34.
30. McCluggage GW. Chapter 7. Benign diseases of the endometrium. In: Kurman RJ, Ellenson LH, Ronnett BM, editors. Blaustein's pathology of the female genital tract. 6th ed. Chicago: Springer; 2010. p. 305–58.
31. Girling JE, Rogers PA. Recent advances in endometrial angiogenesis research. Angiogenesis. 2005;8(2): 89–99.
32. Mandala M, Osol G. Physiological remodelling of the maternal uterine circulation during pregnancy. Basic Clin Pharmacol Toxicol. 2012;110(1):12–8.
33. Matsubara Y, Matsubara K. Estrogen and progesterone play pivotal roles in endothelial progenitor cell proliferation. Reprod Biol Endocrinol. 2012;10:2.
34. Ellensen LH, et al. Chapter 9. Endometrial carcinoma. In: Kurman RJ, Ellenson LH, Ronnett BM, editors. Blaustein's pathology of the female genital tract. 6th ed. Chicago: Springer; 2010. p. 393–452.
35. Tafe LJ, et al. Endometrial and ovarian carcinomas with undifferentiated components: clinically aggressive and frequently underrecognized neoplasms. Mod Pathol. 2010;23(6):781–9.
36. Silva EG, et al. Association of low-grade endometrioid carcinoma of the uterus and ovary with undifferentiated carcinoma: a new type of dedifferentiated carcinoma? Int J Gynecol Pathol. 2006;25(1):52–8.
37. Crum CP, Duska LR, Nucci MR. Chapter 19. Adenocarcinoma, carcinosarcoma and other epithelial tumors of the endometrium. In: Crum CP, Nucci MR, Lee KR, editors. Diagnostic gynecologic and obstetric pathology. Philadelphia: Saunders/Elsevier; 2011. p. 517–81.
38. Quade BJ, Nucci MR. Chapter 20. Uterine mesenchymal tumors. In: Crum CP, Nucci MR, Lee KR, editors. Diagnostic gynecologic and obstetric pathology. Philadelphia: Saunders/Elsevier; 2011. p. 582–639.
39. Gong J, et al. Correlation of thrombomodulin expression and occlusion of the uterine artery for the treatment of leiomyoma. Eur J Obstet Gynecol Reprod Biol. 2011;154(2):192–5.
40. Chen CL, et al. Characteristics of vascular supply to uterine leiomyoma: an analysis of digital subtraction angiography imaging in 518 cases. Eur Radiol. 2013; 23(3):774–9.
41. Chiang S, Oliva E. Recent developments in uterine mesenchymal neoplasms. Histopathology. 2013;62(1): 124–37.
42. Zaloudek CJ, Hendrickson MR, Soslow RA. Mesenchymal tumors of the uterus. In: Kurman RJ, Ellenson LH, Ronnett BM, editors. Blaustein's pathology of the female genital tract. New York: Springer; 2011. p. 453–528.
43. Palma GA, et al. Biology and biotechnology of follicle development. Sci World J. 2012;2012:9138138.
44. Orisaka M, et al. Oocyte-granulosa-theca cell interactions during preantral follicular development. J Ovarian Res. 2009;2(1):9.
45. Hummitzsch K, et al. A new model of development of the mammalian ovary and follicles. PLoS One. 2013; 8(2):e55578.
46. Okamura H, et al. Structural changes and cell properties of human ovarian surface epithelium in ovarian pathophysiology. Microsc Res Tech. 2006;69(6): 469–81.
47. Auersperg N. Ovarian surface epithelium as a source of ovarian cancers: unwarranted speculation or evidence-based hypothesis? Gynecol Oncol. 2013; 130(1):246–51.
48. Worley MJ, et al. Endometriosis-associated ovarian cancer: a review of pathogenesis. Int J Mol Sci. 2013;14(3):5367–79.
49. Akahane T, et al. The origin of stroma surrounding epithelial ovarian cancer cells. Int J Gynecol Pathol. 2012;32(1):26–30.
50. Schauer IG, et al. Cancer-associated fibroblasts and their putative role in potentiating the initiation and development of epithelial ovarian cancer. Neoplasia. 2011;13(5):393–405.
51. Lai D, Ma L, Wang F. Fibroblast activation protein regulates tumor-associated fibroblasts and epithelial ovarian cancer cells. Int J Oncol. 2012;41(2):541–50.
52. Seidman JD, Cho KR, Ronnett BM, Kurman RJ. Chapter 14. Surface epithelial tumors of the ovary. In: Kurman RJ, Ellenson LH, Ronnett BM, editors. Blaustein's pathology of the female genital tract. 6th ed. Chicago: Springer; 2010. p. 393–452.
53. Nucci MR, Curm CR, Lee KR. Chapter 27. The pathology of pelvic-ovarian epithelial (epithelial-stromal) tumors. In: Crum CP, Nucci MR, Lee KR, editors. Diagnostic gynecologic and obstetric pathology. Philadelphia: Saunders/Elsevier; 2011. p. 818–95.
54. Lerwill MF, Young RH. Chapter 18. Metastatic tumors of the ovary. In: Kurman RJ, Ellenson LH, Ronnett BM, editors. Blaustein's pathology of the female genital tract. 6th ed. Chicago: Springer; 2010. p. 929–98.
55. Hirsh MS. Chapter 31. Metastatic tumors to the ovary. In: Crum CP, Nucci MR, Lee KR, editors. Diagnostic gynecologic and obstetric pathology. Philadelphia: Saunders/Elsevier; 2011. p. 972–88.
56. Ribe A, Larrosa C, Carasus L, Palacios J, Prat J. Brenner tumors but not transitional cell carcinomas of the ovary show dysregulation of cell cycle G1-S phase transition. Mod Pathol. 2006;19S1:194A.
57. Prat J. Chapter 25. Ovarian Endometrioid, Clear Cell, Brenner and Rare Epithelial Stromal Tumors. In: Robboy SJ et al., editors. Robboy's Pathology of the Female Reproductive Tract. Philadelphia: Churchill Livingstone/Elsevier; 2009. p. 655–92.

58. Riedel I, et al. Brenner tumors but not transitional cell carcinomas of the ovary show urothelial differentiation: immunohistochemical staining of urothelial markers, including cytokeratins and uroplakins. Virchows Arch. 2001;438(2):181–91.
59. Cuatrecasas M, et al. Transitional cell tumors of the ovary: a comparative clinicopathologic, immunohistochemical, and molecular genetic analysis of Brenner tumors and transitional cell carcinomas. Am J Surg Pathol. 2009;33(4):556–67.
60. Young RH, Scully RE. Ovarian Sertoli-Leydig cell tumors. A clinicopathological analysis of 207 cases. Am J Surg Pathol. 1985;9(8):543–69.
61. Nakashima N, Young RH, Scully RE. Androgenic granulosa cell tumors of the ovary. A clinicopathologic analysis of 17 cases and review of the literature. Arch Pathol Lab Med. 1984;108(10):786–91.
62. Sternberg WH. The morphology, androgenic function, hyperplasia, and tumors of the human ovarian hilus cells. Am J Pathol. 1949;25(3):493–521.

7 Gastrointestinal System, Pancreatobiliary Tract and Liver

Esophagus

Key Morphological Features of Well-Differentiated Esophageal Squamous Cell Carcinoma

- Dyskeratotic squamous cells
- Narrow-based infiltrative or pushing border (Fig. 7.1)

Discussion

The bland squamous cells of well-differentiated squamous cells demonstrate dyskeratosis characterized by early keratinization (keratin pearls in the basal and parabasal layers) and excessive cytoplasmic keratinization. This important feature has been largely overlooked by the surgical pathologists since it is shared by the perfect mimicker of squamous cell carcinoma and pseudoepitheliomatous hyperplasia. A careful survey of the adjacent tissue in the latter, however, usually reveals an underlying infection, inflammation, trauma, or nonsquamous neoplasm [1, 2].

With the exception of the exceedingly rare variant of esophageal verrucous squamous cell carcinoma, squamous cell carcinomas typically show an infiltrative pattern. The infiltrative fronts are usually narrow based with no surface connection. Pseudoepitheliomatous hyperplasia poses a diagnostic problem as in the skin and manifests an infiltrative front as a result of benign epithelial–mesenchymal transition induced by a predisposing lesion [1, 2]. Disruption of the basement integrity results from decreased production of laminin and type IV collagen rather than increased activities of the MMPs. The infiltrative front, however, has a jagged contour with sharp tips which are connected to a broad base. Usually, a connection of the elongated thick invasive projections to the surface can be traced (Fig. 7.2).

Caveat: The rare variant of esophageal verrucous squamous cell carcinoma has the characteristic morphological features as in the skin. It is composed of exophytic and endophytic components which possess different cytological and architectural changes. The cells have low proliferation activity which is restricted to the basal layer.

Differential Diagnosis

Pseudoepitheliomatous Hyperplasia

Pseudoepitheliomatous hyperplasia has both features of well-differentiated squamous cell carcinoma: dyskeratosis and invasive border. However, the adjacent tissue usually shows signs of infection, inflammation, trauma, or other nonsquamous neoplasm. The hyperplastic squamous projections are usually connected to the surface with a broad base and have a jagged contour with pointed tips.

In difficult cases, a panel of immunostainings (p53, MMP-1, and Ki67) should help make the distinction. The neoplastic squamous cells show

X. Sun, *Well-Differentiated Malignancies: New Perspectives*, Current Clinical Pathology,
DOI 10.1007/978-1-4939-1692-4_7,

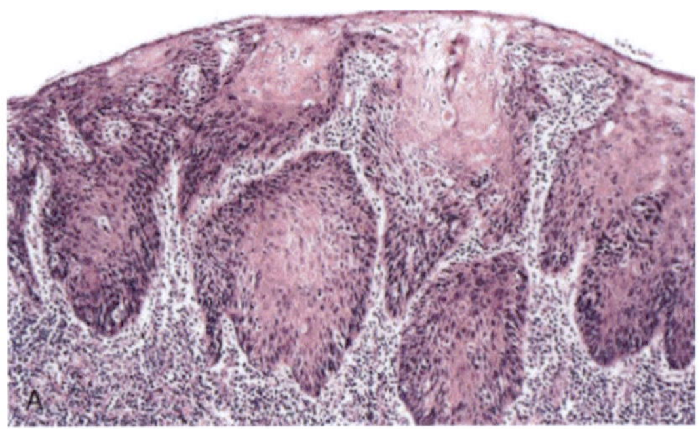

Fig. 7.1 Well-differentiated squamous cell carcinoma. Note narrowly based or detached squamous nests with pushing or infiltrative border. Dyskeratotic cells are noted (Surgical Pathology of the GI tract, Liver, Biliary Tract and Pancreas, *Elsevier/Saunders*, 2009 with permission)

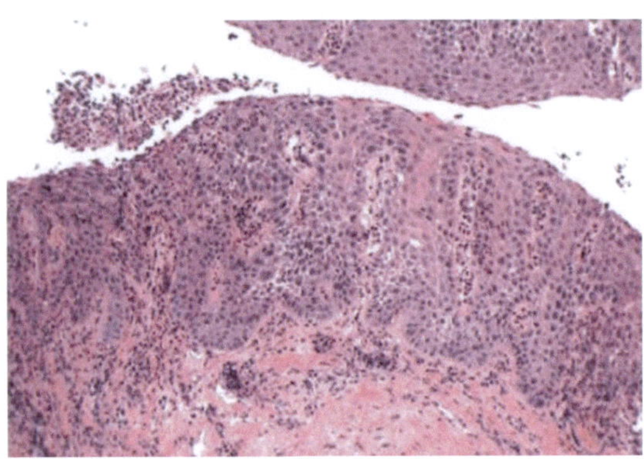

Fig. 7.2 Pseudoepitheliomatous hyperplasia. Note lack of dyskeratosis (Surgical Pathology of the GI tract, Liver, Biliary Tract and Pancreas, *Elsevier/Saunders*, 2009 with permission)

diffuse positivity for the three markers, whereas the hyperplastic epithelium shows only basal staining. In addition, MMP-1 also shows strong stromal staining in squamous cell carcinoma.

Squamous Dysplasia Involving Mucosal Gland Ducts

The seemingly invasive component has similar cytologic features as the surface dysplastic cells which are usually immature. It lacks an infiltrative or pushing border.

Esophageal Diverticula

Esophageal intramural pseudodiverticulosis can resemble squamous cell carcinoma not only pathologically but also clinically and radiologically [3]. Their involvement of the mucosa and submucosa as well as their irregular shapes simulate invasive squamous cell carcinoma. However, neither dyskeratosis nor an invasive border is present. Other clues of their benignity are their association with the submucosal glandular system and the presence of heavy chronic inflammation.

Squamous Papilloma

It lacks dyskeratosis and an infiltrative front. Even in the endophytic growth pattern, a well-circumscribed appearance is discernible. The epithelial cells might have reactive changes but no dyskeratosis.

Key Morphological Feature of Well-Differentiated Esophageal Adenocarcinoma

- Irregularly shaped and sized glands with no serration
- Lack of a layer of periglandular myofibroblasts or myoepithelial cells (Fig. 7.3)

Discussion

Esophageal adenocarcinomas are believed to follow the intestinal metaplasia–dysplasia–carcinoma pathway. The metaplastic glandular epithelium is lined by a layer of periglandular myofibroblastic cells which regulate many aspects of the epithelial cells like in the intestine (refer to the intestine section for more detailed discussion) [4]. Due to the presence of the periglandular myofibroblastic sheath, benign intestinal epithelial proliferations have a characteristic serrated appearance. Except for the rare serrated adenocarcinomas in the colon which possess other easily discernible characteristic features, genuine serration is rarely seen in gastrointestinal epithelial malignancies. This important feature can be very useful in the diagnosis of well-differentiated carcinomas where invasion is insidious and desmoplasia is not evident.

Corresponding to the lack of a serrated appearance in epithelial malignancies is the progressively decreasing presence of periglandular myofibroblastic cells along the spectrum of intestinal hyperplasia to dysplasia and adenocarcinoma

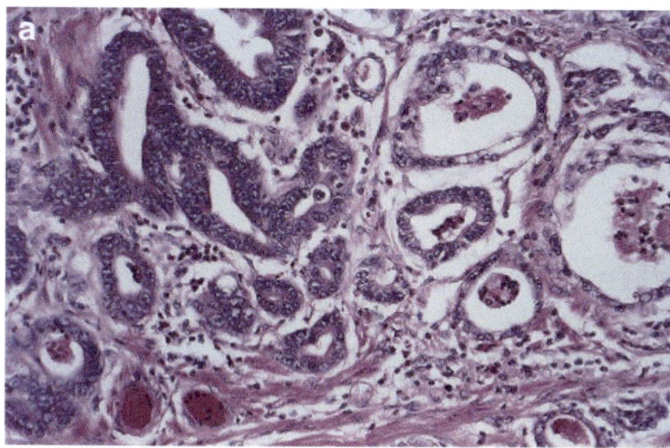

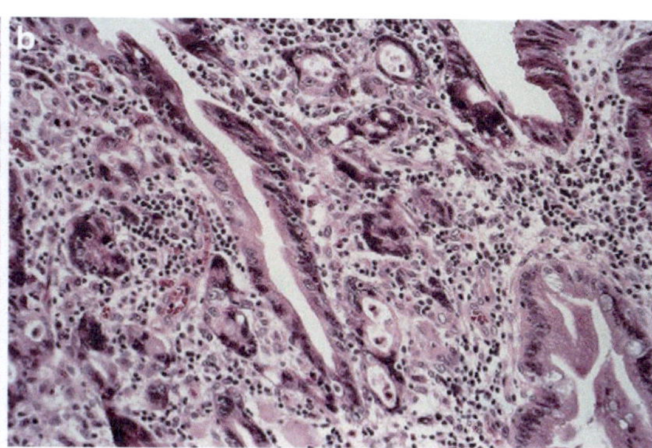

Fig. 7.3 Esophageal adenocarcinoma. Irregularly shaped and sized glands with serration. Lack of a rim of periglandular myofibroblasts (Surgical Pathology of the GI tract, Liver, Biliary Tract and Pancreas, *Elsevier/Saunders*, 2009 with permission)

[5, 6]. In the evaluation of periglandular myofibroblasts, the pathologist should be aware of a common phenomenon in Barrett's esophagus: thickening of the muscularis mucosa and even the muscularis propria [7–9]. The hypertrophic muscle fibers can extend into the lamina propria or even form a new layer of muscular mucosa (duplication of muscularis mucosa). The upward extending muscle fibers, however, do not go around the glands in an accommodating fashion as the periglandular myofibroblasts. To help light up the periglandular myofibroblasts, immunostaining for SMA can be used. The other related issue is to avoid making an erroneous diagnosis of muscle invading adenocarcinoma when the hypertrophic muscle fibers are adjacent to benign or malignant glands in the lamina propria. Attention to the location of the hypertrophic muscle fibers is useful in this regard.

Differential Diagnosis

Benign or Dysplastic Glands Entrapped in Fibrotic Tissue

Fibrosis of the lamina propria and submucosa with entrapment of benign or even dysplastic glands is a common occurrence in metaplastic (Barrett's) esophagus. The entrapped glands usually show cystic dilation and glandular serration. Periglandular myofibroblasts are appreciable.

In difficult cases, panel stains of CD44, E-cadherin, p53, and Ki67 should help in the distinction.

Esophageal Gland Duct Adenoma

Esophageal gland duct adenomas are well circumscribed and located in the submucosa [10]. They resemble their salivary counterpart, sialadenoma papilliferum, which contains a mixture of tubules, cysts, and papillary structures. A key feature is the presence of a two-cell-layer epithelium with the outer layer being myoepithelial cells.

Benign or Dysplastic Glands with Hyperplasia of Muscularis Mucosa

Attention to glandular serration and periglandular fibroblasts should point to the right direction.

Non-adenomatous-Type Dysplasia

While most Barrett's-associated dysplasia present as a flat lesion with predominantly adenomatous (intestinal-type) histopathology, foveolar and serrated types of dysplasia may occur in the esophagus. The importance of recognition of these two uncommon types of dysplasia lies more in their associated clinical outcome than in differentiating them from well-differentiated adenocarcinomas since they have a serrated or foveolar appearance and presumably an extenuated layer of periglandular myofibroblasts. Even though they are cytologically bland, foveolar and serrated dysplasia are believed to have a natural history similar to the high-grade traditional adenomatous dysplasia [11, 12].

Pyloric Gland Adenoma

Rarely, pyloric gland adenomas are present in the esophagus. Barrett's-associated dysplasia may also show a pyloric glandular phenotype. Recognizing their bland dysplastic features as well as their association with severe dysplasia or adenocarcinomas has important clinical significance as with the non-adenomatous dysplasia (refer to stomach section for more discussion).

Stomach

Key Morphological Features of Well-Differentiated Gastric Type Adenocarcinoma

- Variation in glandular shapes and sizes in a non-foveolar/serrated and nonlobular pattern
- Lack of periglandular myofibroblasts (Fig. 7.4)

Discussion

Most gastric adenocarcinomas resemble their esophageal counterparts in that they follow the same intestinal metaplasia to dysplasia to carcinoma pathway. Metaplastic glands also have a layer of periglandular myofibroblasts, and a similar progressively decreasing existence pattern for them exists along the metaplasia–dysplasia–carcinoma spectrum as in the intestine [13] (Figs. 7.5 and 7.6).

The fact that gastric foveolae, hyperplastic polyps, and adenomas share striking morphological similarities with their intestinal equivalents suggests that a similar type of periglandular myofibroblasts should be present around normal nonmetaplastic gastric glands. Our unpublished data indicate that this is the case even though it appears that the lower portions of glands have an attenuated layer of myofibroblast which surrounds several rather than individual glandular lumens. The rapidly proliferative upper portions have a sheath of periglandular myofibroblasts. This layer of myofibroblasts is supposed to play a vital role in the normal glandular morphogenesis and maintenance like their intestinal counterparts. Presumably, their presence in the upper portions of glands contributes to the foveolar appearance of normal and hyperplastic mucosa. This might explain why some benign gastric epithelial lesions such as oxyntic gland polyp/adenomas and pyloric gland adenomas do not have or have only a focal foveolar appearance. Fortunately, these two rare entities can be differentiated from well-differentiated adenocarcinomas by their overall lobular pattern and other cytological features.

Judicious use of the two morphological features is particularly useful in the distinction of

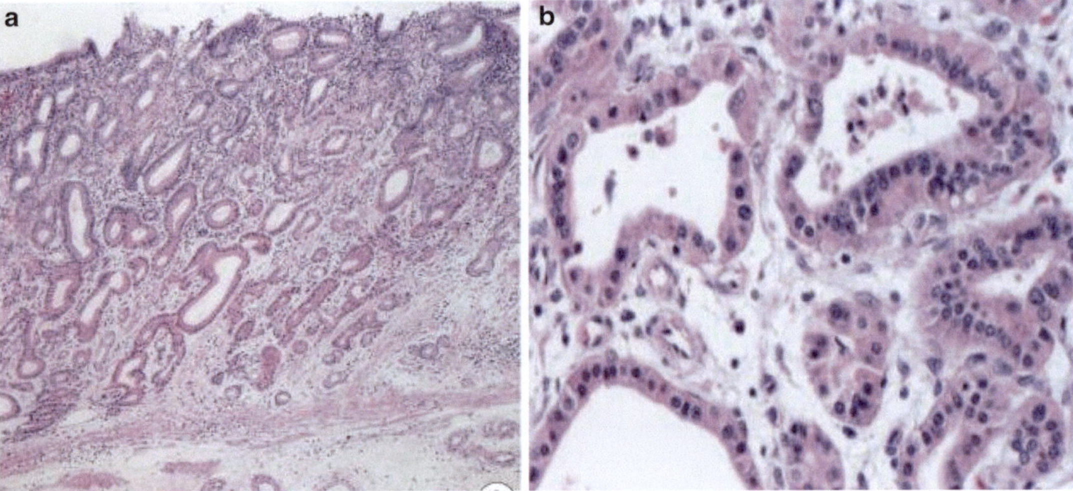

Fig. 7.4 Well-differentiated gastric-type adenocarcinoma. Note lack of periglandular myofibroblast (The Korean Journal of Pathology, *Korean Society of Pathology*, 2012 with permission)

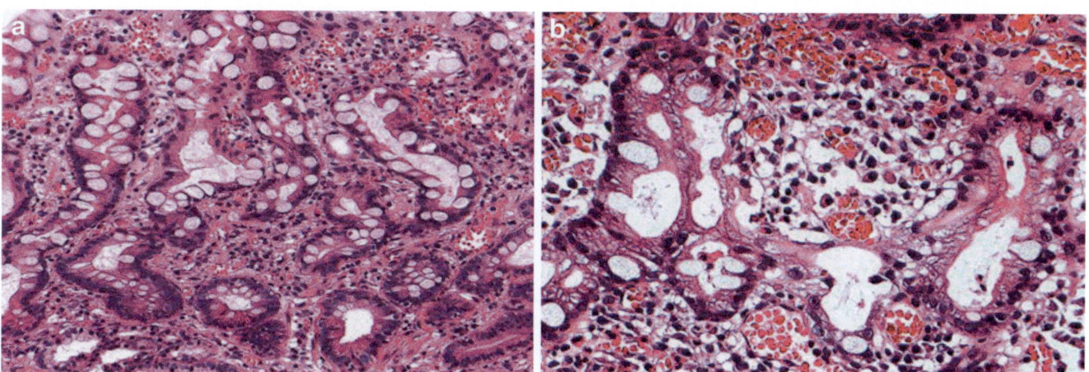

Fig. 7.5 Extremely well-differentiated gastric-type adenocarcinoma. Note deep penetrating irregular bland glands

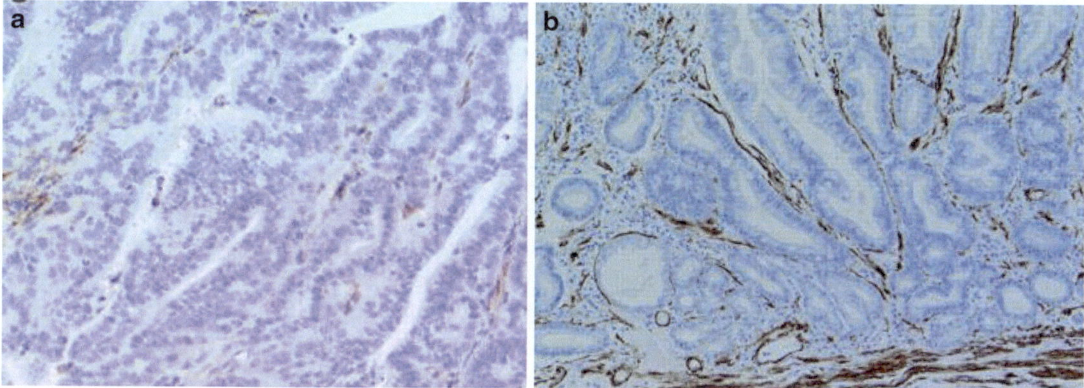

Fig. 7.6 Gastric intestinal-type adenocarcinoma (Gut, *BMJ Publishing Group, Ltd*, 2005 with permission)

well-differentiated gastric adenocarcinomas from most benign proliferations in small biopsy specimens where invasion is not obvious. In the evaluation of periglandular myofibroblasts, a strict criterion should be applied as in the esophagus and intestine. The spindle cells should closely embrace the contours of the corresponding glands to be considered periglandular myofibroblasts. This is to avoid mistaking tumor stromal myofibroblasts for periglandular myofibroblasts since the former can get close to the malignant glands. The tumor stromal cells, however, do not accommodate their arrangement to the shape of the glands and they lack a connection to the muscularis mucosa. Like in the Barrett's esophagus, many benign gastric polyps and reactive lesions have a characteristic smooth muscle component in their lamina propria. These muscle fibers can be traced down to the muscularis mucosa [14]. They might get close to the benign glands; however, they do not show the characteristic embracing pattern. Instead, a perpendicular relationship to the mucosa can be appreciated. In the case of gastritis cystica polyposa/funda, the muscle fibers can be traced up to the muscularis mucosa, and due to their entrapped nature, they can become disorganized. Pancreatic heterotopia also has hypertrophic, disorganized smooth muscle fibers emanating from the muscularis mucosa. The disorganized bundles often mix with pancreatic acini and duct. The importance of appreciating the smooth muscle components and their presenting features lies mainly in avoiding a diagnosis of muscle invading adenocarcinoma especially when reactive changes are present in the epithelial component.

The so-called gastric-type well-differentiated adenocarcinomas have been slowly recognized,

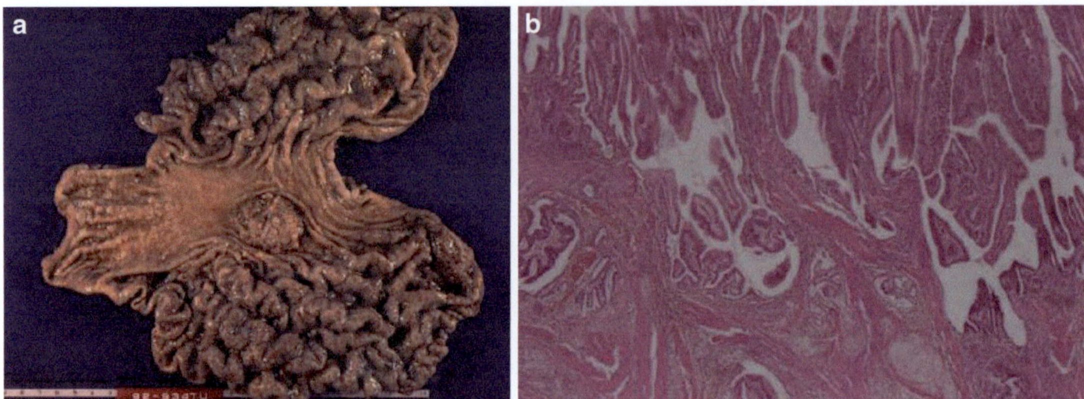

Fig. 7.7 Gastric intestinal-type adenocarcinoma. Pericryptal fibroblasts are absent (**a**, alpha smooth muscle actin stain). Pericryptal fibroblasts are present in intestinal metaplastic glands (**b**)

particularly in Europe and Japan [15]. They consist of cuboidal to columnar cells with mucinous cytoplasm. Characteristically, papillary and villous projections are prominent in the upper portion and irregularly branching and fusing glands are present in the middle and bottom portions of the tumor. This branching and fusion pattern has been interpreted as stromal invasion. In addition to the unique architectural feature, the tumor cells lack surface maturation and show cytological atypia (small nuclei with nucleoli, lack of apical mucinous cap).

A very small fraction of gastric adenocarcinomas are extremely well differentiated [16–18]. The gastric phenotype is easily confused with hyperplastic polyps or even normal gastric mucosa, whereas the intestinal phenotype is more likely mistaken for intestinal metaplasia. The presence of a foveolar appearance in some of the glands indicates that there probably exists at least partially operative interaction between the malignant epithelium and periglandular myofibroblasts. The tumor cells are generally benign looking, slowly proliferative, and p53 negative. However, the malignant nuclei are obviously larger and more hyperchromatic at least focally when comparison with the adjacent normal gastric mucosal cells is made. The only definitive sign of their malignancy is deep location and/or metastasis (Fig. 7.7). In the exercise of identifying deep invasion, we propose that attention be paid to the relationship of the beguilingly benign glands with the adjacent smooth muscle fibers as benign gastric polypoid lesions often contain prominent hypertrophic smooth muscle fibers. The invasive glands should be splitting the horizontally arranged smooth muscle fibers. An emanating relationship with the muscularis mucosa is nonexistent since the invaded fibers are part of the muscularis propria.

Differential Diagnosis

Benign Lesions with Non-foveolar Appearance

Pancreatic Heterotopia

When pancreatic heterotopia is involved by acute and chronic pancreatitis with necrosis and fibrosis with a reactive overlying gastric mucosa, distinction from malignancy is in order. An overall lobulated appearance with squamous metaplasia of the ducts as well as hypertrophic smooth muscle fiber between glands and duct is an important diagnostic feature.

Intestinal-Type Adenoma

Low-grade intestinal-type adenomas can resemble well-differentiated adenocarcinoma both cytologically and architecturally. They, however, show periglandular myofibroblasts and lack desmoplasia.

Rare cases of intestinal-type adenoma with neuroendocrine cell proliferation can mimic invasive adenocarcinoma. The neuroendocrine cells appear to be budding off from angulated glands and infiltrating to the muscularis mucosa or submucosa. The neuroendocrine features of the cells are evident.

Brunner's Gland Nodule

Submucosal Brunner's gland nodule can be seen in the prepyloric region of the stomach. They are composed of benign-looking glands with a lobular arrangement and embraced with layer periglandular myofibroblasts.

Neuroendocrine Tumor

Gastric neuroendocrine tumors can show occasional rosette, tubule, and acinar structures. Attention to their cytological features as well as the presence of other typical growth patterns should help in the distinction.

Oxyntic Gland Polyp/Adenoma

Oxyntic gland polyp/adenomas are rare and present as a deep mucosal lesion with tightly packed irregular glands and anastomosing cords composed of chief cells with nuclear polymorphism and anisonucleosis [19]. They tumors have a low proliferative index corresponding to a benign prognosis. The presence of thin wisps of smooth muscle fibers can mimic a submucosal invading adenocarcinoma. Immunostaining for pepsinogen can help.

Benign Gastric Lesions with Foveolar or Partially Foveolar Morphology

Foveolar Hyperplasia and Dysplasia

Foveolar hyperplasia contains tightly packed foveolar glandular components which can be affected by regenerative atypia (mucin depletion, hyperchromasia, prominent nucleoli, and mitotic figures). The regenerative atypia should be differentiated from foveolar-type dysplasia (adenoma) which lacks stratification [20, 21]. Regenerative atypia, however, usually begins halfway within the gastric mucosa and then extends to the surface with sparing of the bottom portion. Therefore, a full thickness mucosal atypia remains the most reliable criterion for foveolar-type dysplasia. Of course, the presence of active inflammation favors the former.

When accompanied by upward extending smooth muscle fibers, they can be confused with invasive carcinoma. The presence of a foveolar appearance and periglandular myofibroblasts helps make the distinction. In difficult cases, a panel of immunostainings for p53, Ki67, CD44, and LgL2 could be used.

Gastritis Cystic Polyposa/Profunda

Exuberant proliferation of benign mucosa entrapped in deep portions of the gastric wall can resemble invasive adenocarcinoma [14, 22]. Important distinguishing features include a rim of normal lamina propria with an intact myofibroblast layer, foveolar glands arranged in a lobular pattern, and stromal changes such as inflammation, hemorrhage, and fibrosis. The overlying mucosa always shows hyperplastic changes.

Hyperplastic Polyp, Peutz–Jeghers Polyp, Juvenile Polyp, Cronkhite–Canada Syndrome Associated Polyp

All polyps under this heading have a characteristic foveolar component. Except for Cronkhite–Canada syndrome-associated polyps which usually show no prominent muscle proliferation, all the other types have associated muscular proliferation and inflammatory lamina propria.

Nevertheless, the presence of a foveolar-type proliferation does automatically rule out malignancy as dysplasia, and invasive adenocarcinoma can arise from such benign milieu. The intestinal type of dysplasia has the classic nuclear elongation, pseudostratification, and hyperchromasia. As discussed previously, awareness of the criterion for foveolar-type dysplasia is necessary in its distinction from regenerative reactive changes [20, 21]. An invasive component lacks foveolar formation and periglandular myofibroblasts. Other features of malignancy include haphazard glands with greater variation in shape and size, sometimes desmoplasia.

Fundic Gland Polyp

Characteristic morphological features of fundic gland polyps include irregular glands with cystic dilation, budding, flattening of cyst lining cells, as well as presence of chief and parietal cells. The surface and foveolar epithelium can show both hypertrophic and atrophic changes. Because of their small size, well circumscription, and morphological features, distinction from invasive carcinomas is usually straightforward. The issue lies mainly in the distinction between reactive changes and true dysplasia which might involve the surface and foveolar epithelium.

Pyloric Gland Adenoma

This often underappreciated entity contains closely packed glands composed of a monolayer of cuboidal to low columnar epithelial cells with ground cytoplasm, but no mucin cap [15, 23]. Occasional foveola-like structures and cellular blandness and minimally stratified nuclei make it more likely to be mistaken for gastric hyperplastic polyps than for gastric carcinomas. The distinction from the former is, however, clinically significant since 20–30 % of them have been reported to progress to severe dysplasia and/or adenocarcinomas. Furthermore, pyloric adenomas contain p53 positivity and similar chromosomal abnormalities to those of gastric-type adenocarcinomas. Attention to the lack of an apical mucin cap and positivity for both MUC5AC and MUC6 should help clinch the diagnosis.

Colorectum

Key Morphological Features of Well-Differentiated Colorectal Adenocarcinoma

- Glandular proliferation with non-serrated appearance
- Absence of pericryptal myofibroblasts (Figs. 7.8 and 7.9)

Discussion

Well-differentiated colorectal adenocarcinomas are characterized by predominantly well-formed

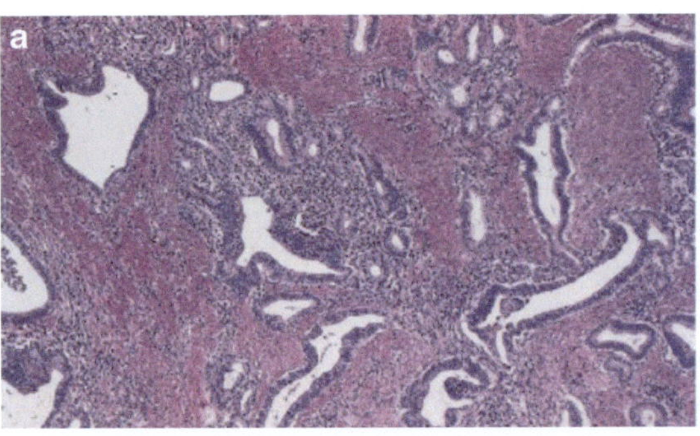

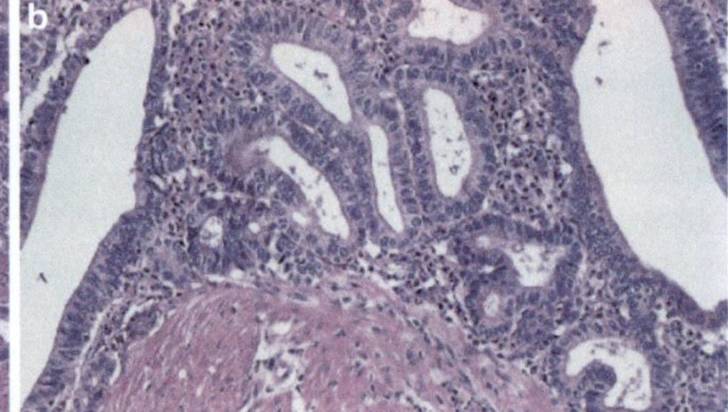

Fig. 7.8 Well-differentiated colonic adenocarcinoma

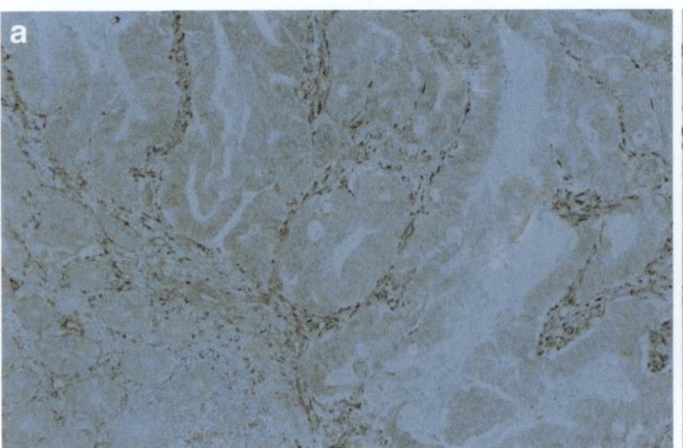

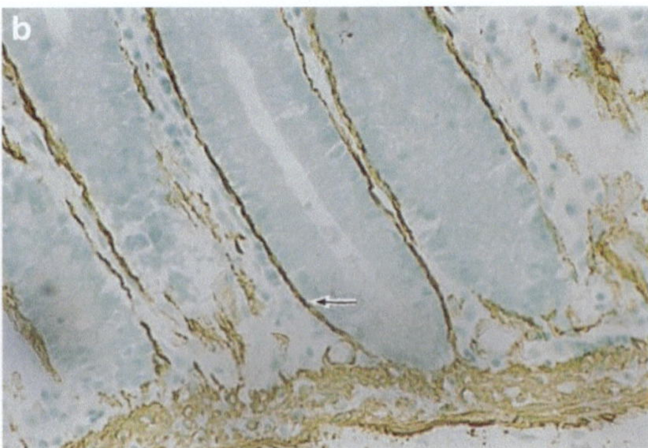

Fig. 7.9 Well- to moderately differentiated colonic adenocarcinoma. Lack of pericryptal myofibroblasts (alpha smooth muscle actin stain) (Surgical Pathology of the GI tract, Liver, Biliary Tract and Pancreas, *Elsevier/Saunders*, 2009 with permission)

glands with smooth and regular lumens. Except for the rare entity of serrated adenocarcinoma which has its characteristic cytological and architectural features, genuine serration is lacking in colorectal adenocarcinomas. Serrations are not to be confused with papillations or pseudoserrations in necrotic complex tubular or cribriform structures. They should contain epithelial tufts composed of only epithelium or epithelium and basement membrane material [24].

The serrated appearance of benign colorectal proliferations is believed to result from a decreased apoptosis/proliferation ratio and delayed cell migration which still follows the normal bottom to surface route [25–27]. Whereas the pericryptal fibroblasts might very well provide some trophic factors for the epithelial growth, their physical presence along with the basement membrane as a component of a complex framework constitutes a powerful restraining force in preventing a full-blown expansion of the crypts and stratification.

The pericryptal fibroblastic sheath in the intestinal tract is a unique syncytium of specialized fibroblasts which extend laterally into the lamina propria to connect with other fibroblasts and downward to associate with the muscularis mucosa [6, 28–32]. Through gap and tight adherence, they are even connected to the overlying epithelial cells. Thus, formed complex network provides the framework for the normal cryptal formation, maintenance, and function. In fact, not only are they a very important component of the stem cell niche located at the bottom of the crypts; the pericryptal fibroblasts also play an essential role in the proliferation, maturation, and upward migration of the epithelial cells. Furthermore, this epithelial–mesenchymal (pericryptal fibroblast) interaction appears to be bidirectional [33]. An excellent example in highlighting this interactive nature is the so-called perineuroma-like proliferation in which the pericryptal fibroblasts are believed to undergo perineural differentiation and demonstrate their characteristic pericryptal whirling growth pattern. Some focal perineuroma-like proliferations are associated with sessile serrated adenomas.

The pericryptal fibroblasts are likely to play an important role in intestinal epithelial tumorigenesis. For instance, pericryptal fibroblasts of colorectal adenomas express high concentrations of cyclooxygenase (COX-2) [34]. Disturbance in their cell adhesion molecule expression has been associated with concurrent neoplasia in patients with ulcerative colitis [35]. More importantly, corresponding to the colorectal hyperplasia–dysplasia–carcinoma spectrum is the progressively decreasing presence of the pericryptal fibroblasts with absence or rarity of pericryptal fibroblast around carcinomatous glands [28, 36, 37]. While it is still premature to conjecture how changes in the pericryptal fibroblasts contribute to epithelial tumorigenesis, the following statement holds true: this is total disruption of a healthy, harmonious nature of the epithelial–mesenchymal interaction with resultant absence or rarity of pericryptal fibroblasts around malignant glands. The diagnostic importance of this observation is analogous to that of the absence of basal cells in prostatic adenocarcinomas and lack of myoepithelial cells in mammary malignancies. It would prove to be very helpful in surgical pathology sign-outs (particularly small biopsies) when other signs of malignancy are not salient.

The nature of dysplasia in serrated lesion differs significantly from that of the conventional adenomas in that apoptosis is largely inhibited and the increased proliferative activity is still restricted to the lower portion of the crypt [25, 26]. Presumably, the epithelial–mesenchymal interaction in serrated adenomas and even serrated adenocarcinomas is better preserved than in their conventional counterparts. The serrated neoplastic cells have a low nuclear/cytoplasmic ratio with preservation of cell polarity and abundant eosinophilic cytoplasm, and they still retain their cell-to-cell adhesion with stratification restricted largely to the tufted areas [25, 26, 38]. This is in contrast to the conventional adenomas where proliferation activity is no longer restricted to the crypt bottom. Instead, they manifest a diffuse, top heavy proliferation pattern. We speculated that a change (disturbance of cell adhesion molecules) similar to that of ulcerative colitis associated pericryptal fibroblasts might happen here, allowing for epithelial stratification and loss of polarity.

It is believed that serrated adenocarcinoma occurs as a result of loss of inhibition on the apoptotic pathways [25–27, 39]. Published diagnostic criteria for differentiating it from non-serrated adenocarcinomas include serrated morphology, mucinous differentiation, eosinophilic cytoplasm, vesicular nuclei, and absence of dirty necrosis. In well-differentiated serrated adenocarcinomas, genuine serration with well-polarized cells is evident. However, information is lacking on the status of periglandular fibroblasts in serrated tumors.

As in the evaluation of gastric and esophageal periglandular fibroblasts, strict criteria must be followed so that tumor stromal myofibroblasts and hypertrophic smooth muscle fibers are not confused for pericryptal fibroblasts. The spindle cells should closely embrace the contours of the corresponding glands/crypts, and a connection to the muscularis mucosa is usually possible.

Finally, a small fraction of inflammatory bowel disease-associated colorectal adenocarcinomas present as the so-called very well-differentiated adenocarcinoma (low-grade tubuloglandular adenocarcinoma) of the colon [40]. They are composed of cells with low-grade nuclei. Some of the glands have round or tubular profiles, while some have branching glands. They lack both serration and pericryptal fibroblasts.

Differential Diagnosis

Adenoma with Pseudoinvasion

Importantly, these misplaced epithelial cells are usually surrounded by a rim of lamina propria (with pericryptal sheath fibroblasts) and have a well-circumscribed or lobular overall appearance [41]. Cytologically, they are similar to their mucosal counterparts with which communication can sometimes be found. The adjacent stroma usually contains hemorrhage or hemosiderin. When mucin pools are present, they lack the features of malignant mucin (irregular, dissecting pools with floating malignant cells).

Colitis Cystica Polyposa/Profunda

The benign herniated or misplaced glands often present as well-circumscribed lobules. Presence of a rim of lamina propria (with pericryptal fibroblast) can be found. Evidence of previous injury is often discernible.

Sessile Serrated Adenoma

They are characterized by irregular crypts with a dilated base which might extend laterally in parallel to the muscularis mucosa. Sometimes, the crypts can be herniated through the muscularis mucosa, giving the erroneous impression of invasive adenocarcinoma. The telltale signs are serration and maturation at the base of the crypts.

Benign Polyp

Hyperplastic polyps are rarely confused with well-differentiated adenocarcinomas because of their small size and characteristic serration. Inflammatory or hamartomatous polyps can reach a bigger size, and serration is sometimes not prominent. Furthermore, strands of smooth muscle cells can be present next to benign glands, and misplacement of epithelial cells into deeper structures can occur. Attention to the presence of a rim of benign lamina propria (with intact pericryptal fibroblasts) can be very helpful in ruling out invasive carcinoma.

The Small Intestine and Periampullary Region

The vast majority of adenocarcinomas in the small intestine and periampullary area are almost identical to colorectal carcinomas and can be evaluated as such. The so-called pancreatobiliary type makes up less than 20 % of the adenocarcinomas in the periampullary region and is mostly well differentiated. Morphologically they conform to their pancreatic ductal and extrahepatic biliary counterparts and therefore are subjected to their criteria (nonlobular arrangement of glands and tubules, prominent desmoplasia around individual glands).

Differential Diagnosis for Small Intestine Adenocarcinoma

Brunner's Gland Hyperplasia and Hamartoma

Their benignity is usually manifested in lobulation and cellular blandness. The benign glands might extend into the lamina propria and even become pedunculated with resultant hyperplastic fibromuscular stroma and adipose tissue, thus creating an invasive appearance. However, de novo dysplasia and carcinomas of the glands remain to be documented. Instead, rare reported cases of adenoma and adenocarcinoma actually represent secondary involvement by the surface dysplasia or adenocarcinoma. The involved glands remain lobular and presence of periglandular fibroblasts is discernible.

Neuroendocrine Tumor with Acinar Growth Pattern

Duodenal neuroendocrine tumors usually show gland-like formations which can contain secretions. Attention to the cytological features and the lack of true glandular lumens allows for their distinction from well-differentiated adenocarcinoma.

Pancreatic Heterotopia

When involved by regenerative atypia, pancreatic heterotopia might simulate invasive carcinoma. However, its lobulation and lack of desmoplasia give it away.

Gastric Heterotopia with Secondary Mucosal Prolapse

It contains tightly packed benign glands composed of chief and parietal cells with surface epithelial (foveolar) hyperplasia. When pedunculated, arborizing bundles of smooth muscle fibers can be traced to the hyperplastic muscularis mucosa. It is not to be confused with muscle invading adenocarcinoma.

Colitis Cystica Profunda, Misplacement of Adenomatous Epithelium

The misplaced benign epithelium in the submucosal or muscularis can imitate well-differentiated adenocarcinoma. As in colitis cystica polyposa/profunda, the benign glands are well-circumscribed lobules. The presence of a rim of lamina propria (with pericryptal fibroblasts) can be identified.

Differential Diagnosis for Periampullary Adenocarcinoma

Ampullary Adenoma Involving Periampullary Glands

Due to the enmeshment of the periampullary ducts and glands with smooth fibers, a perfect picture of invasive adenocarcinoma is created when adenomatous cells of the ampulla extend into the adjacent glands. Attention to the lobular feature and similar nuclear features as those of the surface adenomatous component should point in the right direction. Moreover, the involved ducts and glands do not elicit desmoplasia.

Colonization of Mucosal Basement Membrane by Underlying Well-Differentiated Invasive Pancreatic or Biliary Duct Adenocarcinoma

The significance of this entity lies mainly in its distinction from primary ampullary adenomas. Instead of having irregular glands with abundant desmoplasia, it closely resembles a primary adenoma. In difficult cases, immunostainings are needed. These adenoma-like cells are positive for CK7 and MUC1 and negative for CDX2 and MUC2.

Paraduodenal Pancreatitis

When located in deeper locations, the pancreatic tissue is usually surrounded by hypertrophic smooth muscle fibers and fibrosis. Differentiation from pancreatobiliary-type adenocarcinomas requires appreciation of a lobular configuration and lack of desmoplasia.

Liver

Key Morphological Features of Well-Differentiated Hepatocellular Carcinoma

- Thick cords with higher cell density (equal or greater than three-cell thick) and or reduced reticulin reduction
- Capillarization of sinusoids (diffuse CD34 positivity) (Figs.7.10, 7.11, and 7.12)

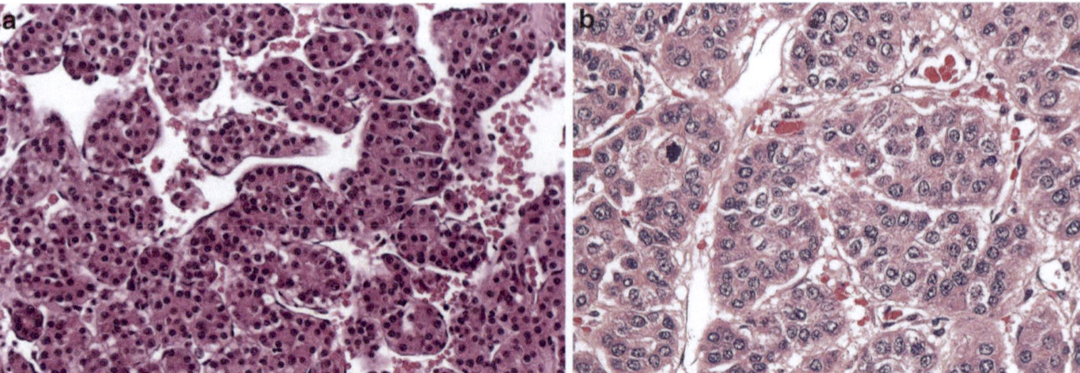

Fig. 7.10 Well-differentiated hepatocellular cell carcinoma. Note thick cords with endothelial wrapping (Atlas of Liver Pathology, *Elsevier/Saunders*, 2011 with permission)

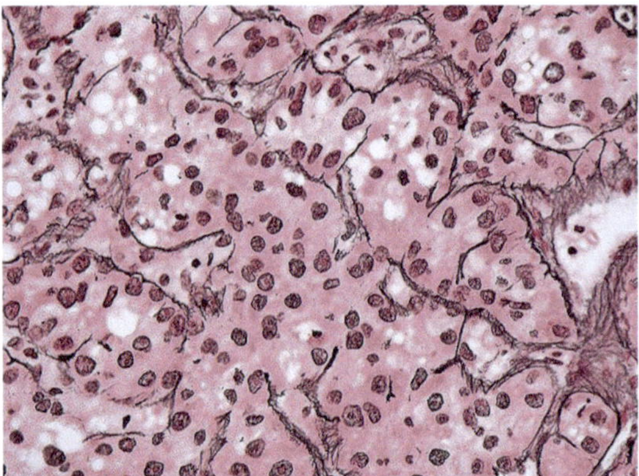

Fig. 7.11 Well-differentiated hepatocellular cell carcinoma. Thick cords are highlighted with reticulin stain (Atlas of Liver Pathology, *Elsevier/Saunders*, 2011 with permission)

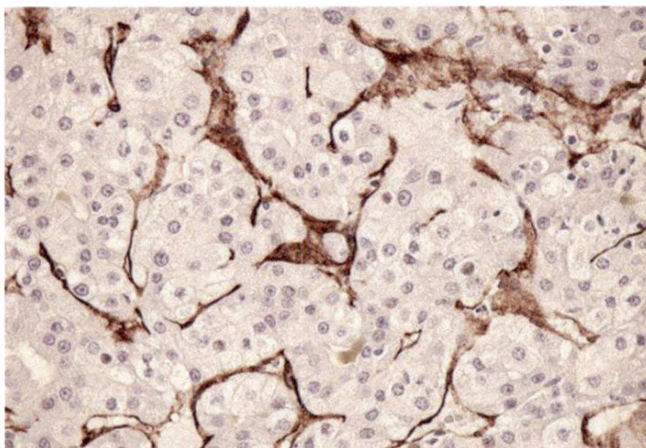

Fig. 7.12 Well-differentiated hepatocellular cell carcinoma. Capillarization of sinusoids is demonstrated by CD31 reactivity of the wrapping endothelial cells (Atlas of Liver Pathology, *Elsevier/Saunders*, 2011 with permission)

Discussion

The normal adult hepatic tissue is ideally crafted for optimal substance transport between the circulation, bile canaliculi, and hepatocytes. The hepatic cords are normally one-cell layer thick with sinusoid vessels lining on each side. Two-cell thick plates and even rosette formations are visible only in regenerative conditions. The normal hepatic structure is maintained by a delicate network of reticulin lining the hepatic sinusoids as a result of normal epithelial–mesenchymal (stellate cells) interaction [42, 43]. Importantly other fibrogenic activity of the organ is kept to the minimum in the functional units with visible fibrous tissue limited to the portal tracts, bile duct and accompanying vascular bundles, and the capsule.

In most hepatocellular carcinomas, the antifibrogenic feature of the hepatoblasts is largely conserved (Fig. 7.13). While reticulin production is still operational or even increased, it seems to be outstripped by the rapidly proliferating tumor cells [43, 44]. Thus [44], thick cords (three or more cells across) lined by attenuated reticulin fibers become evident. This important feature can be appreciated even in the rare fibrolamellar and scirrhous variants in which abundant fibrotic tissue is present. The increased fibrogenic activity in these two variants indicate their cholangiolar differentiation (fibrolamellar variant cells: positive for CK7, EMA, and Hepar1; cirrhotic variant cells: negative for Hepar1 and positive for CK7) [45–49]. The pseudoglandular variant can also be viewed as having thickened plates if one can men-

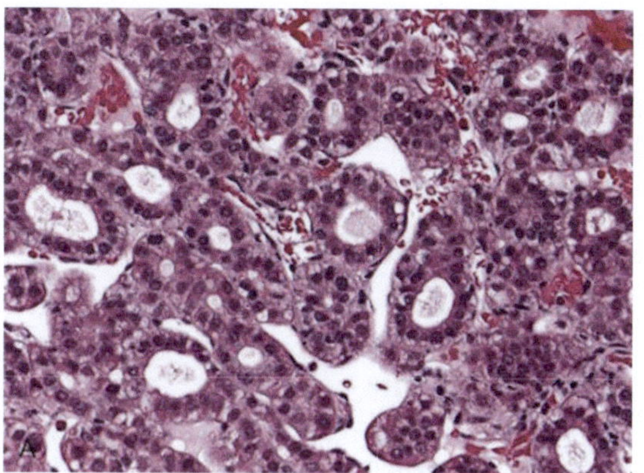

Fig. 7.13 Well-differentiated hepatocellular cell carcinoma, pseudoglandular variant. Note endothelial wrapping and lack of desmoplastic stroma (Atlas of Liver Pathology, *Elsevier/Saunders*, 2011 with permission)

tally cut the lumen open and spread the cells out. The normal canaliculi are lined by only two to three hepatocytes, and when spread out, the cords are no more than three cells thick. The imaginary cords in hepatocellular carcinomas seem to be more cellular and more diffuse than those derived from rosettes in hepatic adenomas and hepatitis.

In evaluating reticulin stain, it is important to pick areas uncompromised by steatosis. It is known that steatosis can impair the production of reticulin to an extent comparable to that of the hepatocellular carcinoma [50]. Moreover, hepatocellular carcinomatous cells can have steatotic changes.

Another important feature of hepatocellular carcinomatous cells is that they maintain the capability to induce brisk angiogenesis and obtain abundant blood supply like their hepatoblast counterparts [51–53]. The difference is, however, that the former tend to derive their nutrients from the arterioles, while the latter is supplied by both portal veins and arterioles. Thus, the tumor microvessels are subjected to higher perfusion pressures leading to capillarization. The normal sinusoids are negative for CD34 and CD31. Capillarized microvessels become positive for the two markers. This important feature has also been employed widely in the daily surgical pathology sign-out.

In the utility of both the reticulin and CD34/CD31 stains for the differentiation of hepatic nodules, it is advisable that they are considered in tandem. Rare cases of hepatocellular carcinoma with increased reticulin production have been reported and the increased reticulin production presents in the form of monolayer trabecular pattern [44]. Disturbance in the blood supply is common in benign hepatic nodules, and focal capillarization of the microvessels can occur. When the two stains seem to conflict with each other, careful attention to the distribution of CD34/CD31 positivity and finding a non-steatotic area can be very helpful. For instance, in cirrhotic nodule, the CD34/CD31 positivity is largely restricted to the periphery while focal nodular hyperplasia has its positivity near the fibrous septa [54, 55]. Variable staining patterns have been reported for hepatic adenomas. However, they have intact or only focally reduced reticulin framework with cords less than three cells across [54, 55].

Differentia Diagnosis

Macroregenerative Nodules, Dysplastic Nodule, and Early Hepatocellular Carcinoma

Large regenerative nodules measure 0.8 cm or greater and have intact reticulin framework with cell plates no more than two-cell thick. CD34 or CD31 stain may show some peripheral staining and reveal some unpaired arterioles. When large cell dysplasia or small cell dysplasia occur, a dysplastic nodule is formed.

Early hepatocellular carcinomas have been increasingly evaluated by surgical pathologists. Defined as nodules less than 2 cm in diameter, they lack a tumor capsule and grow by replacing the existing hepatocyte cords [56–58]. Stromal invasion with various numbers of portal tracts can be present within the nodule. The reticulin framework is usually reduced but not totally lost. Increased CD34 sinusoidal staining and unpaired arterioles are present.

Focal Nodular Hyperplasia

This lesion contains cell plates of normal or slightly increased thickness with sinusoidal vessels. It can show CD34-/Cd31-positive microvessels which are adjacent to the fibrous septa. Other diagnostic features include a central fibrous area connecting with multiple well-circumscribed nodules. The central area contains large arterial vessels with no accompanying large bile ducts and portal veins.

Nodular Regenerative Hyperplasia

Nodular regenerative hyperplasia contains small nodules with minimal fibrous septation. Its cell plates are less than two cells thick and areas of atrophy with reticulin condensation are common between the nodules. The sinusoids might be arterialized; therefore, focal CD34 positivity can be seen.

Hepatic Adenoma

Hepatic adenomas can have thickened plates, but their thickness is usually less than 3 cells across. Reticulin stain reveals intact or only focally reduced reticulin staining. Diffuse CD34 positivity has been reported in some cases; however, majority of cases show negativity or focal positivity.

The tumors usually lack a capsule and occur as a result of oral contraceptive or anabolic steroid use or other metabolic disorders. This is in contrast to classical hepatocellular carcinomas which develop largely in cirrhotic liver and rarely arise from hepatic adenomas. In difficult cases, immunostainings for glypican-3 and AFP can be applied to make the distinction.

Epithelioid Angiomyolipoma

Hepatic angiomyolipomas usually contain a scant fat component. Problems might arise when the tumor cells show trabecular formation with abundant eosinophilic cytoplasm. However, spider web-like cytoplasm and presence of thick-walled vessel should arouse doubt about a hepatocellular carcinoma. Immunostainings for HMB45 and smooth muscle actin light up the tumor cells.

Pancreas

Key Morphological Features of Well-Differentiated Ductal Adenocarcinoma

- Nonlobular arrangement of glands and tubules
- Prominent desmoplasia around individual glands (Figs. 7.14)

Discussion

The pancreatic exocrine morphogenesis/organogenesis follows the classic paradigm for glandular formation with a resultant lobular appearance. In chronic pancreatitis, the most common mimicker of well-differentiated ductal adenocarcinomas, this lobular pattern is still largely preserved even though the benign ducts are often atrophic and deprived of acinar structures. In contrast, carcinomatous glands are nonlobular and randomly distributed.

Reviewing this vital organ of the human body, one would not help but wonder at the ingenuity of Mother Nature in devising various safety mechanisms in order to prevent and limit the dreadful event of activating or leaking destructive digestive enzymes to adjacent tissues or organs.

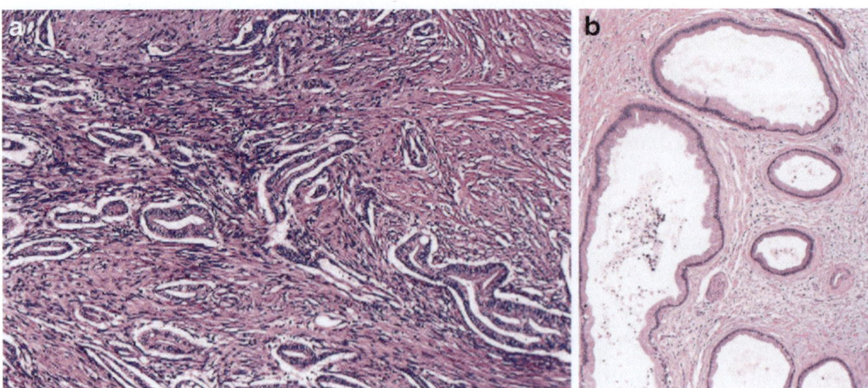

Fig. 7.14 Well-differentiated pancreatic ductal carcinoma. Note nonlobular arrangement of irregular glands and prominent desmoplasia (Surgical Pathology of the GI tract, Liver, Biliary Tract and Pancreas, *Elsevier/Saunders*, 2009 with permission)

First of all, rather than obtaining its blood flow from a single source, the pancreas derives its arterial supply from rich anastomoses around the organ with many contributing components [59, 60]. Second, benign pancreatic ductal structures containing digestive enzymes are structurally separated from muscular vessels and are surrounded by acini and fibrous tissue [61, 62]. In doing so, the risk of lethal hemorrhage due to corrosion into the large arteries by digestive enzymes is reduced. This vessel shunning property of ductal epithelium has been illustrated by developmental biology research showing that early endothelial cells are essential for the onset of pancreatic budding and endocrine specification, but later on they inhibit further branching and exocrine differentiation [63–66].

The pancreatic interlobular lymphatics are channeled into a surface network which facilitates the drainage of its lymph fluid which might contain destructive enzymes [67]. The pancreas lacks a capsule which might cut off its blood supply or hinder lymphatic or venous outflow when the organ becomes inflamed. At the cellular level, a delicate check and balance system is instituted to prevent enzyme activation and self-destruction [68–70].

To further protect from self-destruction, the pancreas is equipped with specialized fibroblasts: pancreatic stellate cells. These fibroblasts are present around the acini [71, 72], small pancreatic ducts, and blood vessels and play a very important intermediary role in the epithelial–endothelial cross talk, ameliorate inflammation, and fill in structural void [73, 74].

This close epithelial–mesenchymal (stellate cells) interaction has been taken advantage of by transformed malignant ductal epithelial cells to form a strong alliance which gives rise to prominent desmoplasia characteristically associated with pancreatobiliary adenocarcinomas [74]. This resultant desmoplasia along with the inherent epithelial abhorrence for blood vessels makes pancreatic ductal adenocarcinoma one of the most hypovascularized tumors [75, 76]. Actually, pancreatic adenocarcinomas contain even less vessels than chronically inflamed pancreatic tissue. To circumvent growth hindrance by hypovascularity, not only the malicious alliance between the ductal epithelium and the stellate cells in the stroma provides each other with necessary proliferative factors and antiapoptotic stimuli, but it also instructs the tumor cells to employ the unconventional survival mechanism of autophagy in this seemingly less desirable environment [71, 72, 74, 77–79].

Molecular studies indicate that the stellate cells in desmoplasia demonstrate similar but elevated gene expressions to those in fibrosis in chronic pancreatitis (21). Histologically, desmoplasia differs from usual fibrosis by higher cellularity and presence of young collagen. However, in the pancreatic pathology, the distinction is sometimes difficult. This problem can be alleviated if attention is paid to the relationship between the fibrous proliferation and the epithelial cells and the arrangement of the latter. In chronic pancreatitis, the fibrosis is mainly around atrophic lobules, whereas active desmoplasia is abundant between individual malignant glands which are randomly scattered [61].

Other morphological clues reportedly helpful in making a diagnosis of well-differentiated pancreatic ductal carcinoma include naked glands in fatty tissue, presence of glands near muscular vessels (not tumor stroma vessels), and perineural invasion [61, 80]. Their utility is, however, of limited practical significance particularly in a biopsy specimen because their presence is infrequent.

Because of its bland cytological features and lack of abundant desmoplasia, the rare foamy gland variant of pancreatic adenocarcinoma is easily missed by the unwary [61]. This variant can also mix with ordinary ductal adenocarcinoma in variable portions. The malignant glands sometimes are present between normal pancreatic lobules with minimal or no desmoplastic reaction. Appreciation of the unique cytological features of this variant is essential in avoiding underdiagnosis. The cells contain abundant pale, microvesicular cytoplasm with small irregular and hyperchromatic nuclei. The apical cytoplasm is sharply demarcated from the brush border-like zone. It is believed that foamy gland cells differentiate toward endocervical or gastric foveolar

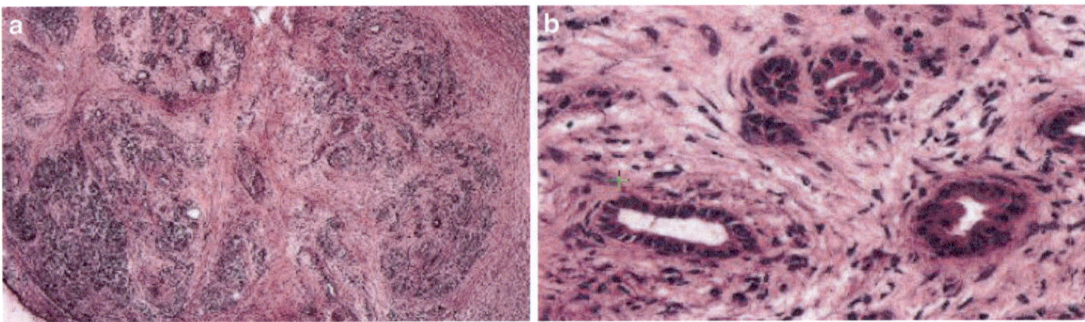

Fig. 7.15 Chronic pancreatitis. Note lobulation and interlobular fibrosis (Surgical Pathology of the GI tract, Liver, Biliary Tract and Pancreas, *Elsevier/Saunders*, 2009 with permission)

cells, and this differentiation probably weakens the symbiotic relationship between the malignant epithelial cells and the stellate cells leading to a paucicellular and myxoid stroma. When in doubt, a panel of confirmatory immunostaining can be performed. The brushlike zone of the neoplastic glands shows strong positivity for B72.3, CEA, and MUC1.

Differential Diagnosis

Chronic Pancreatitis

Chronic pancreatitis is intricately entangled with ductal carcinoma in several aspects. It can present a mass lesion making it necessary to rule out malignancy. Chronic pancreatic inflammation predisposes the tissue to malignancy. Furthermore, chronic inflammation might also superimpose on a ductal carcinoma as a result of mass effect of the latter. Lastly, histopathologic differentiation between chronic pancreatitis and well-differentiated ductal carcinoma poses a challenge even for the experienced.

Nevertheless, chronic pancreatitis contains atrophic acini with retention of ducts and islets of Langerhans. Even though there may be prominent fibrosis, an overall lobular arrangement can be appreciated at low power (Fig. 7.15). The location of fibrosis in alcohol-related pancreatitis is mainly perilobular, and the lobules are more regular and less angulated than the malignant glands which are separated by abundant desmoplasia (high cellularity, young collagen) [81]. Chronic obstructive pancreatitis shows both interlobular and intralobular fibrosis, and the presence of lobular arrangement sets it apart from malignant glands [81]. Other morphological clues of benignity include less dense cytoplasm, shunning from muscular vessels, nerves, and even adipose tissue.

Lymphoplasmacytic Sclerosing Pancreatitis

This type of pancreatitis is characterized by a cuff-like periductal fibrosis which shows a storiform pattern of fibroblasts admixed with inflammatory cells. A suspicion can be confirmed by IgG4 immunostaining which lights up the plasma cells.

Key Morphological Features of Pancreatic Acinar Cell Carcinoma

- High cellularity with no desmoplasia
- Moderate to abundant eosinophilic cytoplasm with prominent nucleoli (Fig. 7.16)

Discussion

The wnt/beta-catenin signaling plays an essential role in the expansion and differentiation of the acinar linage during organogenesis. Activating mutations of beta-catenin or truncating mutations of the APC genes have been reported in acinic cell carcinomas. In some cases, nuclear localization of beta-catenin has also been observed. Therefore, acinic cell carcinomas probably represent unbridled acinic proliferation and differentiation [82, 83].

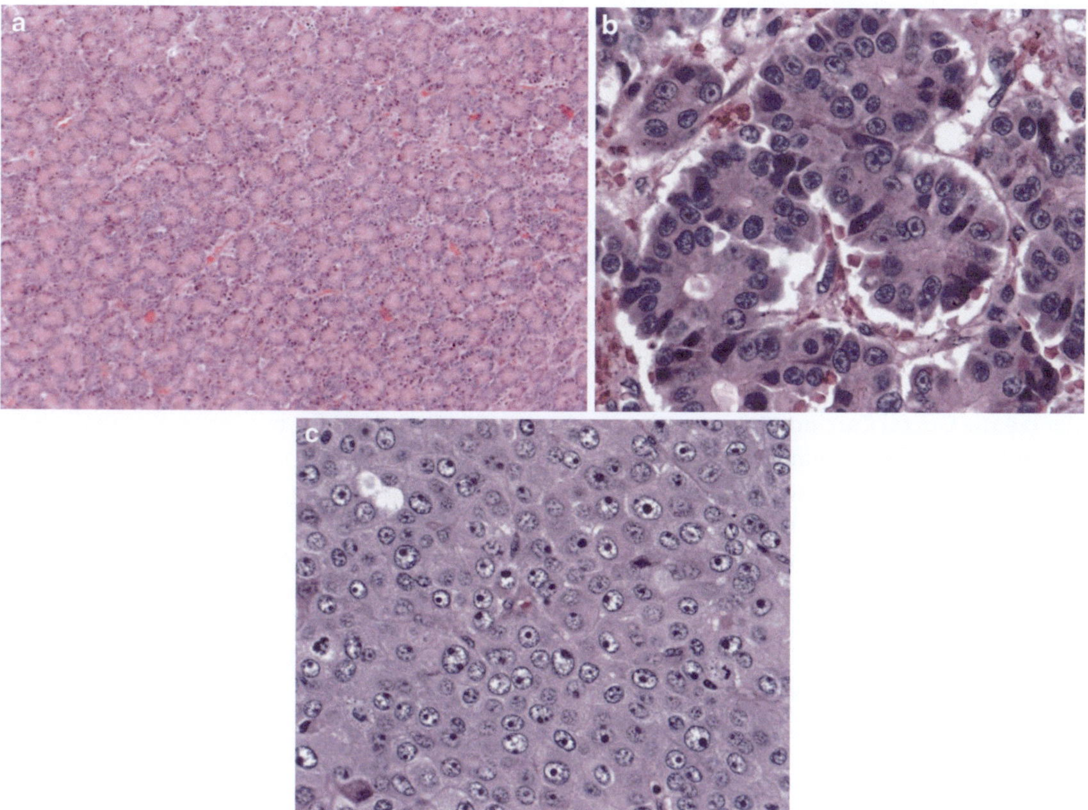

Fig. 7.16 Pancreatic acinic cell carcinoma. There is hypercellularity. Tumor cells have moderate to abundant eosinophilic cytoplasm with prominent nucleoli. Minimal stromal component is evident (Tumor of the Pancreas, *Armed Force Institute of Pathology/American Registry of Pathology*, 2007 with permission)

In stark contrast to their ductal counterparts, acinic cell carcinomas are well circumscribed and even encapsulated and contain high cellularity and no desmoplasia. The malignant cells are characterized by uniformity, abundant eosinophilic granules, and prominent nucleoli.

Most cases have a paucity of fibrous stroma. Even though in some cases, abundant fibrous tissue is present, it is mainly in the septa rather than in close proximity of individual acinar structures. Tumor extension into the fibrous capsule is common. However, the possibility of mixed acinar–ductal carcinoma should be considered when individual acinar structures invade the fibrous stroma [83].

The pancreatic acinic cells are equipped with a repertoire of mechanisms in dealing with intracellular activation of destructive enzymes. This probably is the reason why they become less associated with the stellate cells than their ductal counterparts and why no powerful symbiosis as seen in ductal adenocarcinomas develops in acinic cell carcinomas. Presumably, this lack of symbiosis along with beta-catenin alterations contributes to more frequent necrosis and cystic degeneration even though acinic cell carcinomas are much more vascularized than ductal adenocarcinomas.

Differential Diagnosis

Benign Acinar Proliferations

Acinic cell nodules are microscopic and therefore are unlikely to be confused with acinic cell carcinomas even though they might show some dysplastic features.

Rare cases of acinic cell cystadenoma have been reported and the main concern is to differentiate it from acinic cell cystadenocarcinoma.

Presence of prominent nucleoli, solid areas, more complex epithelial structures, necrosis, and infiltration of the stroma indicate malignancy.

Pancreatic Neuroendocrine Neoplasm

Pancreatic neuroendocrine neoplasms are characterized by classical trabecular or gyriform pattern with salt–pepper chromatin features. They lack prominent nucleoli, basal nuclear polarity, eosinophilic granular cytoplasm, widespread glandular formation, and frequent mitotic figures.

Pancreatic Ductal Carcinoma

Pancreatic ductal carcinomas have characteristic stromal desmoplasia and lack eosinophilic granular cytoplasm. Problems might arise when an acinic cell carcinoma shows a solid sheet growth pattern with abundant septal stroma. Attention to the location of fibrotic stroma and even immunostainings might be needed to rule out poorly differentiated ductal carcinoma. Rare cases of acinic cell carcinoma with abundant intracellular and extracellular mucin have been reported. Cursive examination might lead to an erroneous diagnosis of mucinous ductal carcinoma.

Solid Pseudopapillary Neoplasm

Solid pseudopapillary neoplasms are featured by loosely cohesive, polygonal cells with nuclear grooves. While mitotic figures and true tumor necrosis are uncommon, degenerative changes are significant.

Key Morphological Features of Solid Pseudopapillary Carcinoma

- Solid areas with rich vasculature and areas with significant degenerative changes
- Loosely cohesive, uniform polygonal cells with frequent longitudinal nuclear grooves (Figs. 7.17 and 7.18)

Discussion

This unique entity represents a malignancy of botched acinic differentiation with endocrine transdifferentiation by default [84, 85]. Disturbances in the wnt/beta-catenin signaling system seem to be more pervasive than what is seen in acinic cell carcinomas. Importantly, there is concurrent nuclear translocation of both beta-catenin and E-cadherin molecules (Fig. 7.19). The translocation of E-cadherin from the cell membrane to the nucleus disrupts the cell skeleton structure and cell-to-cell adhesion apparatus and might account for the cytological features of tumor cells: polygonal shape, loose cohesiveness, and longitudinal nuclear grooves.

Compared to the ductal carcinomas, solid pseudopapillary carcinomas are hypervascular and blood lakes are frequently present at the tumor periphery. Whereas tumor necrosis is uncommon, they are characterized by remarkable degenerative changes such as cytoplasmic vacuoles, myxoid stroma, foamy macrophages, and cholesterol crystals. Cystic and pseudopapillary

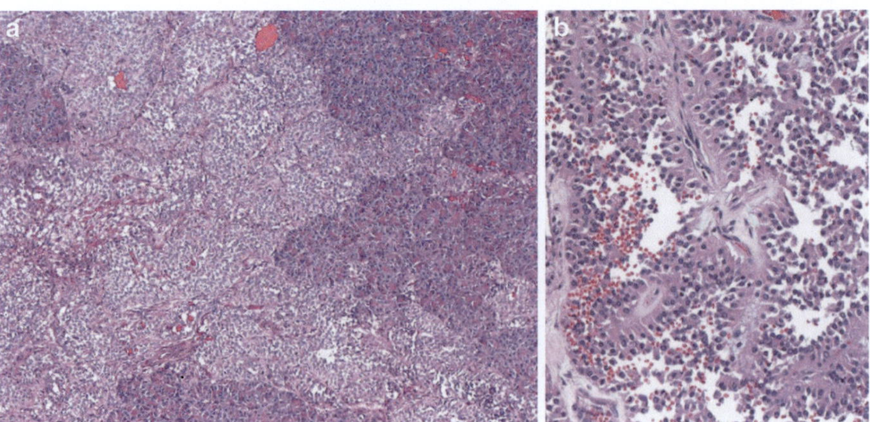

Fig. 7.17 Pseudopapillary carcinoma. Note that solid areas have rich vasculature and adjacent degenerating areas (**a**). Pseudopapillary formation due to degeneration (**b**) (Tumor of the Pancreas, *Armed Force Institute of Pathology/ American Registry of Pathology*, 2007 with permission)

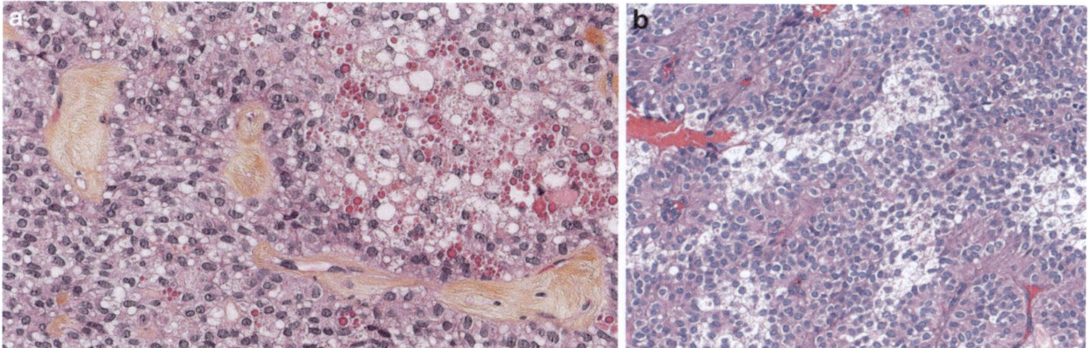

Fig. 7.18 Pseudopapillary carcinoma. Hyaline globules, nuclear grooves, and foamy cells are some important morphological features (Tumor of the Pancreas, *Armed Force Institute of Pathology/American Registry of Pathology*, 2007 with permission)

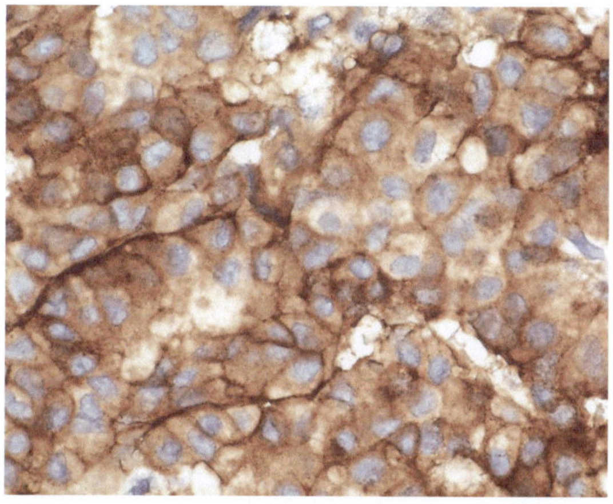

Fig. 7.19 Pseudopapillary carcinoma. Tumor cells are diffusely positive for beta-catenin (Tumor of the Pancreas, *Armed Force Institute of Pathology/American Registry of Pathology*, 2007 with permission)

structures are frequently present. Along with the cytological features, these changes could be attributed to the functional loss of function of the catenin/E-cadherin complex. Some tumor cells contain so-called hyaline globules which are condensed alpha-1 antitrypsin, an indication of their acinar differentiation.

Differential Diagnosis

Well-Differentiated Pancreatic Endocrine Neoplasm

Well-differentiated pancreatic endocrine neoplasms lack pseudopapillae, diffuse degenerative changes, and loosely cohesive polygonal cells with nuclear grooves. In difficult cases, immunostainings are required to make the distinction. Importantly, both entities are positive for CD56 and NSE. Solid pseudopapillary neoplasms are, however, negative for synaptophysin but only focally and weakly positive for chromogranin. Beta-catenin and E-cadherin stains might be useful.

Acinar Cell Carcinoma

Acinar cell carcinomas contain cohesive cuboidal cells with prominent nucleoli and eosinophilic granular cytoplasm. Mitosis, necrosis, and luminal formation are more common.

Pseudocyst

They lack an epithelial lining and other features of solid pseudopapillary neoplasms.

Features of Well-Differentiated Pancreatic Endocrine Neoplasm (Grade II Neuroendocrine Tumor)

- Ki67 index of 3 to 30 % or mitotic count of 2 to 20/10 HPF

Discussion

The 2010 WHO classification has replaced the term “well-differentiated neuroendocrine carcinoma” with neuroendocrine tumor grade II [86]. In conformity to the scheme for gastrointestinal tract neuroendocrine tumors, it adopts mitotic count as the sole index for grading, leaving out functionality, necrosis, and cellular atypia. Information on tumor size, extent of adjacent tissue involvement, and large vessel invasion has been incorporated into the staging system. In an apparent effort to improve data collection on this relatively rare entity, it has been recommended that all pancreatic neuroendocrine tumors be reported to the cancer registries.

Relative to well-differentiated neuroendocrine neoplasms in other organs, pancreatic endocrine neoplasms are characterized by a much wider variation from the classical neuroendocrine theme [87, 88]. Variants include cells with foamy or clear cytoplasm, oncocytic and cystic degeneration, widespread glandular formation, and even marked nuclear atypia with prominent nucleoli. Awareness with these variants avoids mistaking them for other lesions. This is particularly the case with the last variant which could be easily passed off as poorly differentiated endocrine carcinoma (NET III) or ductal carcinoma [88].

Differential Diagnosis

Microcystic Serous Adenoma

The solid variant of serous adenomas can resemble pancreatic endocrine neoplasms. They lack characteristic salt–pepper chromatin. In difficult cases, immunostainings for neuroendocrine markers would be useful.

Acinic Cell Carcinoma

Acinic cell carcinomas are characterized by eosinophilic granular cytoplasm with prominent nucleoli.

High-Grade Neuroendocrine Neoplasm or Ductal Carcinoma

The pleomorphic variant of well differentiated pancreatic endocrine neoplasm may have cells with marked nuclear atypia with prominent nucleoli. However, the nuclear changes are usually accompanied by abundant cytoplasm with a low N/C ratio and low mitotic figures. These two features set it apart from poorly differentiated pancreatic neuroendocrine neoplasms (NET GIII). The lack of prominent desmoplasia helps rule out ductal carcinoma.

Extrahepatic Biliary Duct and Gall Bladder

Key Morphological Features of Well-Differentiated Adenocarcinoma

- Nonlobular arrangement of well-formed glands and tubules
- Prominent desmoplasia around individual glands (Fig. 7.20)

Discussion

Developed from the same hepatic diverticulum as the ventral pancreas, the normal bile duct cells are also closely associated with stromal cells (stellate cells) probably to prevent leakage of obnoxious and carcinogenic bile to the adjacent organs [89–94]. And this relationship has also been accentuated in bile duct adenocarcinoma evidenced as abundant desmoplasia formation [95, 96]. Well-differentiated bile duct adenocarcinomas therefore are characterized by widely distributed well-formed but irregular glands with abundant desmoplasia.

The vast majority of adenocarcinomas of the extrahepatic bile duct and gallbladder resemble their pancreatic counterparts. Typically, the tumor cells have ample cytoplasm with variable amount of cytoplasmic mucin. However, some cases can have atrophic glands and a foamy gland variant has also been recognized [97] (Fig. 7.21).

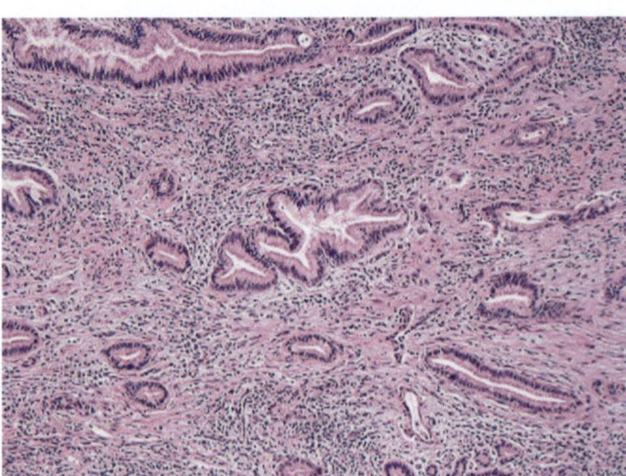

Fig. 7.20 Well-differentiated extrahepatic cholangiocarcinoma. Note nonlobular arrangement of irregular glands (Surgical Pathology of the GI tract, Liver, Biliary Tract and Pancreas, *Elsevier/Saunders*, 2009 with permission)

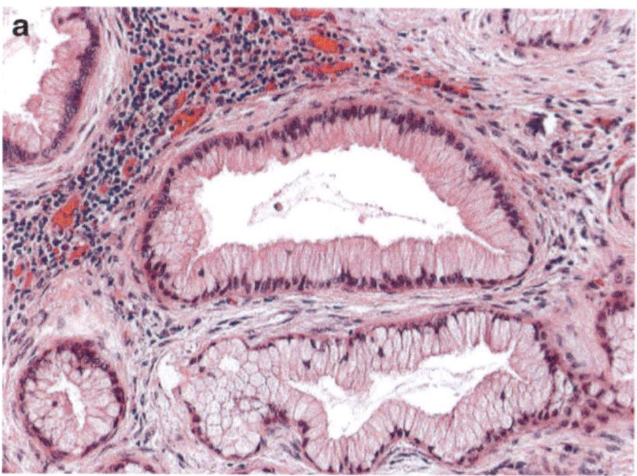

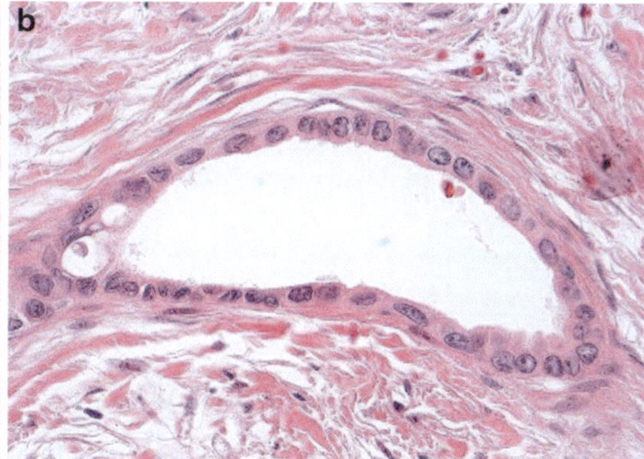

Fig. 7.21 Variants of extrahepatic cholangiocarcinoma. Foamy gland variant (**a**) and atrophic variant (**b**) (Surgical Pathology of the GI tract, Liver, Biliary Tract and Pancreas, *Elsevier/Saunders*, 2009 with permission)

Awareness of such cases is essential to avoid mistaking them for benign lesions. Moreover, desmoplasia in the gallbladder adenocarcinomas is usually not as prominent as in other parts of the pancreatobiliary tract, and prominent desmoplasia like fibrosis can be induced in inflammation-associated cholecystic injuries.

Differential Diagnosis

Rokitansky–Aschoff Sinus

Rokitansky–Aschoff sinuses have a nonlobular configuration and occasional fibrotic stroma mimicking invasive adenocarcinoma. They are composed of, however, less densely populated large spaces with smooth contours and are connected to the surface epithelium with a perpendicular orientation.

Luschka's Ducts

The reactive periductal glands (Luschka's ducts) are uniform and less dispersed with a lobular configuration. No periglandular desmoplasia is present.

Dysplasia Involving Rokitansky–Aschoff Sinuses and Luschka's Ducts

When dysplasia involves these benign lesions, they are more likely to resemble invasive adenocarcinomas. Useful clues to their benignity include connection of dysplastic glands with the surface, contiguity of the dysplastic area with adjacent normal-looking glands, and identification of bile in the lumen.

Benign Fibroepithelial Polyp and Adenomyomatous Hyperplasia

The former is characterized by lobulated pyloric glands separated by muscle fibers, and the latter represents exaggerated Rokitansky–Aschoff sinuses with hypertrophic smooth muscle fibers.

Intrahepatic Bile Ducts

Key Morphological Features of Well-Differentiated Adenocarcinoma of Intrahepatic Bile Duct

Classical

- Nonlobular arrangement of well-formed glands and tubules
- Prominent desmoplasia around individual glands (Fig. 7.22)

Variants

- Nonlobular arrangement of well-formed glands
- Characteristic replacing or infiltrative pattern (Fig. 7.23)

Discussion

Most (classical) intrahepatic bile duct adenocarcinomas resemble their extrahepatic cousins, and they can be evaluated as such.

Nevertheless, there exist two distinctive variants which can be easily passed off as benign bile ductal lesions. Distinction from the benign mimickers requires recognition of their unique growth patterns. The bile ductular variant is characterized by arborizing small tubule or cord-like structures with slit-like lumens [98–100]. The tumor cells exhibit a marked replacing growth pattern with scattered ghostlike structures (preexisting hepatic lobules) or regenerative nodules with fibrotic portal tracts within the tumor.

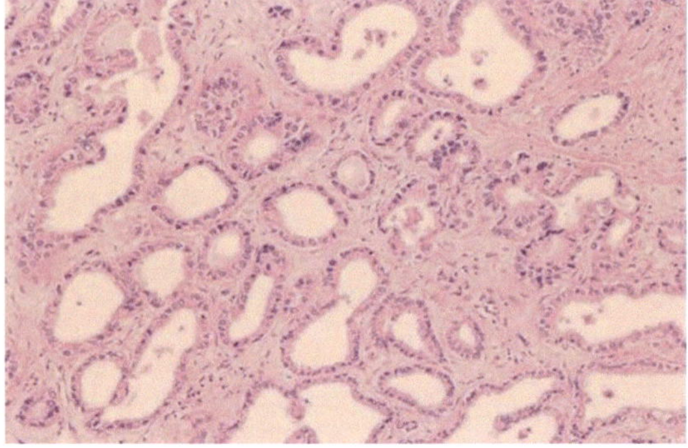

Fig. 7.22 Classic intrahepatic cholangiocarcinoma

The so-called ductal plate malformation type contains characteristic interconnecting benign-looking ductal cells with expanded portal tract mesenchyme [101]. The glandular cells can wrap around the hepatic arterioles in a crescent-like fashion. The telltale sign of malignancy is that it has an infiltrative pattern.

The morphological features of the two variants of intrahepatic bile duct adenocarcinoma indicate that they probably arise from progenitor cells located at the canals of Hering where they are influenced by a hepatogenic environment or they possess intrinsic potency to differentiate somewhat toward hepatocytes. This hepatocytic differentiation can explain their lack of prominent desmoplasia which is the most characteristic feature of classical cholangiocarcinomas.

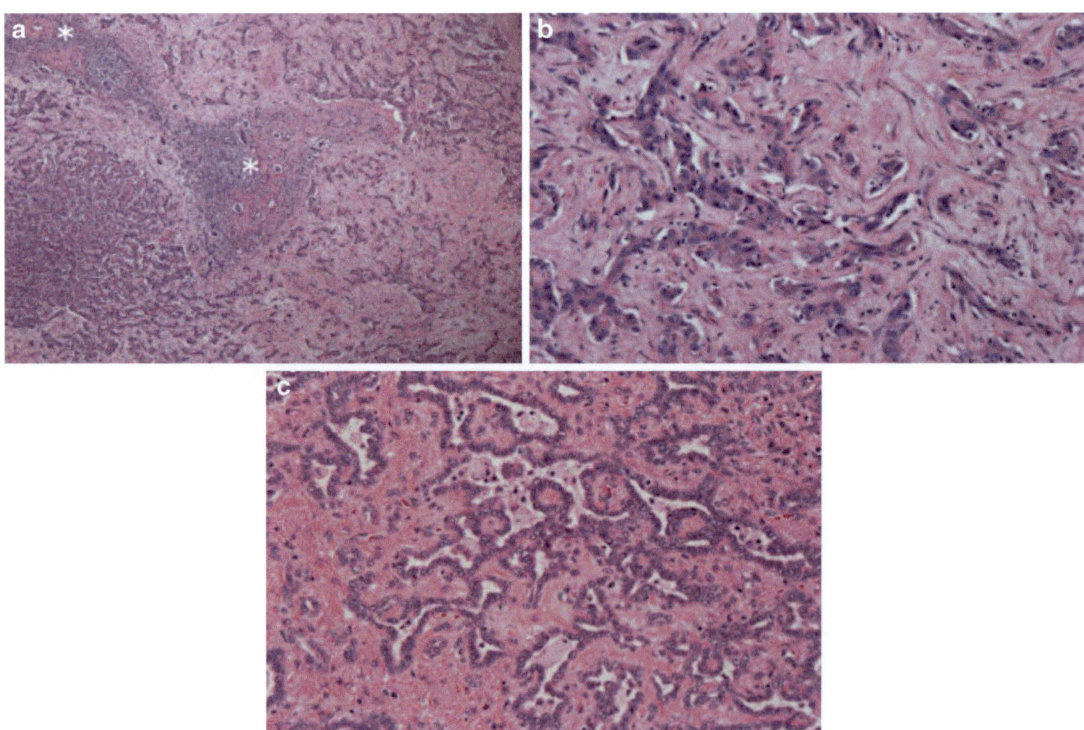

Fig. 7.23 Variants of intrahepatic cholangiocarcinoma. Well-formed tubules replacing parenchyma in a bile ductular variant (**a**, **b**, * portal tract). Ductal plate malformation variant (**c**)

Differential Diagnosis

Bile Duct Hamartoma

Bile duct hamartomas mimic the ductal plate malformation-type cholangiocarcinoma. The key distinguishing features are dilated cysts composed of small cuboidal or even flat cell. Even though the glandular structures are irregular, they lack an infiltrative pattern.

Bile Duct Adenoma

This well-circumscribed lesion contains uniformly sized tubules with intervening fibrous stroma. Residual portal tracts are usually visible in the lesion or at the periphery. In difficult cases, immunostainings for B72.3, Dpc4, and mCEA can help.

Benign Ductular Proliferation

As a sign of the tremendous regenerative capability of the liver, benign ductular proliferation is commonly seen in many hepatic lesions. A common finding in classical hepatocellular carcinomas is the presence of marked bile ductular reaction next to the tumor mass. Appreciation of this finding is critical to avoid mistaking it as the cholangiocarcinomatous component of a combined hepatocellular carcinoma–cholangiocarcinoma [102].

Furthermore, extensive ductular proliferation has been reported in livers which have undergone tumor ablation [102]. Representing a metaplastic reaction, the cirrhotic background is largely preserved (including the native portal tracts). The proliferative/metaplastic glands tend to have a more uniform pattern with no desmoplasia. Atrophy and inflammatory infiltration are common.

Caroli's Disease

This congenital dilatation of large intrahepatic bile ducts is characterized by dilated ducts wrapping around hepatic arteries creating a crescent-like structure. Interconnecting ductular epithelia in an expanded portal mesenchyme is often seen. However, neither infiltrative nor replacing pattern is present.

Appendix

Key Morphological Features of Low-Grade Appendiceal Mucinous Neoplasm (Well-Differentiated Appendiceal Mucinous Adenocarcinoma)

- Circumferential mucosal replacement by mucin-containing cells
- Undulating or flat growth with a broad pushing border (Fig. 7.24)

Discussion

Appendiceal adenocarcinomas are uncommon, and in most cases, they resemble their colonic counterparts in histopathological presentation.

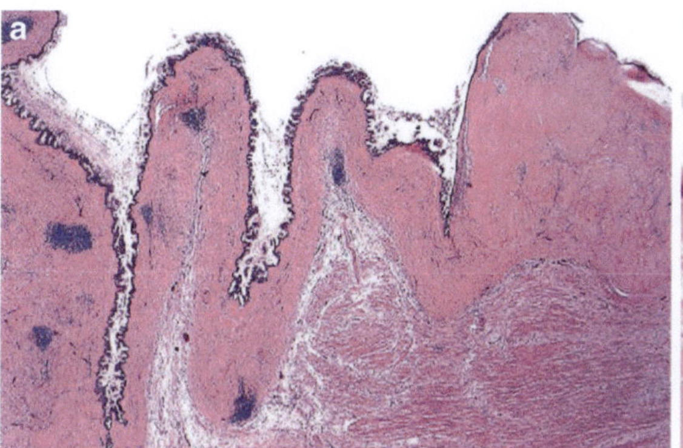

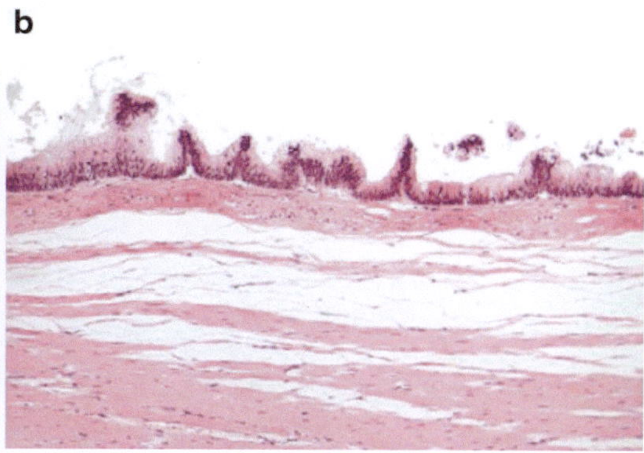

Fig. 7.24 Low-grade appendiceal mucinous neoplasm. Circumferential mucosal replacement by mucin-containing cells. Note undulating (**a**) and flat growth pattern (Surgical Pathology of the GI tract, Liver, Biliary Tract and Pancreas, *Elsevier/Saunders*, 2009 with permission)

Here we discuss a unique entity: low-grade appendiceal mucinous neoplasm (well-differentiated mucinous adenocarcinoma).

Low-grade appendiceal mucinous neoplasms are characterized as a circumferential growth with an undulating or flat surface. The growth enlarges, deforms, or even destroys the appendix [103, 104]. The tumor cells are usually tall, thin with basal nuclei and thin mucin vacuoles. In general, they show a broad pushing border with no overt invasion of the mucosa. However, occasional diverticulum-like protrusions into the deep tissue are present. Denudation of the epithelium is also common. The appendiceal wall is usually fibrotic and lacks lymphoid tissue.

Differential Diagnosis

Simple Mucocele

Simple mucoceles are small cystic spaces lined by atrophic epithelium with associated inflammation. They lack the circumferential involvement pattern.

Adenoma with Mucocele

Adenomas with mucocele formation lack circumferential undulating or flattening of the luminal epithelium characteristic of low-grade appendiceal neoplasms. The cells have typical adenomatous features.

Anus

Key Morphological Features of Well-Differentiated Anal Gland Adenocarcinoma

- Small glands infiltrating the wall
- Lack of a myoepithelial cell layer (Fig. 7.25)

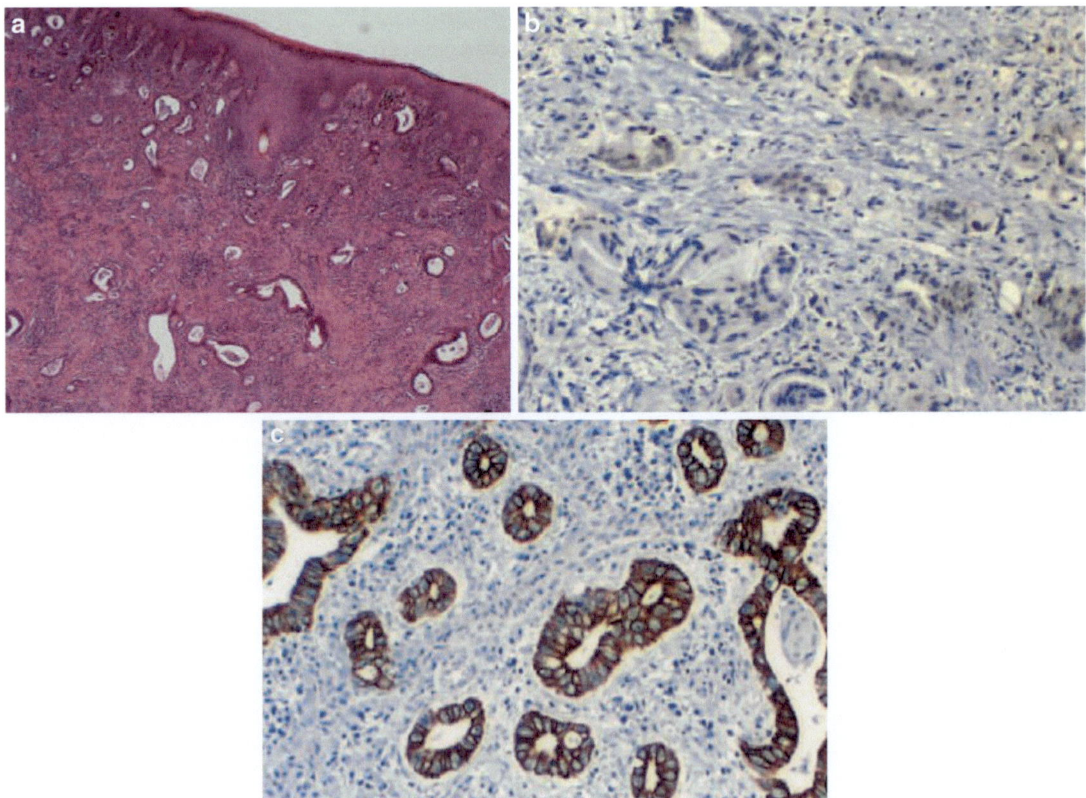

Fig. 7.25 Anal gland carcinoma. There is haphazard infiltration of the wall of the anorectal wall (**a**). Malignant glands lack a layer of myoepithelial cells (**b**) and are reactive with CK7 (**c**) (Archives of Pathology and Laboratory Medicine, *American Society of Clinical Pathology*, 2007 with permission)

Discussion

Most adenocarcinomas of the anal canal are secondary involvement by a primary rectal adenocarcinoma. Primary anal gland adenocarcinomas are characterized by small infiltrative glands without an intraluminal component and surface mucosal dysplasia [105–107]. Instead, the tumors are centered within the anorectal wall. The infiltrative pattern is not to be confused with normal distribution of anal glands in the internal and even external sphincter muscles [108]. In this aspect, immunostaining for p63 might be very useful in making the distinction since malignant glands lack a myoepithelial layer which is present around benign anal glands. Immunostainings for CK7 and CK20 are useful in differentiating them from rectal adenocarcinomas. Primary anal canal adenocarcinomas are positive for CK7 and negative for CK20 [105] (1).

Differential Diagnosis

Tailgut Cyst

Tailgut cysts are well circumscribed, multicystic with the cyst lining cells being mainly stratified squamous epithelium and occasional cuboidal or columnar cells. Disorganized smooth muscle fibers in the cyst wall can be seen.

Anal Duct or Gland Cyst

Anal duct or gland cysts can present in all three anatomical zones of the anus. Characteristically, they form intraepithelial microcysts and contain goblet cell metaplasia. The benign gland might penetrate the internal sphincter muscle or even the external sphincter muscle fibers. Presence of myoepithelial cells distinguishes them from anal gland adenocarcinomas.

Hidradenoma Papilliferum of the Perianal Skin

Hidradenomas papilliferum of the perianal skin is believed to derive from perianal sweat gland and contains well-circumscribed complex papillary structures composed of two layers of epithelial cells. The outer layer cells are myoepithelial in nature.

Squamous Cell Carcinoma with Prominent Mucinous Features (Mucoepidermoid Carcinoma)

Squamous cell carcinomas with prominent mucinous features contain a squamous cell component in addition to mucinous microcysts. It seems that the squamous component is biologically closer to adenocarcinoma than to anal squamous cell carcinomas [109].

Key Morphological Features of Well-Differentiated Anal Squamous Cell Carcinoma

- Dyskeratotic squamous proliferation with infiltrative or pushing border
- Or Complex papillary structure (Fig. 7.26)

Discussion

Squamous cell carcinomas of the anus are etiologically similar to their cervical counterparts. The diagnostic criteria for esophagus apply to both of them (see esophagus section for more discussion). Two locally invasive variants are to be recognized. The giant condyloma acuminatum of Buschke–Lowenstein normally are large (>10 cm in diameter) complex papillary structures with focal invasion identified in only 50 % of reported case series. Verrucous carcinomas have characteristic pushing border front and crater-like keratinization.

Differential Diagnosis

Condyloma

Condylomas are usually less bulky and have shorter papillae and less epithelial atypia than giant condyloma acuminatum. They also lack locally destructive growth pattern of the latter.

Bowenoid Papulosis

Bowenoid papulosis occurs mainly in young adults and is characterized by its circumscription and low-grade epithelial atypia with surface maturation. It lacks complex structures and dermal involvement.

Bowenoid papulosis should not be confused with Bowen's disease which is a variant of squamous cell carcinoma in situ in an older population. The latter shows greater cytological atypia with surface maturation disturbance and occasional involvement of adnexal structures.

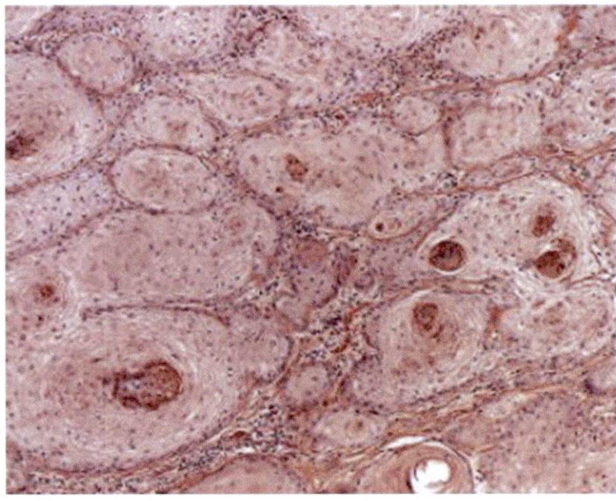

Fig. 7.26 Well-differentiated anal squamous cell carcinoma (Surgical Pathology of the GI tract, Liver, Biliary Tract and Pancreas, Elsevier/Saunders, 2009 with permission)

Squamous Dysplasia Involving Anal Ducts

Squamous dysplasia involving anal ducts manifests a smooth rather than ragged contour. Comparison to adjacent uninvolved ductal structures helps with the appreciation of the smooth outlines of the involved. The nuclear features are the same as those of the dysplastic surface epithelium.

Gastrointestinal Tract Stroma

Key Morphological Features of High-Risk Gastrointestinal Stromal Tumor (GIST)

- Spindle and/or epithelial proliferation in the submucosa
- Mitotic activity > 5/50HPF (Fig. 7.27)

Discussion

The older scheme for separating GISTs into benign and malignant categories has been replaced by a stratification system in which the

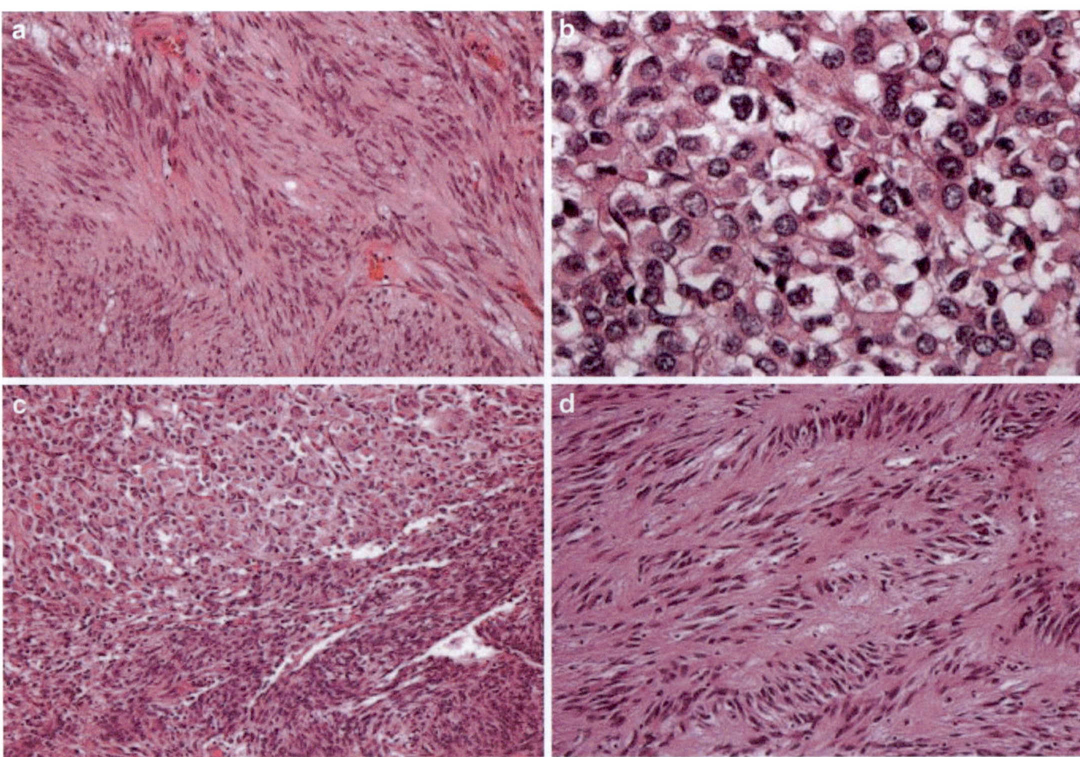

Fig. 7.27 Gastrointestinal stromal tumor. The different histocytological presentations have no prognostic significance

risk of aggressive clinical behavior is predicted based on data from large-scale studies [110, 111]. In the stratification system, hemorrhage, necrosis, and nuclear pleomorphism, tumor size and even infiltrative growth pattern have been excluded. The 2010 AJCC classification uses mitotic rate as the only criterion in separating GISTs into low (grade 1) and high (grade 2) categories. In acknowledgment of the effect of anatomical location on tumor behavior, it recommends different staging criteria for gastric and small intestinal GISTS. The staging criteria for the former also apply to omental GISTs and those for the latter to esophageal, colorectal, mesenteric, and peritoneal GISTs.

Morphologically, most GISTS have a spindle cell pattern with epithelioid, mixed cell patterns accounting for the rest [112, 113]. Typically, the spindle cells are in short fascicles or whorls and contain eosinophilic fibrillary cytoplasm and indistinct cell borders. Epithelioid cells in GISTs are characterized by round cells with eosinophilic to clear cytoplasm arranged in nests or sheets. Cytological atypia is more frequently present than in spindle cells. Counterintuitively, scattered bizarre epithelioid cells are more commonly seen in low-grade gastric GISTs than in high-grade ones. As there are many other entities with spindle and epithelioid morphology in the gastrointestinal tract, the importance of microscopic examination of GISTs lies mainly in differentiating them from other spindle and epithelioid tumors and choosing appropriate fields for mitotic counting [112, 113].

As the database on GISTS expands, future studies might bring into the picture additional stratifying criteria, such as tumor rupture and status of surgical margins. Furthermore, high-grade small bowel GISTs are composed of long fascicles of spindles cells and contain less stromal skeinoid fibers than their benign counterparts. A tightly packed epithelioid appearance has been associated with an adverse clinical outcome in gastric GISTS. The current recommendation is that the presence of such morphological features should prompt at least a more meticulous evaluation of mitotic activity [110].

Differential Diagnosis For Spindle Cell GISTs

Reactive Nodular Fibrous Pseudotumor and Pseudosarcomatous Proliferation

Reactive nodular fibrous pseudotumors occur mainly in the outer layer of the gut in patients with a previous history of abdominal surgery or trauma. Transmural extension, however, is possible. The hypocellular bland spindle and stellar cells are arranged haphazardly or in short fascicles.

Pseudosarcomatous proliferation contains granulation tissue with associated ulceration or polyps. The stromal cells, endothelial cells, and adjacent epithelial cells usually show marked cytological atypia. Overall low cellularity and a prominent inflammatory infiltrate are noticeable.

Leiomyoma

Leiomyomas have characteristic intersecting fascicles composed of cells with abundant eosinophilic cytoplasm, blunt end nuclei, and distinctive cell borders. Relative to GISTs, they have less cellularity. The tumor cells are diffusely negative for CD117 and CD34.

Schwannoma

Gastrointestinal schwannomas occur most frequently in the stomach, and they typically lack or contain inconspicuous trademark components of the tumor: Verocay bodies, nuclear palisading, xanthoma cell, and hyalinized vessels. Instead, they acquire an important feature: presence of a rim of lymphoid tissue with follicular center formation. The spindle cells have elongated, tapering, and often buckled nuclei and are arranged in trabeculae or even sheets. To further confound the matter, gastric and anorectal GISTs are commonly associated with fascicles of spindle cells with prominent nuclear palisading.

Thus accurate distinction between the two entities depends heavily on immunostainings. The tumor cells of the former stain are strongly positive for S100 (both nuclei and cytoplasm) and negative for CD117 and CD34.

Inflammatory Myofibroblastic Tumor

Inflammatory myofibroblastic tumors occur predominantly in the mesentery and omentum of children and young adults. The compact spindle cell variant resembles GISTs. However, the tumors contain a prominent component of inflammatory cells with significant numbers of plasma cells. Tumor cells are positive for ALK-1 and negative for CD117.

Inflammatory Fibroid Polyp

Inflammatory fibroid polyps contain loosely collagenous- or granulation-type stroma, with CD34+fibroblasts distributed in a patternless pattern. Characteristic onion-skin cuffs of perivascular spindle cells and inflammatory infiltration (eosinophils as the prominent component) set them apart from GISTs. The tumor cells are positive for PDGFR and negative for CD117.

Desmoid Fibromatosis

Desmoid fibromatosis is a predominantly mesenteric tumor with possible infiltration of the gut wall. It is characterized by long sweeping fascicles of spindle cells and collagenous matrix (sometimes keloid-like collagen fibers). It lacks high cellularity, nuclear palisading, skeinoid fibers, and epithelioid cell components. Other characteristic features of the tumor include small muscular arteries and thin-walled and often ectatic veins with scant perivascular lymphocytes and scattered mast cells. The tumor cells commonly express beta-catenin and infrequently CD117.

Solitary Fibrous Tumor

Solitary fibrous tumors are located mainly in the peritoneum and retroperitoneum with possible serosal involvement. Characteristic features include a patternless pattern of the spindle cells, alternating hypercellularity and hypocellularity, ropy keloid collagen fibers, and hemangiopericytoma-like vasculature. The tumor cells are CD34 positive and CD117 negative.

Spindle Tumors with Malignant Cytology

The differential diagnosis of spindle GISTs includes melanoma, sarcomatoid carcinoma, leiomyosarcoma, malignant peripheral nerve sheath tumor, clear cell sarcoma, and other rare entities. A detailed discussion of them is out of the scope of this book. Several excellent review papers are available for reference.

For Epithelioid GISTs

Neuroendocrine Tumor

Low-grade neuroendocrine tumors might exhibit both spindle and epithelioid cell patterns. Their characteristic chromatin and growth patterns usually point to the right diagnosis.

PEComa and Glomus Tumor

PEComas are characterized by a perivascular epithelioid cell proliferation which forms sheets or nests. Occasional CD117-positive cases have been reported. Therefore, in difficult cases myomelanocytic markers (HMB-45 or Melan A) should be included.

Glomus tumor cells have a uniform round shape distinctive cell borders and are closely associated with ectatic vessels. They are positive for SMA and negative for CD117.

Paraganglioma

Paragangliomas predominantly involve the duodenum and consist of three types of cells: spindle, epithelioid, and ganglion-like cells. The first two form the so-called Zellballen structure. Interestingly, the spindle cells are S100 positive and the ganglion-like cells stain for synaptophysin. All three of them are positive for NSE.

Epithelioid Tumors with Malignant Cytology

The differential diagnosis of epithelioid GISTs includes melanoma, poorly differentiated carcinoma and neuroendocrine tumors, epithelioid leiomyosarcoma, and other rare entities. A detailed discussion of them is out of the scope of this book. Several excellent review papers are available for reference.

Caution: Variable expression of CD117 has been reported in melanoma, angiosarcomas, and PEComas.

The Gastrointestinal Neuroendocrine Tissue

Key Features of Well-Differentiated Gastrointestinal Neuroendocrine Carcinoma (Net GII)

- Ki67 index of 3 to 20 % or mitotic counter 2 to 20/10 HPF (Fig. 7.28)

Discussion

The 2010 WHO classification replaces the term well-differentiated neuroendocrine carcinoma with neuroendocrine tumor grade 2 (NET GII) [86]. It uses mitotic count as the sole index in the three-tier tumor grading system for the gastrointestinal tract. This is in contrast to the four-tier system for the pulmonary system in which tumor grading is based on both mitotic count and necrosis. Importantly, cytological atypia is left out in both systems. Analogous to pulmonary neuroendocrine tumors, the gastrointestinal neuroendocrine tumors are a heterogeneous population of tumors which most likely can also be divided into two molecular and biological distinct categories with carcinoid (NET G1) and atypical carcinoid (NET G2) tumors manifesting similar genetic changes [114–116]. The two categories have remarkable differences in histopathologic and cytological features which allow their easy separation.

Information on tumor size, location, depth of tissue involvement, and even nodal metastasis has been incorporated into the staging scheme. In acknowledgement of their functional diversity and nonrandom distribution of the various cell types in the gastrointestinal system, a slightly different staging system has been adopted for the foregut, midgut, and hindgut, respectively [117].

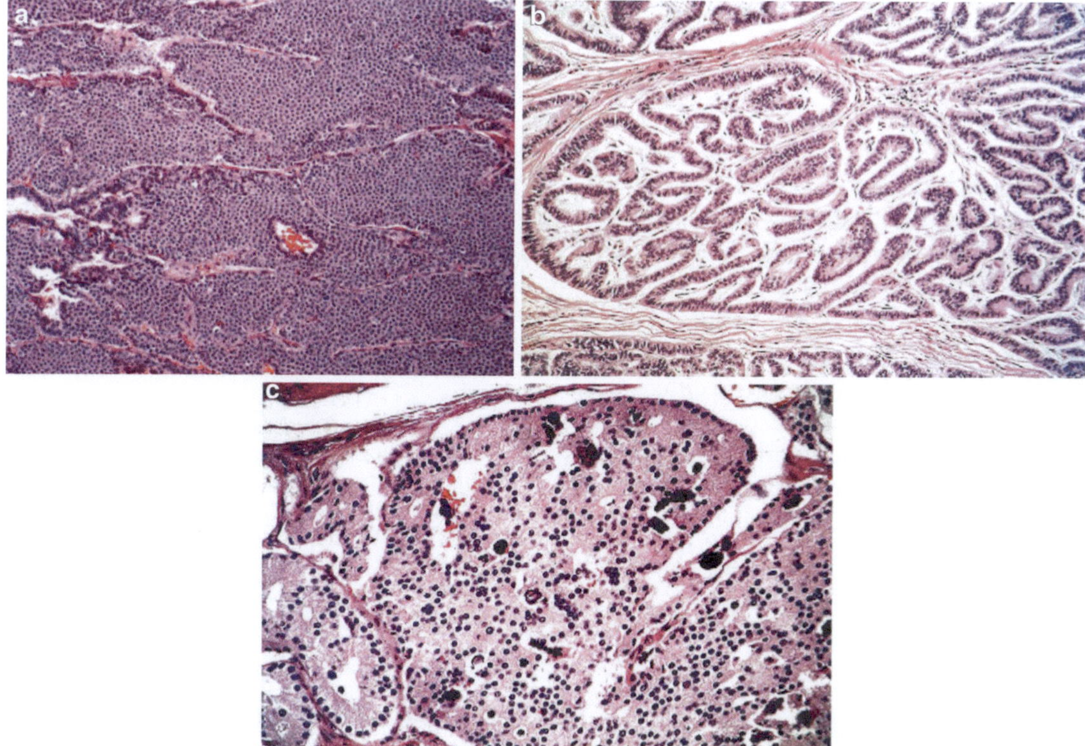

Fig. 7.28 Gastrointestinal neuroendocrine tumor. As for gastrointestinal stromal tumor, the different histological manifestations of the tumor carry no clinical significance. Mitotic index is the sole index in the grading (Surgical Pathology of the GI tract, Liver, Biliary Tract and Pancreas, *Elsevier/Saunders*, 2009 with permission)

Differential Diagnosis

Adenocarcinoma

NET G1 and G2 tumors have their characteristic trabecular, nest-like, or glandular patterns composed of bland-looking cells with uniform central nuclei with salt and pepper chromatin pattern. Therefore, a diagnosis is usually straightforward for typical cases.

Duodenal NET G1 and G2 tumors can have a prominent tumor acinar or glandular pattern with frequent intraluminal psammoma bodies [116]. Cursory low power examination can lead to an erroneous diagnosis of well-differentiated adenocarcinoma.

Appendiceal duodenal NET G1 and G2 tumors can show goblet cell and Paneth cell differentiation and focal glandular formation. The so-called tubular type simulates invasive adenocarcinoma even more in that it presents as teardrop-like tubules in a loosely fibrotic stroma [116]. The tumor cells are negative for chromogranin A (rectal neuroendocrine tumors are negative for chromogranin A).

Glomus Tumor

Glomus tumors are composed of uniform small round cells with lumpy chromatin pattern, and their close association with ectatic vessels is evident. The tumor cells are positive for SMA and negative for chromogranin and synaptophysin.

Lymphoma, Melanoma, and Poorly Differentiated Tumors

Lymphomas, melanomas, or poorly differentiated tumors can present in a nest pattern. However, attention to their cytological and other histological features avoids an erroneous diagnosis. In difficult cases, immunostainings are required.

References

1. Zayour M, Lazova R. Pseudoepitheliomatous hyperplasia: a review. Am J Dermatopathol. 2011;33(2): 112–22. Quiz 123–6.
2. El-Khoury J, Kibbi AG, Abbas O. Mucocutaneous pseudoepitheliomatous hyperplasia: a review. Am J Dermatopathol. 2012;34(2):165–75.
3. Clickman JN, Odze RD. Chapter 20. Epithelilal neoplasms of the esophagus. In: Odze RD, Goldblum JR, editors. Surgical pathology of the GI tract, liver, biliary tract, and pancreas: an expert consult title. Philadelphia: Saunders/Elsevier; 2009. p. 535–62.
4. Ochicha O, Pringle JH, Mohammed AZ. Immunohistochemical study of epithelialmyofibrblast interaction in Barrett metaplasia. Indian J Pathol Microbiol. 2010;53(2):262–6.
5. Li A et al. Immunohistochemical analysis of pericryptal fibroblast sheath and proliferating epithelial cells in human colorectal adenomas and carcinomas with adenoma components. Pathol Int. 1999;49(5):426–34.
6. Yao T, Tsuneyoshi M. Significance of pericryptal fibroblasts in colorectal epithelial tumors: a special reference to the histologic features and growth patterns. Hum Pathol. 1993;24(5):525–33.
7. Faragalla HF et al. Immunohistochemical staining for smoothelin in the duplicated versus the true muscularis mucosae of Barrett esophagus. Am J Surg Pathol. 2011;35(1):55–9.
8. Rubio CA, Riddell R. Musculo-fibrous anomaly in Barrett's mucosa with dysplasia. Am J Surg Pathol. 1988;12(11):885–9.
9. Lewis JT, Wang KK, Abraham SC. Muscularis mucosae duplication and the musculo-fibrous anomaly in endoscopic mucosal resections for Barrett esophagus: implications for staging of adenocarcinoma. Am J Surg Pathol. 2008;32(4):566–71.
10. Harada O et al. Esophageal gland duct adenoma: immunohistochemical comparison with the normal esophageal gland and ultrastractural analysis. Am J Surg Pathol. 2007;31(3):469–75.
11. Brown IS, Whiteman DC, Lauwers GY. Foveolar type dysplasia in Barrett esophagus. Mod Pathol. 2010;23(6):834–43.
12. Mahajan D et al. Grading of gastric foveolar-type dysplasia in Barrett's esophagus. Mod Pathol. 2010;23(1):1–11.
13. Mutoh H et al. Pericryptal fibroblast sheath in intestinal metaplasia and gastric carcinoma. Gut. 2005;54(1):33–9.
14. Tuner JR, Odze RD. Chapter 17. Polyps of the stomach. In: Odze RD, Goldblum JR, editors. Surgical pathology of the GI tract, liver, biliary tract, and pancreas: an expert consult title. Philadelphia: Saunders/ Elsevier; 2009. p. 415–46.
15. Kushima R et al. Gastric-type well-differentiated adenocarcinoma and pyloric gland adenoma of the stomach. Gastric Cancer. 2006;9(3):177–84.
16. Yao T et al. Extremely well-differentiated adenocarcinoma of the stomach: clinicopathological and immunohistochemical features. World J Gastroenterol. 2006;12(16):2510–6.
17. Lee WA. Gastric extremely well differentiated adenocarcinoma of gastric phenotype: as a gastric counterpart of adenoma malignum of the uterine cervix. World J Surg Oncol. 2005;3:28.

18. Yamamoto J et al. Extremely well differentiated adenocarcinoma of the stomach diagnosed preoperatively as esophageal achalasia: report of a case. Surg Today. 2005;35(6):488–92.
19. Singhi AD, Lazenby AJ, Montgomery EA. Gastric adenocarcinoma with chief cell differentiation: a proposal for reclassification as oxyntic gland polyp/adenoma. Am J Surg Pathol. 2012;36(7):1030–5.
20. Park do Y et al. Adenomatous and foveolar gastric dysplasia: distinct patterns of mucin expression and background intestinal metaplasia. Am J Surg Pathol. 2008;32(4):524–33.
21. Lauwers GY, Riddell RH. Gastric epithelial dysplasia. Gut. 1999;45(5):784–90.
22. Odze RD et al. Gastritis cystica profunda versus invasive adenocarcinoma. Am J Surg Pathol. 2012;36(2):316.
23. Chen ZM et al. Pyloric gland adenoma: an entity distinct from gastric foveolar type adenoma. Am J Surg Pathol. 2009;33(2):186–93.
24. Makinen MJ. Colorectal serrated adenocarcinoma. Histopathology. 2007;50(1):131–50.
25. Parfitt JR, Driman DK. Survivin and hedgehog protein expression in serrated colorectal polyps: an immunohistochemical study. Hum Pathol. 2007; 38(5):710–7.
26. Horkko TT, Makinen MJ. Colorectal proliferation and apoptosis in serrated versus conventional adenoma-carcinoma pathway: growth, progression and survival. Scand J Gastroenterol. 2003;38(12): 1241–8.
27. Cunningham KS, Riddell RH. Serrated mucosal lesions of the colorectum. Curr Opin Gastroenterol. 2006;22(1):48–53.
28. Adegboyega PA et al. Immunohistochemical study of myofibroblasts in normal colonic mucosa, hyperplastic polyps, and adenomatous colorectal polyps. Arch Pathol Lab Med. 2002;126(7):829–36.
29. Yeung TM et al. Regulation of self-renewal and differentiation by the intestinal stem cell niche. Cell Mol Life Sci. 2011;68(15):2513–23.
30. Shaker A, Rubin DC. Intestinal stem cells and epithelial-mesenchymal interactions in the crypt and stem cell niche. Transl Res. 2010;156(3):180–7.
31. Sappino AP et al. Colonic pericryptal fibroblasts. Differentiation pattern in embryogenesis and phenotypic modulation in epithelial proliferative lesions Virchows. Arch A Pathol Anat Histopathol. 1989;415(6):551–7.
32. Kaye GI, Lane N, Pascal RR. Colonic pericryptal fibroblast sheath: replication, migration, and cytodifferentiation of a mesenchymal cell system in adult tissue. II. Fine structural aspects of normal rabbit and human colon. Gastroenterology. 1968;54(5):852–65.
33. Pai RK et al. Histologic and molecular analyses of colonic perineurial-like proliferations in serrated polyps: perineurial-like stromal proliferations are seen in sessile serrated adenomas. Am J Surg Pathol. 2011;35(9):1373–80.
34. Adegboyega PA et al. Subepithelial myofibroblasts express cyclooxygenase-2 in colorectal tubular adenomas. Clin Cancer Res. 2004;10(17):5870–9.
35. Okayasu I et al. Mucosal remodeling in long-standing ulcerative colitis with colorectal neoplasia: significant alterations of NCAM+or alpha-SMA+subepithelial myofibroblasts and interstitial cells. Pathol Int. 2009;59(10):701–11.
36. Radovic S et al. Demonstration of perycriptal fibroblasts in inflammatory-regenerative and dysplastic epithelial lesions of the flat colonic mucosa. Adv Clin Path. 2001;5(4):139–45.
37. Higaki S et al. Immunohistological study to determine the presence of pericryptal myofibroblasts and basement membrane in colorectal epithelial tumors. J Gastroenterol. 1999;34(2):215–20.
38. Fu X et al. Retained cell-cell adhesion in serrated neoplastic pathway as opposed to conventional colorectal adenomas. J Histochem Cytochem. 2010;59(2):158–66.
39. Noffsinger AE. Serrated polyps and colorectal cancer: new pathway to malignancy. Annu Rev Pathol. 2009;4:343–64.
40. Okayasu I. Development of ulcerative colitis and its associated colorectal neoplasia as a model of the organ-specific chronic inflammation-carcinoma sequence. Pathol Int. 2012;62(6):368–80.
41. Redston M. Chapter 23. Epithelial neoplasms of the large intestine polyps. In: Odze RD, Goldblum JR, editors. Surgical pathology of the GI tract, liver, biliary tract, and pancreas: an expert consult title. Philadelphia: Saunders/Elsevier; 2009. p. 481–534.
42. Kanel GC, Korula J. Atlas of liver pathology. 3rd ed. Philadelphia: Elsevier/Saunders; 2011.
43. Burt AD, Portmann BC, Ferrell LD. MacSween's pathology of the liver. 5th ed. Philadelphia: Churchill Livingstone/Elsevier; 2007.
44. Hong H, Patonay B, Finley J. Unusual reticulin staining pattern in well-differentiated hepatocellular carcinoma. Diagn Pathol. 2011;6:15.
45. Ward SC, Waxman S. Fibrolamellar carcinoma: a review with focus on genetics and comparison to other malignant primary liver tumors. Semin Liver Dis. 2011;31(1):61–70.
46. Krings G et al. Immunohistochemical pitfalls and the importance of glypican 3 and arginase in the diagnosis of scirrhous hepatocellular carcinoma. Mod Pathol. 2013;26(6):782–91.
47. Okamura N et al. Cellular and stromal characteristics in the scirrhous hepatocellular carcinoma: comparison with hepatocellular carcinomas and intrahepatic cholangiocarcinomas. Pathol Int. 2005;55(11):724–31.
48. Seok JY et al. A fibrous stromal component in hepatocellular carcinoma reveals a cholangiocarcinoma-like gene expression trait and epithelial-mesenchymal transition. Hepatology. 2012;55(6):1776–86.
49. Ward SC et al. Fibrolamellar carcinoma of the liver exhibits immunohistochemical evidence of both hepatocyte and bile duct differentiation. Mod Pathol. 2010;23(9):1180–90.

50. Singhi AD et al. Reticulin loss in benign fatty liver: an important diagnostic pitfall when considering a diagnosis of hepatocellular carcinoma. Am J Surg Pathol. 2012;36(5):710–5.
51. Zhu AX et al. HCC and angiogenesis: possible targets and future directions. Nat Rev Clin Oncol. 2011;8(5):292–301.
52. Matsumoto K et al. Liver organogenesis promoted by endothelial cells prior to vascular function. Science. 2001;294(5542):559–63.
53. Yang ZF, Poon RT. Vascular changes in hepatocellular carcinoma. Anat Rec (Hoboken). 2008;291(6): 721–34.
54. Goodman ZD, Terraciano L. In: Burt AD, Portmann BC, Ferrell LD, editors. MacSween's pathology of the liver. Philadelphia: Churchill Livingstone/ Elsevier; 2007. p. 761–814. Chapter 15: Tumors and tumor-like lesions of the liver.
55. Kanel GC, Korula J. Chapter 10. Neoplasms and related lesions. In: Atlas of liver pathology. Philadelphia: Saunders/Elsevier; 2010. p. 249–320.
56. Jin SY, Choi IH. Early hepatocellular carcinoma. Korean J Hepatol. 2011;17(3):238–41.
57. Kondo F. Histological features of early hepatocellular carcinomas and their developmental process: for daily practical clinical application: hepatocellular carcinoma. Hepatol Int. 2009;3(1):283–93.
58. Park YN. Update on precursor and early lesions of hepatocellular carcinomas. Arch Pathol Lab Med. 2011;135(6):704–15.
59. Ibukuro K. Vascular anatomy of the pancreas and clinical applications. Int J Gastrointest Cancer. 2001;30(1–2):87–104.
60. Okahara M et al. Arterial supply to the pancreas; variations and cross-sectional anatomy. Abdom Imaging. 2010;35(2):134–42.
61. Hruban RH, Bishop PM, Klimstra DS. In: Silverberg SG, editor. Tumors of the pancreas, AFIP atlas of tumor pathology series 4. Washington, DC: ARP, AFIP; 2007.
62. Hruban RH, Pitman MB, Klimstra DS. Chapter 1. The normal pancreas. In: Tumors of the pancreas. Washington, DC: ARP press; 2007. p. 1–26.
63. Villasenor A, Cleaver O. Crosstalk between the developing pancreas and its blood vessels: an evolving dialog. Semin Cell Dev Biol. 2012;23(6):685–92.
64. Magenheim J et al. Blood vessels restrain pancreas branching, differentiation and growth. Development. 2011;138(21):4743–52.
65. Cleaver O, Dor Y. Vascular instruction of pancreas development. Development. 2012;139(16):2833–43.
66. Pierreux CE et al. Epithelial: endothelial cross-talk regulates exocrine differentiation in developing pancreas. Dev Biol. 2010;347(1):216–27.
67. O'Morchoe CC. Lymphatic system of the pancreas. Microsc Res Tech. 1997;37(5–6):456–77.
68. Sah RP, Garg P, Saluja AK. Pathogenic mechanisms of acute pancreatitis. Curr Opin Gastroenterol. 2012;28(5):507–15.
69. Sah RP, Saluja A. Molecular mechanisms of pancreatic injury. Curr Opin Gastroenterol. 2011;27(5):444–51.
70. Chen JM, Ferec C. Genetics and pathogenesis of chronic pancreatitis: the 2012 update. Clin Res Hepatol Gastroenterol. 2012;36(4):334–40.
71. Luo G et al. Stroma and pancreatic ductal adenocarcinoma: an interaction loop. Biochim Biophys Acta. 2012;1826(1):170–8.
72. Pandol S et al. Desmoplasia of pancreatic ductal adenocarcinoma. Clin Gastroenterol Hepatol. 2009;7(11 Suppl):S44–7.
73. Omary MB et al. The pancreatic stellate cell: a star on the rise in pancreatic diseases. J Clin Invest. 2007;117(1):50–9.
74. Apte MV, Pirola RC, Wilson JS. Pancreatic stellate cells: a starring role in normal and diseased pancreas. Front Physiol. 2012;3:344.
75. Olive KP et al. Inhibition of Hedgehog signaling enhances delivery of chemotherapy in a mouse model of pancreatic cancer. Science. 2009;324(5933): 1457–61.
76. Olson P et al. Imaging guided trials of the angiogenesis inhibitor sunitinib in mouse models predict efficacy in pancreatic neuroendocrine but not ductal carcinoma. Proc Natl Acad Sci U S A. 2011;108(49):E1275–84.
77. Le A et al. Conceptual framework for cutting the pancreatic cancer fuel supply. Clin Cancer Res. 2012;18(16):4285–90.
78. Kang R, Tang D. Autophagy in pancreatic cancer pathogenesis and treatment. Am J Cancer Res. 2012;2(4):383–96.
79. Feig C et al. The pancreas cancer microenvironment. Clin Cancer Res. 2012;18(16):4266–76.
80. Hruban RH, Pitman MB, Klimstra DS. Chapter 7. Ductal adenocarcinoma. In: Tumors of the pancreas. Washington, DC: ARP press; 2007. p. 111–218.
81. Wenig BM, Heffers CS. Chapter 34. Inflammtory, infectious and other non-neoplastic disorders of the pancreas. In: Odze RD, Goldblum JR, editors. Surgical pathology of the GI tract, liver, biliary tract, and pancreas: an expert consult title. Philadelphia: Saunders/Elsevier; 2009.
82. Lowery MA et al. Acinar cell carcinoma of the pancreas: new genetic and treatment insights into a rare malignancy. Oncologist. 2011;16(12):1714–20.
83. Stelow EB et al. Pancreatic acinar cell carcinomas with prominent ductal differentiation: mixed acinar ductal carcinoma and mixed acinar endocrine ductal carcinoma. Am J Surg Pathol. 2010;34(4):510–8.
84. El-Bahrawy MA et al. E-cadherin/catenin complex status in solid pseudopapillary tumor of the pancreas. Am J Surg Pathol. 2008;32(1):1–7.
85. Serra S, Chetty R. Revision 2: an immunohistochemical approach and evaluation of solid pseudopapillary tumour of the pancreas. J Clin Pathol. 2008;61(11):1153–9.
86. Kloppel G. Classification and pathology of gastroenteropancreatic neuroendocrine neoplasms. Endocr Relat Cancer. 2011;18 Suppl 1:S1–16.

87. Asa SL. Pancreatic endocrine tumors. Mod Pathol. 2011;24 Suppl 2:S66–77.
88. Hruban RH, Pitman MB, Klimstra DS. Chapter 12. Endocrine neoplasms. In: Tumors of the pancreas. Washington, DC: ARP press; 2007. p. 251–304.
89. Ando H. Embryology of the biliary tract. Dig Surg. 2010;27(2):87–9.
90. Strazzabosco M, Fabris L. Development of the bile ducts: essentials for the clinical hepatologist. J Hepatol. 2012;56(5):1159–70.
91. Dai J et al. Impact of bile acids on the growth of human cholangiocarcinoma via FXR. J Hematol Oncol. 2011;4:41.
92. Xia X et al. Bile acid interactions with cholangiocytes. World J Gastroenterol. 2006;12(22): 3553–63.
93. Perez MJ, Briz O. Bile-acid-induced cell injury and protection. World J Gastroenterol. 2009;15(14): 1677–89.
94. Bernstein H et al. Bile acids as endogenous etiologic agents in gastrointestinal cancer. World J Gastroenterol. 2009;15(27):3329–40.
95. Sirica AE, Campbell DJ, Dumur CI. Cancer-associated fibroblasts in intrahepatic cholangiocarcinoma. Curr Opin Gastroenterol. 2011;27(3): 276–84.
96. Leyva-Illades D et al. Cholangiocarcinoma pathogenesis: role of the tumor microenvironment. Transl Gastrointest Cancer. 2012;1(1):71–80.
97. Adsay VN, Klimstra DS. Benign and malignant tumors of the gallbladder and extrahepatic biliary tract. In: Odze RD, Goldblum JR, editors. Surgical pathology of the GI tract, liver, biliary tract, and pancreas: an expert consult title. Philadelphia: Saunders/ Elsevier; 2009. p. 845–76.
98. Nakanuma Y et al. Pathological spectrum of intrahepatic cholangiocarcinoma arising in non-biliary chronic advanced liver diseases. Pathol Int. 2011; 61(5):298–305.
99. Nakanuma Y et al. Pathological classification of intrahepatic cholangiocarcinoma based on a new concept. World J Hepatol. 2010;2(12):419–27.
100. Sempoux C et al. Intrahepatic cholangiocarcinoma: new insights in pathology. Semin Liver Dis. 2011;31(1):49–60.
101. Nakanuma Y et al. Intrahepatic cholangiocarcinoma with predominant “ductal plate malformation” pattern: a new subtype. Am J Surg Pathol. 2012;36(11): 1629–35.
102. Yeh MM. Pathology of combined hepatocellular-cholangiocarcinoma. J Gastroenterol Hepatol. 2010;25(9):1485–92.
103. Panarelli NC, Yantiss RK. Mucinous neoplasms of the appendix and peritoneum. Arch Pathol Lab Med. 2011;135(10):1261–8.
104. Carr NJ, Emory TS, Sobin LH. Chaper 24. Epithelial neoplasm of the appendix. In: Odze RD, Goldblum JR, editors. Surgical pathology of the GI tract, liver, biliary tract, and pancreas: an expert consult title. Philadelphia: Saunders/Elsevier; 2009. p. 639–52.
105. Lisovsky M et al. Immunophenotypic characterization of anal gland carcinoma: loss of p63 and cytokeratin 5/6. Arch Pathol Lab Med. 2007;131(8):1304–11.
106. Longacre TA, Kong CS, Welton ML. Diagnostic problems in anal pathology. Adv Anat Pathol. 2008;15(5):263–78.
107. Shia J. An update on tumors of the anal canal. Arch Pathol Lab Med. 2009;134(11):1601–11.
108. Tanaka E et al. Morphology of the epithelium of the lower rectum and the anal canal in the adult human. Med Mol Morphol. 2012;45(2):72–9.
109. Kondo R et al. Mucoepidermoid carcinoma of the anal canal: an immunohistochemical study. J Gastroenterol. 2001;36(7):508–14.
110. Zhao X, Yue C. Gastrointestinal stromal tumor. J Gastrointest Oncol. 2012;3(3):189–208.
111. Chapter 16. Gastrointestinal stromal tumor. In: Edge SB, et al, editors. AJCC cancer staging handbook. 7th ed. Chicago: Springer; 2010. p. 219–226.
112. Abraham SC. Distinguishing gastrointestinal stromal tumors from their mimics: an update. Adv Anat Pathol. 2007;14(3):178–88.
113. Kirsch R, Gao ZH, Riddell R. Gastrointestinal stromal tumors: diagnostic challenges and practical approach to differential diagnosis. Adv Anat Pathol. 2007;14(4):261–85.
114. Swarts DR, Ramaekers FC, Speel EJ. Molecular and cellular biology of neuroendocrine lung tumors: evidence for separate biological entities. Biochim Biophys Acta. 2012;1826(2):255–71.
115. Rekhtman N. Neuroendocrine tumors of the lung: an update. Arch Pathol Lab Med. 2010;134(11): 1628–38.
116. Graeme-Cook F. Chapter 25. Neuroendocrine tumors of the GI tract and appendix. In: Odze RD, Goldblum JR, editors. Surgical pathology of the GI tract, liver, biliary tract, and pancreas: an expert consult title. Philadelphia: Saunders/Elsevier; 2009. p. 653–93.
117. American Joint Committee on Cancer. Chapter 17. Neuroendocrine tumors. In: Edge SB, editor. AJCC cancer staging handbook. 7th ed. Chicago: Springer; 2010. p. 227–36.

8 Lung and Pleura

Lung

Key Morphological Features of Well-Differentiated Adenocarcinoma

- Ragged glandular/papillary structures
- Expansive growth pattern (Figs. 8.1 and 8.2)

Discussion

Most pulmonary adenocarcinomas present with a mixed histological and cytological picture. Traditionally, they have been graded depending on the degree of gland or papilla formation. In 2011, the International Association for the Study of Lung Cancer/American Thoracic Society/European Respiratory Society recommends that pulmonary adenocarcinomas should be graded based on the predominant growth pattern rather than the least differentiated components as for most other carcinomas [1]. The glandular structures of well-differentiated pulmonary adenocarcinomas resemble more clefts or slits than genuine glands. Reflecting the tremendous plasticity of pulmonary stem cells which eventually give rise to more than 40 different cell types in adult lungs, adenocarcinomatous cells can assume many different cellular shapes which might be present in a single tumor [2, 3]. The vast majority of well-differentiated pulmonary adenocarcinomas show features indicating Clara cell or type II pneumocyte differentiation. The tumor cells are bland with ample cytoplasm except for prominent nucleoli. Characteristically, they have protruding and frizzy luminal surface (papillary) borders [3–5]. Consistent with their Clara cell differentiation, this cellular characteristic of adenocarcinomas contributes to the cleft/slit appearance of malignant glands.

Rather than having an infiltrative growth pattern, pulmonary adenocarcinomas are well circumscribed with an overall irregularly lobular appearance [6]. Presumably, the circumscription and cleft-like morphology result from a unique epithelial–mesenchymal interaction evidenced in the lung organogenesis in which the fetal respiratory epithelium seems to adapt and fill available spaces created in the mesenchyme [7–9]. Thus, tumor growth and invasion are dependent on the myofibroblasts at the invasive fronts. The fibrous front at the periphery of the adenocarcinomas might be the driving force in tumor invasion instead of being a restraining force for tumor growth as the traditional dogma stipulates. Supporting evidence is emerging that the activated pulmonary myofibroblasts play an important role in cancer invasive nests in that they lead and cheer the epithelial cells on in the process of invasion [8] (Fig. 8.3).

Thus, in the lungs, primary malignant tumor invasion is not manifested as an infiltrative process. Instead, it is defined as an expansive, destructive growth pattern in which the normal, highly differentiated alveolar structures are replaced by tumor structures. Except for rare cases of colloid adenocarcinoma which are characterized by mucin pools distending alveolar

X. Sun, *Well-Differentiated Malignancies: New Perspectives*, Current Clinical Pathology,
DOI 10.1007/978-1-4939-1692-4_8, © Springer Science+Business Media New York 2015

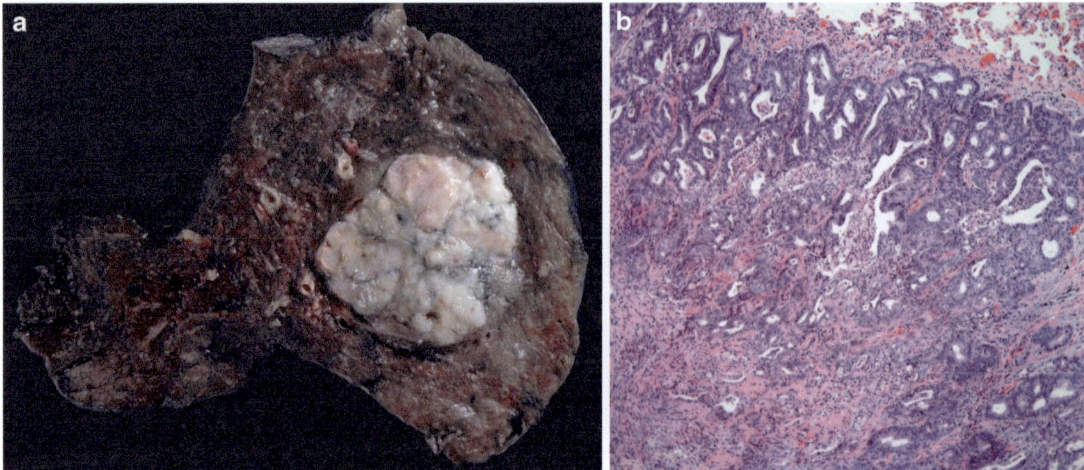

Fig. 8.1 Adenocarcinoma. Well circumscription at both gross and microscopic levels (Tumors and Tumor – Like Conditions of the Lung and Pleura, *Elsevier/Saunders*, 2010 with permission)

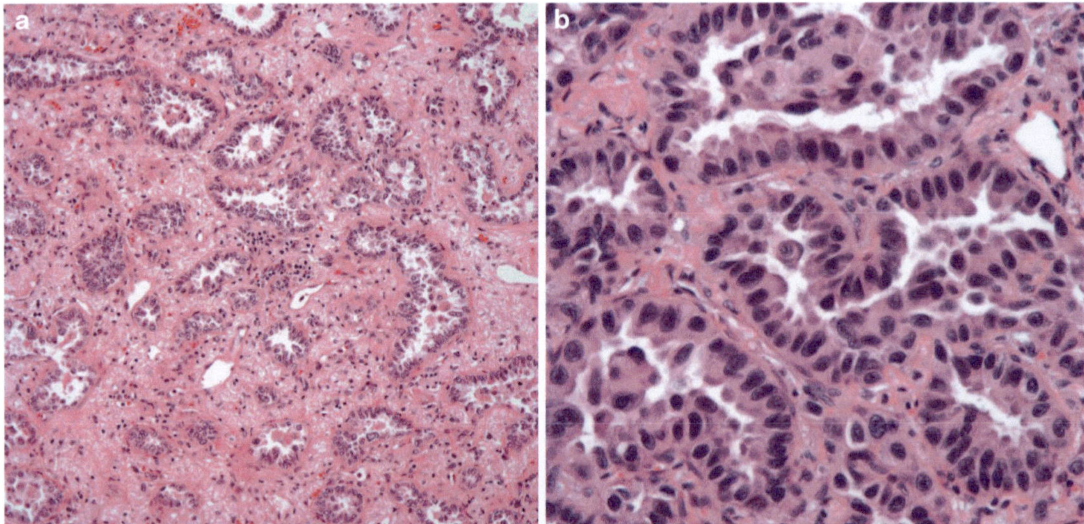

Fig. 8.2 Well-differentiated adenocarcinoma. Expansive (destructive) growth pattern. Note ragged glandular structures (Tumors and Tumor – Like Conditions of the Lung and Pleura, *Elsevier/Saunders*, 2010 with permission)

spaces and dissecting the alveolar walls, alveolar structures should not be present in the tumor body. Importantly, alveolar filling (aerogenic spread) and lepidic growth patterns are not considered evidence of invasion. And interstitial thickening which can be present in metastatic carcinomas is uncharacteristic of primary pulmonary carcinomas. This claim is in line with the 2011 International Association for the Study of Lung Cancer/American Thoracic Society/ European Respiratory Society Recommendation [1]. The society recommends discontinuation of the term of bronchoalveolar carcinoma (BAC). Instead it spits the former BACs into four entities: adenocarcinoma in situ, minimally invasive adenocarcinoma, invasive mucinous adenocarcinoma, and lepidic predominant non-mucinous adenocarcinoma depending on the tumor cell type and size and the size of the invasive component. If vascular or pleural invasion or necrosis is present, the tumor should be called lepidic predominant adenocarcinoma rather than minimally invasive adenocarcinoma regardless of the size of the invasive component.

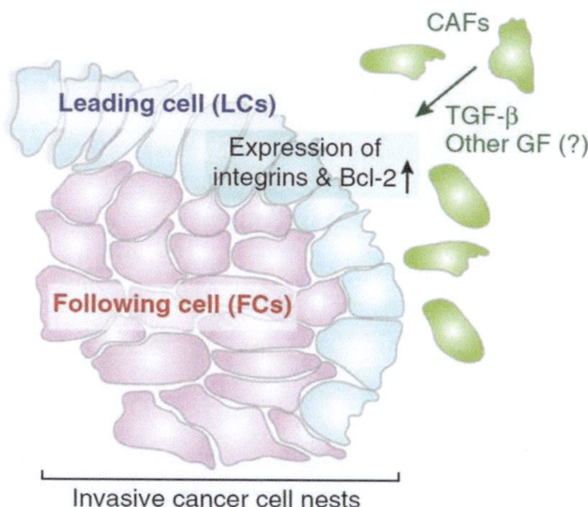

Fig. 8.3 The leading role of stromal myofibroblasts in tumor advance

Differential Diagnosis

Benign Mucus Gland Adenoma

Mucous gland adenomas are rare and present as endobronchial masses. Even though they can form complex cystic, tubular, and papillary structures, no invasion of the bronchial wall is evident. The cells are cytological benign.

Because pulmonary adenocarcinomas rarely present as an endophytic mass, the main issue here is to rule out low-grade mucoepidermoid carcinomas. Benign mucous gland adenomas do not have squamous and intermediate cells.

Alveolar Adenoma

Present as a peripheral nodule, alveolar adenomas contain dilated alveolar spaces filled with eosinophilic material. The septa are thickened by spindle cell-rich mesenchyme. They lack a destructive invasion pattern.

Mesothelioma and Adenomatoid Tumor of the Pleura

Mesotheliomas rarely present as a well-circumscribed mass, and pseudomesotheliomatous adenocarcinomas are fairly uncommon. A panel of immunostainings (CEA, B72.3, MOC31, and TTf-1) are required to make the distinction in difficult cases.

Rare cases of adenomatoid-like adenocarcinomas can be differentiated from adenomatoid tumors by lack of expansive invasion in the latter.

Squamous Cell Carcinoma

Primary pulmonary squamous cell carcinoma variants can have cystic, adenomatoid-like, or syringomatous patterns. They usually lack the slit-like appearance with protruding and frizzy luminal borders characteristic of adenocarcinomas.

Salivary Gland-Type Tumor

Because of their rarity in the lung, they are frequently misdiagnosed as non-small cell carcinomas particularly in small biopsies. Importantly, they present as a well-circumscribed, endobronchial mass. Familiarity with their characteristic growth patterns facilitates their recognition.

Key Features of Well-Differentiated Pulmonary Squamous Cell Carcinoma

- Well-circumscribed squamous mass
- Expansive growth pattern (Fig. 8.4)

Discussion

With the exception of rare exophytic variant of squamous cell carcinoma in which no invasion of the bronchial wall is present, the vast majority of pulmonary squamous cell carcinomas share with their adenocarcinoma counterparts two important morphological features: well circumscription and expansile invasion pattern. As discussed in the preceding section, these shared features are probably resultant from the employment of an embryonic/fetal mechanism in tumor growth and invasion [7–9]. In a form of so-called collective migration in which the tumor cells migrate in a whole group rather than in single cells, the leading cells in the invasive cell nests are guided and cheered on by the activated myofibroblast vanguard [9]. Like in adenocarcinomas, alveolar filling, lepidic spreading, and septal thickening are incompatible with such an alliance.

Whereas pulmonary adenocarcinomas show features indicating differentiation toward Clara cells and/or type II pneumocytes, squamous cell carcinomas are believed to arise from basal cells located in the human bronchus and bronchioles and differentiate along the squamous linage.

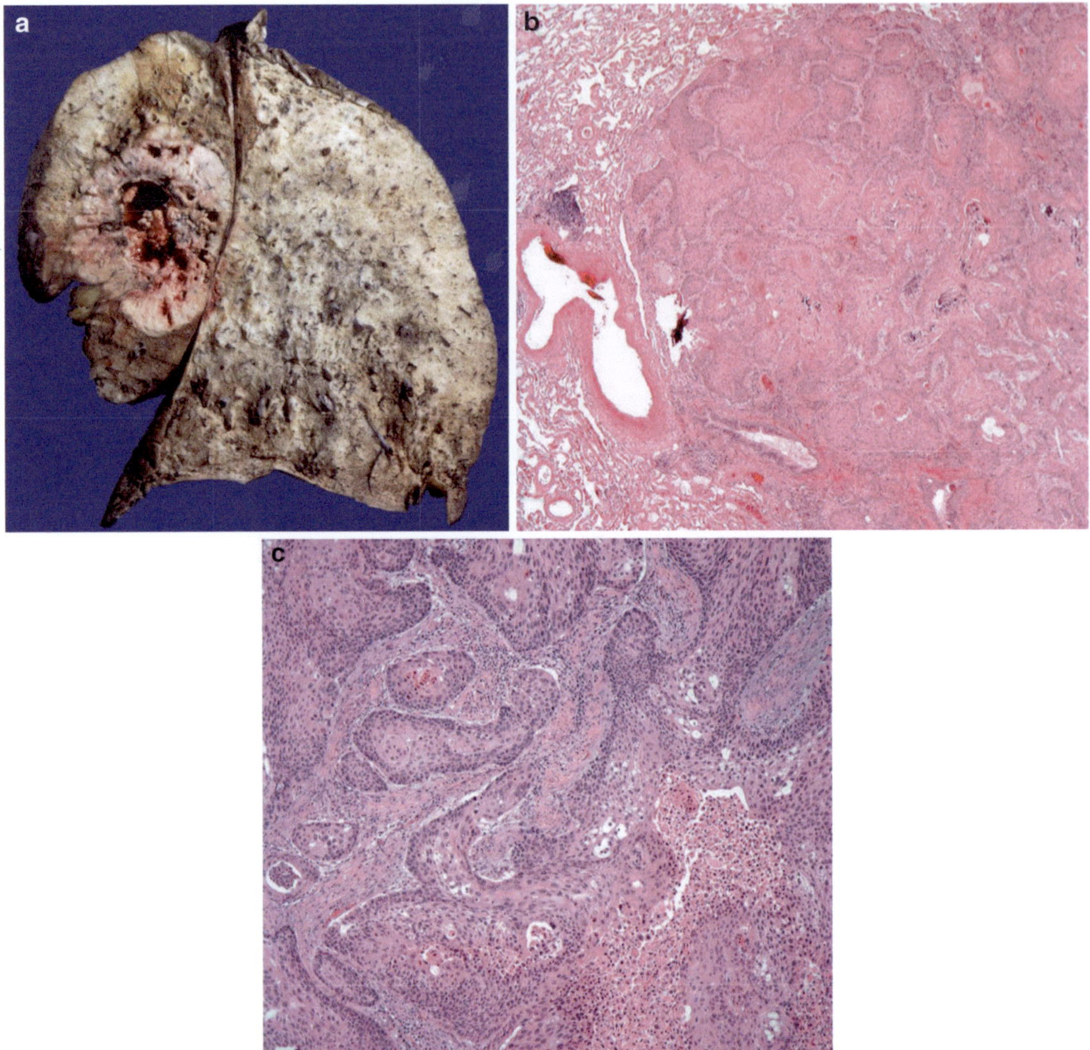

Fig. 8.4 Squamous cell carcinoma with well circumscription and expansive growth pattern (Tumors and Tumor – Like Conditions of the Lung and Pleura, *Elsevier/Saunders*, 2010 with permission)

Unlike the former in which in situ lesions are usually absent, squamous cell carcinomas frequently contain precursor lesions. And this feature can be used in the distinction between primary and metastatic squamous cell carcinomas.

Awareness of the variety of different growth patterns of squamous cell carcinomas is important in order not to mistake them for adenocarcinomas or adenosquamous carcinomas. The variants can have cystic formation and adenoid and syringomatous structures and even clear cells. When in doubt, a panel of immunostainings (p63, keratin 5/6, TTF-1) should be applied.

Differential Diagnosis

Squamous Papilloma, Papillomatosis, Invasive Papillomatosis

Pulmonary squamous papillomas are rare endobronchial proliferations and are associated with human papilloma virus. Typically, they present as an exophytic mass with only mild cytological atypia. Problem arises when the lesion is affected by dysplasia or even carcinoma in situ and when there is involvement of the underlying glands. With papillomatosis, there is a greater degree of cytological atypia and a greater tendency to show an inverted growth pattern (inverted papilloma)

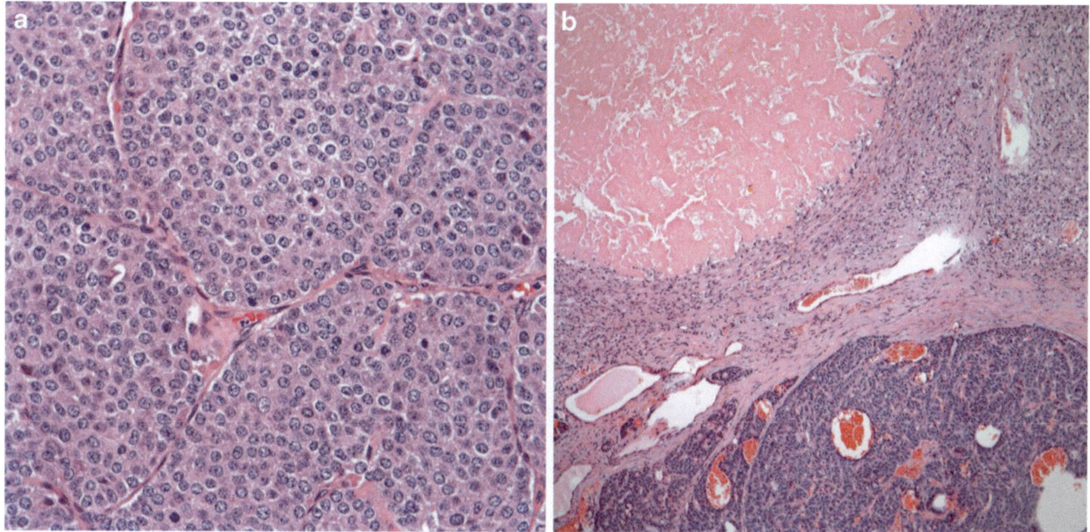

Fig. 8.5 Atypical carcinoid. Note mitotic figures (**a**) and necrosis (**b**) (Tumors and Tumor – Like Conditions of the Lung and Pleura, *Elsevier/Saunders*, 2010 with permission)

and alveolar space involvement (invasive papillomatosis) [10]. These lesions are differentiated from squamous cell carcinoma by their smooth outlines and lack of bronchial and/or parenchymal invasion (destruction).

Squamous Metaplasia or Dysplasia Involving Glands

These lesions do not form a mass and the involved glands have a smooth outline. No destruction of the bronchial wall and/or pulmonary parenchyma is evident.

Primary Pulmonary Adenocarcinoma and Adenosquamous Carcinoma

As discussed in the adenocarcinoma section, primary adenocarcinomas have a slit appearance with ragged luminal borders. This feature allows their distinction from squamous cell carcinoma with prominent cystic changes and adenomatoid/pseudoglandular or syringomatous patterns.

Key Morphological Features of Atypical Carcinoid Tumor of the Lung

- Mitotic figures 2 to 10/10 HPF
- Necrosis (Fig. 8.5)

Discussion

In contrast to the three-tier classification for gastrointestinal neuroendocrine tumors in which mitotic activity is the only criteria for the distinction of NET G1 and NET G2 tumors, pulmonary neuroendocrine tumors are divided into four tiers: carcinoid, atypical carcinoid, small cell carcinoma, and large cell carcinoma [11]. Carcinoids and atypical carcinoids apparently share similar molecular changes which are different from small cell carcinomas and large cell neuroendocrine carcinomas. They have been called well-differentiated and moderately differentiated neuroendocrine carcinomas respectively even though they share virtually identical histopathological and cytological presentations. Histopathologically, they manifest as organoid, trabecular, insular palisading, ribbon, rosette, and even glandular patterns. Typically, the tumor cells are uniformly small to medium size with moderate amount of cytoplasm and contain round nuclei with characteristic salt–pepper chromatin pattern and occasionally small nucleoli. They can also present as variants which are composed of spindle, oncocytic, mucinous, clear, and even melanocytic cells.

The differentiation between carcinoid tumor and atypical carcinoid is the mitotic activity greater than 2 to 10/10 HPF and/or necrosis in the latter

[12, 13]. The necrosis can be punctuate or infarct-like. Most of atypical carcinoids meet the two criteria. Cases of with necrosis, but containing less than 2 mitotic figures/per 10 high power fields are called atypical carcinoid. Importantly cellular pleomorphism (neuroendocrine atypia) has no place in the differentiation and they are separated from tumorlets by their size of greater than 0.5 cm in greatest dimension. The high neuroendocrine tumors have their characteristic histological and cytological features allowing their differentiation from carcinoids and atypical carcinoids.

Key Morphological Feature of Low-Grade (Well-Differentiated) Salivary Gland-Type Carcinoma of the Lung

Pulmonary salivary gland-type tumors are rare and most of them are malignant. They usually present as a well-circumscribed, endobronchial mass. Refer to the section on salivary gland tumors for histopathological features for different types of malignancy.

Pleura

Key Morphological Features of Malignant Mesothelioma

- Diffuse involvement of the pleura or expansive fibrous interlobular septa
- Stromal invasion (Figs. 8.6, 8.7, 8.8, and 8.9)

Discussion

Rather than being a passive barrier layer, the mesothelium actively participates in the transmesothelial transportation of solutes and fluid, immunosurveillance, regulation of inflammation, and wound healing [14]. One important feature of the mesothelial cells is their capability to undergo epithelial–mesenchymal transition (EMT) in both reactive (reversible) and malignant processes. This transition allows cells to gain locomotiveness and become more involved in regulation of the inflammation, production, and remodeling of the extracellular matrix [14].

Malignant mesotheliomas rarely present as well-defined masses. Even if a mass lesion is accompanied by diffuse pleural involvement, the lesion is more likely to be an adenocarcinoma [15]. The typical presentation of malignant mesothelioma is a diffusely thickened pleura encasing the whole lung. However, in rare cases of desmoplastic mesothelio-

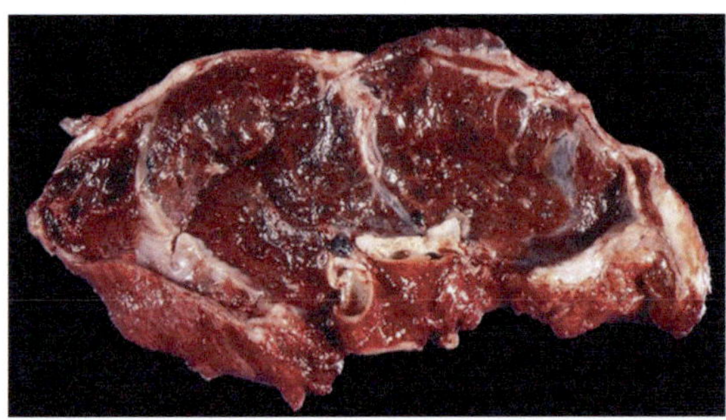

Fig. 8.6 Malignant mesothelioma. Encasing growth pattern (Tumors and Tumor – Like Conditions of the Lung and Pleura, *Elsevier/Saunders*, 2010 with permission)

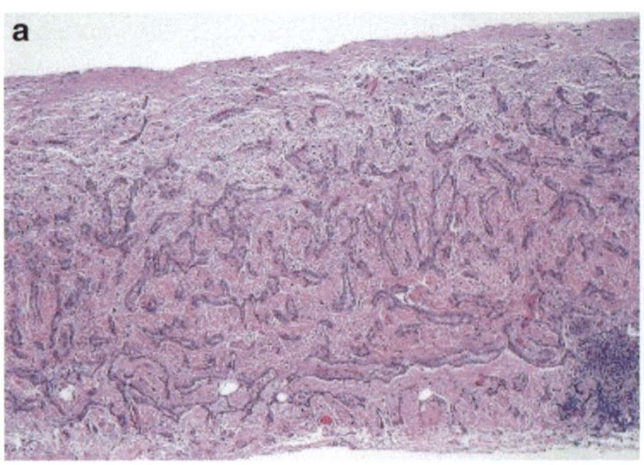

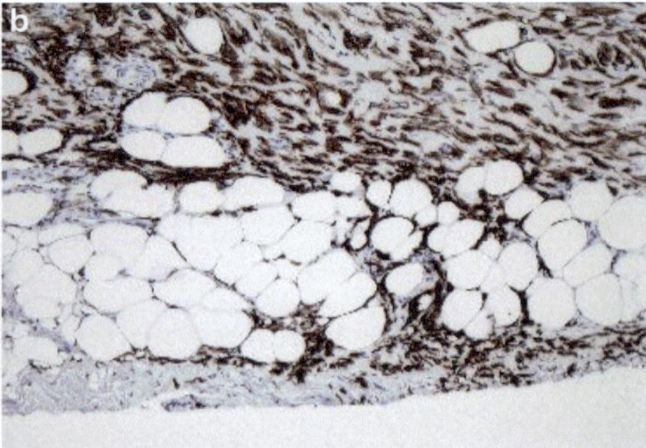

Fig. 8.7 Through and through extension of malignant mesothelioma (**a**). Fat involvement is evident (**b**, keratin stain) (Archives of Pathology and Laboratory Medicine, *American Society of Clinical Pathology*, 2012 with permission)

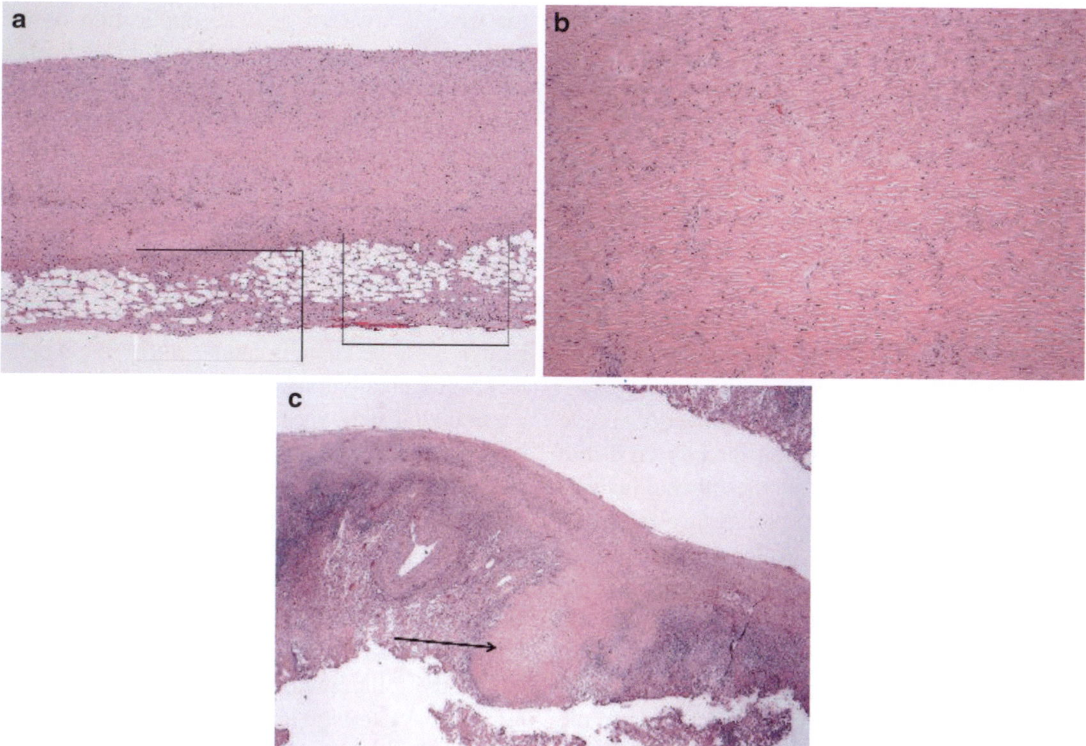

Fig. 8.8 Malignant mesothelioma. Thin desmoplastic malignant mesothelioma with fat invasion (**a**). Characteristic storiform pattern (**b**) and thickened septum (**c**) (Archives of Pathology and Laboratory Medicine, *American Society of Clinical Pathology*, 2012 with permission)

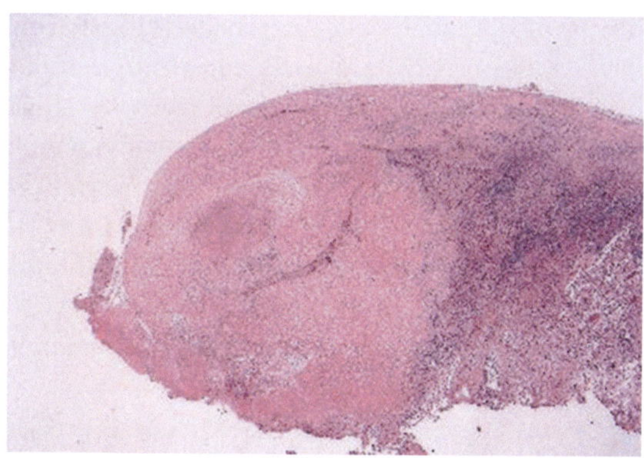

Fig. 8.9 Malignant mesothelioma. Nodular growth pattern (Archives of Pathology and Laboratory Medicine, *American Society of Clinical Pathology*, 2012 with permission)

mas, the pleura can be thin. The tumor instead manifests as expansive fibrous proliferation of the pulmonary interlobular septae [15]. This non-mass-forming propensity of malignant mesothelioma can be attributed, at least partially to the easy activation of the cellular EMT machinery. Other possible contributors might include the rhythmic, stretching mechanical force exerted on the pleura by respiration and limited free space between the visceral and parietal pleuras (pleural cavity).

One of the most common mesothelioma mimicker is fibrinous pleuritis/fibrous pleurisy. The natural course of pleurisy is as follows: first, fibrinous exudates appear on top of the pleural surface. The exudates are then replaced by granulation tissue which matures to fibrous tissue when the inciting agent gets cleared [15–18]. EMT is likely to play an important role in the granulation tissue formation. In the process, polarized mesothelial cells lose cell polarity and adhesiveness and gain locomotive ability. The upward migrating fibroblast-like (mesothelial) cells not only participate in the regulation of inflammation, extracellular matrix production, and remodeling but also play an important role in the new vessel formation in the granulation layer atop of the original mesothelial layer. One important but often neglected feature of fibrinous pleuritis is that it contains parallel vessels which are perpendicular to the pleural surface [15]. One plausible explanation for the unique vascular arrangement is that angiogenesis occurs following a parallel framework provided by the upward migratory transitioned mesothelial cells which also secrete angiogenic factors. Because adult mesothelial cells are known to retain much of the plasticity and vasculogenesis potential evidenced in embryonic mesothelial cells, it is also possible that the vascular arrangement could result from direct mesothelial vasculogenesis (by the transitioned mesothelial cells in the granulation tissue) [19–21].

The normal serosa is lined by a layer of simple flat mesothelial cells which sit directly on a thin submesothelial layer. The submesothelial layer is composed of few fibroblasts, collagen, elastin, and other extracellular matrix protein. Most surgical specimens, however, show a reactive mesothelium which runs the whole gamut of cytological and architectural atypia. Many of the reactive mesothelial changes closely mimic malignant mesothelioma and yet bear little resemblance to the simple structureless nonreactive mesothelial lining. Furthermore, most of epithelioid mesothelioma cells are bland looking. Except for conspicuous nucleoli, they show little nuclear atypia, minimal mitotic activity, infrequent hemorrhage, and necrosis. These might well be the reasons why malignant mesotheliomas are not graded by a well-established scheme as most sarcomas and carcinomas. Therefore, the two features we discuss here apply to all malignant mesotheliomas.

Instead, malignant mesotheliomas are categorized into epithelioid, spindle cell, and biphasic variants. This categorization calls into attention the mesenchymal origin of the mesothelial cells and their capacity for EMT. Familiarity with the variants and subvariants facilitates a proper differential diagnosis.

Stromal invasion has been recognized as the most reliable mesothelial malignancy yardstick. However, due to the unique anatomical and cellular characteristics of the pleura and other serosal surfaces, stroma invasion needs to be specifically defined in order to avoid confusion. Importantly, it is neither basement membrane breach nor deep location in the pleura. Even transgressing of the elastic layer cannot be used as the golden criterion for stromal invasion because duplication of the layer can occur in reactive processes [21].

The first criterion for stromal invasion is through and through extension of mesothelial proliferation in a greatly thickened pleura [15, 17, 18]. The emphasis on through and through extension as an unequivocal evidence for stromal invasion takes into account that both benign and malignant mesothelial cells are capable of producing copious extracellular matrix material and the fact that benign mesothelial cells can be entrapped at deep levels of a greatly thickened pleura. It is therefore paramount that the specimen is properly orientated to avoid en face or tangential sectioning.

Reactive lesions can have both epithelioid and spindle cells at deep levels. Additional qualifiers are needed to exclude these benign cells as deep extending malignant cells. Benign, entrapped epithelioid mesothelial cells can show both proliferative changes and cytological atypia due to the inflammatory stimuli. However, they have a characteristic linear pattern in which they are parallel to the pleural surface. Their deep location simply is resultant from the original mesothelial surface being buried by a granulation and/or subsequent organizing process. In cases of repeated cycles of effusion, layers of linear mesothelial cells can occur. Moreover, these entrapped cells usually form only simple tubules, and a sharp demarcation from the adjacent fibrous can be appreciated. A pancytokeratin stain can help light up their circumscription feature. Thus, to satisfy the through and through extension criterion, the epithelioid cells should lack linearity and circumscription and form longer and more complex structures than benign reactive counterparts.

Organizing pleuritis can have marked proliferation of fibroblasts, spindle mesothelial cells and endothelial cells. An important clue to the benign nature of this spindle proliferation is zonation in that the cellularity is greatest toward the surface and the number tapers off in the underneath tissue. This zonation might simply be a reflection on a concentration gradient of the pro-inflammatory agents in the pleura. As discussed earlier, the vascular arrangement (parallel to each other but perpendicular to the surface) can be a very useful hint for its benignity. Therefore, the modifier for through and through extension criterion for spindle cell mesothelioma is randomness in the cellular and vascular distribution.

The second criterion of stromal invasion is involvement of the fat or skeletal muscle or the adjacent organ parenchyma [15, 17, 18]. If one thinks of the mesothelium and the submesothelial layer as the equivalent of epithelium and lamina propria, respectively, "the stroma" here could be likened to the submucosa and even the muscularis propria in other tubular organs. In the evaluation of fat invasion, several points are worthwhile pointing out. First, pleuritis can extend into the chest wall adipose tissue. Attention to the infiltrative component, however, reveals mainly inflammatory cells and blood vessels. This is in contrast to the mesothelial nature of the infiltrates in malignant mesotheliomas. A cytokeratin stain can highlight this feature in difficult cases. Second, the so-called fake fat phenomenon in organizing pleuritis can be a source of overdiagnosis of fat invasion [22]. Thought to derive from the biopsy or processing procedure, these fatlike spaces can be deep in the pleura. Characteristically, these spaces have their long axis in parallel with the pleural surface, and the seemingly infiltrative cells manifest either horizontal (epithelioid) or zonational (spindle cells) features. Fat invasive mesotheliomatous cells typically present a downward growth pattern. In difficult cases, immunostaining of S100 can help.

The third criterion is nodular stromal expansion [15, 17]. Whereas malignant mesotheliomas rarely present as well-defined grossly identifiable masses, they can induce microscopic nodular proliferation of the stroma irrespective of tumor cell morphology (spindle or epithelioid). This nodular stroma expansion has excellent specificity and corresponds well with significantly increased TGF expression in mesotheliomatous cells [23]. However, its frequency particularly in small biopsy specimens could limit its use.

For both epithelioid and spindle lesions, sometimes, the pathologist has to use the term atypical mesothelial proliferation when definitive evidence of stromal invasion is elusive. This is particularly true for frozen section and small biopsy specimens.

Differential Diagnosis

Epithelioid Variant

Mesothelial Hyperplasia

Depending on the nature of the inciting agent, benign mesothelial hyperplasia can be diffuse or focal. As mentioned above, organization of fibrin and inflammatory exudates atop of mesothelial cells and subsequent formation of a new layer of mesothelium can cause an impression of stromal invasion. The linearity, well circumscription, and simplicity of the mesothelial proliferation are important features. In general, cellular atypia is more common and apparently related to the concurrent inflammation. Necrosis, when present, is accompanied by cellular debris and inflammation rather than in the form of bland necrosis characteristic of mesotheliomas.

Well-differentiated papillary mesotheliomas are a rare entity, which typically behave as benign tumors [24]. They generally present multifocal nodules and their papillae have broader central fibrovascular core than that of their malignant counterparts. Even though shallow submesothelial invasion has been reported in some cases, no deep invasion is present.

Multicystic mesotheliomas or multilocular inclusion cysts most commonly occur in the peritoneum. They present as a single mass with no stromal invasion.

Adenomatoid Tumor

Usually presented as small solitary cystic nodules, multiple nodules have been reported in some cases. They have their characteristic histological features such as cords and sheet of vacuolated cells with displaced peripheral nuclei separated by thin fibrocollagenous tissue. Clinical and radiological information is important to differentiate them from the adenomatoid subvariant of malignant mesothelioma.

Metastatic Malignancies

Metastatic lesions are more frequently encountered than primary pleural malignancies. Although they can induce pleural effusion and thickening, the typical picture is a pleural-based mass rather than a diffuse involvement of the pleura (localized malignant mesotheliomas are extremely rare). The patient's clinical–radiological

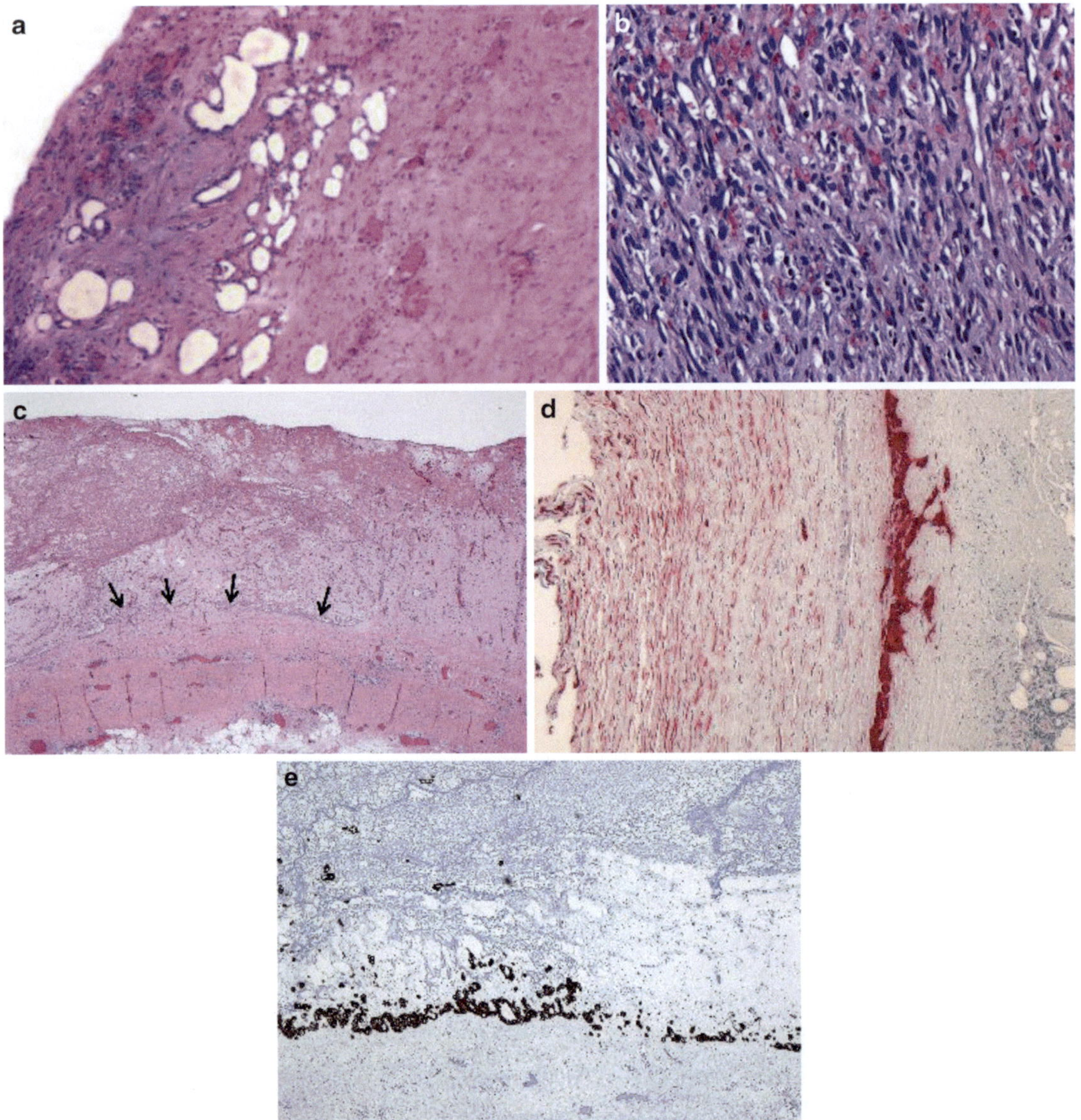

Fig. 8.10 Reactive pleuritis. Zonation (**a**), parallel vessels which are perpendicular to the surface (**b**), and layering (**c**, **d**, **e**, keratin stain) (Color Atlas and Text of Pulmonary Pathology, *Wolters Kluwer/Lippincott Williams & Wilkins*, 2008 with permission)

information as well as the tumor's morphological features constitute an important basis on which the differential diagnosis is rendered and a panel of immunostainings is employed.

Spindle Cell Variant

Fibrinous Pleuritis, Fibrous Pleurisy, Fibrous Plaque

Fibrinous pleuritis and pleurisy remain the most challenging entities in the pleural pathology because there can be diffuse thickening of the pleura and marked spindle cell proliferation. As discussed above, several clues are very useful in differentiating them from malignant mesotheliomas. They include zonation, parallel vessels perpendicular to the surface, mixed inflammatory infiltrates, and dirty necrosis (Fig. 8.10). Furthermore, there seems to have a zonal arrangement of cytological atypia with the cells close to the surface showing more severe atypia than those underneath [24].

Desmoplastic mesotheliomas are easily passed off as plaque or pleurisy because they are paucicellular, and in some cases, the pleura remains thin. In those cases with a thin pleura, the tumor cells proliferate as fibrous expansion of the interlobular septae or bearing resemblance to bronchiolitis obliterans organizing pneumonia [25]. High index of suspicion followed by careful sectioning and reviewing to identify stroma invasion (criterion 2) and expansive proliferation of the interlobular septae is essential in arriving to a right diagnosis. Immunostainings are not very helpful in this situation because the neoplastic cell might not stain for calretinin and both entities may stain positive for keratin 5/6 [25].

Solitary Fibrous Tumor, Sarcoma

The entities are generally not difficult to differentiate from malignant mesotheliomas since they are localized spindle cell lesions. It would be useful to know that fibrosarcomatous subvariant has features indistinguishable from those of fibrosarcomas and sarcomatoid mesotheliomas can have heterologous elements such osteosarcomatous or chondrosarcomatous components. Immunostainings might be needed in difficult cases.

References

1. Travis WD et al. International association for the study of lung cancer/American thoracic society/European respiratory society international multidisciplinary classification of lung adenocarcinoma. J Thorac Oncol. 2011;6(2):244–85.
2. Farver CF, Zander DS. In: Goldblum JR, editor. Pulmonary pathology, Foundations in diagnostic pathology. Philadelphia: Churchill Livingstone/Elsevier; 2008.
3. Warburton D et al. Lung organogenesis. Curr Top Dev Biol. 2010;90:73–158. Chapter 26: Usual lung cancers.
4. Tan D, Alrawi S. Chapter 26. Usual lung cancer. In: Dani CFF, Zander S, Zander S, editors. Pulmonary pathology. Philadelphia: Churchill Livingstone/Elsevier; 2008. p. 544–62.
5. Cesar A, Moran SS. Tumors and tumor-like conditions of the lung and pleura. Philadelphia: Elsevier; 2010.
6. Moran CA, Suster S. Chapter 3. Nonsmall cell carcinomas of the lung. In: Tumors and tumor-like conditions of the lung and pleura. Philadelphia: Saunders/Elsevier; 2010. p. 51–110.
7. Blanc P et al. A role for mesenchyme dynamics in mouse lung branching morphogenesis. PLoS One. 2012;7(7):e41643.
8. An J et al. Significance of cancer-associated fibroblasts in the regulation of gene expression in the leading cells of invasive lung cancer. J Cancer Res Clin Oncol. 2013;139(3):379–88.
9. Bremnes RM et al. The role of tumor stroma in cancer progression and prognosis: emphasis on carcinoma-associated fibroblasts and non-small cell lung cancer. J Thorac Oncol. 2011;6(1):209–17.
10. Flieder DB. Chapter 26. Benign neoplasms of the lung. In: Zander DS, Farver CF, editors. Pulmonary pathology. Philadelphia: Churchill Livingstone/Elsevier; 2008. p. 669–92.
11. Travis WD et al. Diagnosis of lung adenocarcinoma in resected specimens: implications of the 2011 international association for the study of lung cancer/American thoracic society/European respiratory society classification. Arch Pathol Lab Med. 2012;137(5):685–705.
12. den Bakker MA, Thunnissen FB. Neuroendocrine tumours – challenges in the diagnosis and classification of pulmonary neuroendocrine tumours. J Clin Pathol. 2013;66(10):862–9.
13. Rekhtman N. Neuroendocrine tumors of the lung: an update. Arch Pathol Lab Med. 2010;134(11):1628–38.
14. Yung S, Chan TM. Intrinsic cells: mesothelial cells – central players in regulating inflammation and resolution. Perit Dial Int. 2009;29 Suppl 2:S21–7.
15. Oviedo SP, Cagle PT. Diffuse malignant mesothelioma. Arch Pathol Lab Med. 2012;136(8):882–8.
16. Zander DS, Farver CF. Chapter 35. Inflammatory and fibrosing pleural processes. In: Zander DS, Farver CF, editors. Pulmonary pathology. Philadelphia: Churchill Livingstone/Elsevier; 2008. p. 733–44.
17. Anttila S. Epithelioid lesions of the serosa. Arch Pathol Lab Med. 2012;136(3):241–52.
18. Cagle PT, Allen TC. Pathology of the pleura: what the pulmonologists need to know. Respirology. 2011;16(3):430–8.
19. Munoz-Chapuli R et al. Cellular precursors of the coronary arteries. Tex Heart Inst J. 2002;29(4):243–9.
20. Wilm B et al. The serosal mesothelium is a major source of smooth muscle cells of the gut vasculature. Development. 2005;132(23):5317–28.
21. Kawaguchi M, Bader DM, Wilm B. Serosal mesothelium retains vasculogenic potential. Dev Dyn. 2007;236(11):2973–9.
22. Churg A et al. The fake fat phenomenon in organizing pleuritis: a source of confusion with desmoplastic malignant mesotheliomas. Am J Surg Pathol. 2011;35(12):1823–9.
23. Vehvilainen P et al. Latent TGF-beta binding proteins (LTBPs) 1 and 3 differentially regulate transforming growth factor-beta activity in malignant mesothelioma. Hum Pathol. 2011;42(2):269–78.
24. Moran CA, Suster S. Chapter 13. Tumors of pleura. In: Tumors and tumor-like conditions of the lung and pleura. Philadelphia: Saunders/Elsevier; 2010. p. 387–436.
25. Wright JL. Chapter 35. Inflammatory and fibrosing pleural processes. In: Zander DS, Farver CF, editors. Pulmonary pathology. Philadelphia: Churchill Livingstone/Elsevier; 2008. p. 733–44.

9 Thyroid Gland, Salivary Gland, and Thymus

Thyroid Gland

Key Morphological Features of Papillary Carcinoma

- Highly infiltrative borders
- Predominantly branching papillary structures composed of cells with unique nuclear changes (nuclear enlargement, overlapping, crowding, chromatin clearing, irregular nuclear contours, nuclear grooves, and pseudoinclusion) (Figs. 9.1, 9.2, 9.3, and 9.4)

Discussion

Papillary carcinomas are the most common thyroid malignancies. If the encapsulated follicular variant is left out as a distinct entity (precursor or borderline) as they show molecular and immunochemical features between follicular adenomas and papillary carcinomas, it is safe to say that vast majority of papillary carcinomas lack a capsule (exception: the rare macrofollicular variant) which is the trademark of follicular adenomas and carcinomas [1, 2]. Instead, they have infiltrative borders.

The characteristic morphological of papillary carcinomas is papillae admixed with a variable portion of follicular structures. The neoplastic papillary structures are characterized by a branching structure composed of a delicate fibrovascular core lined by a one layer of atypical cells. The cliché "not all papillary carcinomas have a papillary growth pattern and not all papillary patterned thyroid lesions are papillary carcinoma" serves as a useful reminder for surgical pathologist but has led to the de-emphasis of the evaluation of the papillary structures in thyroid pathology. Actually the papillary structures in papillary carcinoma are more branching and contain more fibrovascular tissue than the simpler nonbranching papillae present in benign thyroid lesions such as nodular goiters and follicular adenomas [3]. The lining cells of the former are arranged in a nonpolar, haphazard pattern while the latter contains cells with basally located nuclei [3].

It is known that papillary carcinomas show wide variation not only in growth pattern but in cell morphology as well. The only unifying characteristic feature among all of papillary variants is the nuclear changes. They include nuclear enlargement and crowding and overlapping, nuclear clearing, irregular nuclear contours, nuclear grooves, and nuclear pesudoinclusion. Studies have attributed these changes to RET/PTC mutations with the nuclear translocation of beta-catenin playing an important role (with the help of vimentin amassed adjacent to the nuclear membrane) [4, 5].

Because many other benign lesions can have focal nuclear changes similar to those of papillary carcinomas and currently there is no consensus as to how many of them and how extensive they should be in order to qualify for papillary carcinoma, it is highly advisable that other features such as lack of encapsulation, infiltrative borders, fibrous bands, complexity of papillae, as

X. Sun, *Well-Differentiated Malignancies: New Perspectives*, Current Clinical Pathology,
DOI 10.1007/978-1-4939-1692-4_9, © Springer Science+Business Media New York 2015

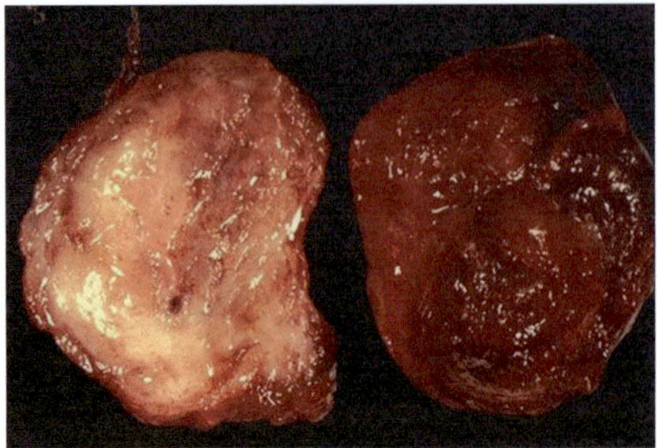

Fig. 9.1 Papillary carcinoma. Infiltrative growth pattern (Diagnostic Pathology and Molecular Genetics of the Thyroid: A comprehensive Guide for Practicing Thyroid Pathology, *Wolters Kluwer/Lippincott Williams & Wilkins*, 2009 with permission)

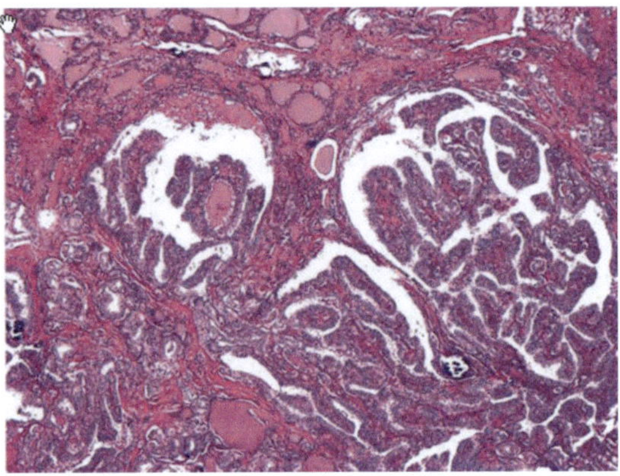

Fig. 9.2 Papillary carcinoma. Infiltrative border (Diagnostic Pathology and Molecular Genetics of the Thyroid: A comprehensive Guide for Practicing Thyroid Pathology, *Wolters Kluwer/Lippincott Williams & Wilkins*, 2009 with permission)

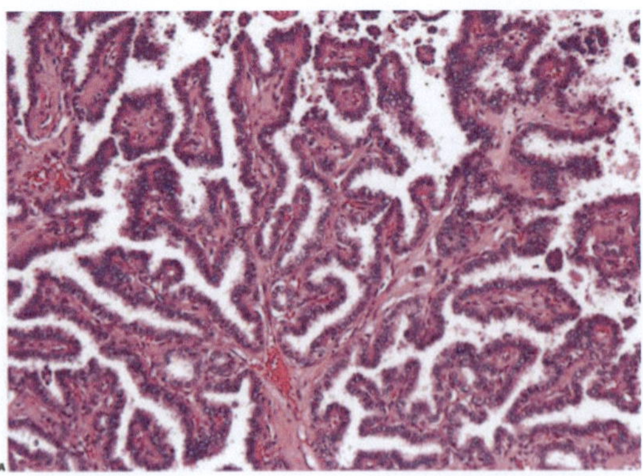

Fig. 9.3 Papillary carcinoma with branching papillary structures (Diagnostic Pathology and Molecular Genetics of the Thyroid: A comprehensive Guide for Practicing Thyroid Pathology, *Wolters Kluwer/Lippincott Williams & Wilkins*, 2009 with permission)

well as clinical information are taken into consideration (Fig. 9.5). In difficult cases, several promising immunostainings could be used (galectin-3, HBME-1, CITED1, and vimentin).

Differential Diagnosis

Benign Papillary Proliferation

The papillary structures are usually nonbranching. The cells maintain polarity and lack the typical nuclear features.

Lymphocytic/Autoimmune Thyroiditis

The infiltrative lymphocytes can induce nuclear clearing and intranuclear grooves and focal fibrosis. To distinguish a micropapillary carcinoma from reactive changes associated with thyroiditis, it is essential to choose areas lacking inflammatory infiltrates and require that all the nuclear changes are present before making a diagnosis of papillary carcinoma arising from lymphocytic/autoimmune thyroiditis

Grave's Disease and Toxic Nodular Goiter

They may have papillary formations with cells exhibiting chromatin clearing, intranuclear grooves, and pesudonuclear inclusions. However, the former is a diffuse lesion involving the whole gland with areas of lymphocytic infiltration. Close examination of the papillae reveals infoldings within follicles. Complex arborization is not the theme. The lining cells maintain their polarity and lack nuclear overlapping. Similar changes can be seen in toxic nodular goiters.

Hyalinizing Trabecular Adenoma

Characterized by a trabecular growth pattern with intermixed hyaline material, the tumor cells show many nuclear changes of papillary carcinoma. Papillary carcinomas, however, rarely present as a trabecular growth pattern containing prominent stromal hyalinization. In difficult cases HBME-1 and galectin-3 stains can be employed to make the distinction.

Hurthle Cell Lesions

They may contain nuclear elongation and nuclear grooves, and some degree of nuclear clearing and contour irregularity can be seen. Hurthle cells contain centrally located round nuclei with prominent central nucleoli but lack nuclear overlapping

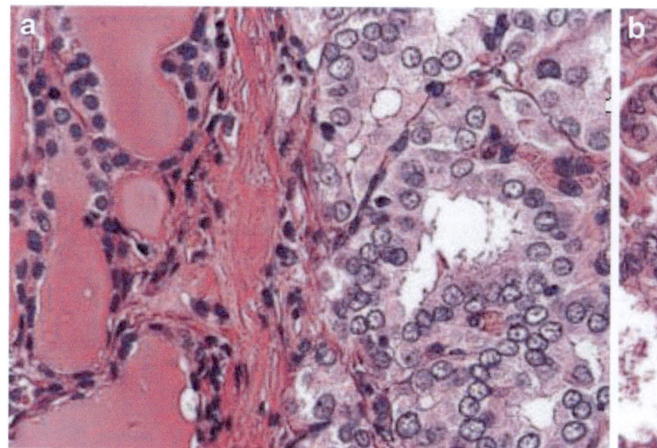

Fig. 9.4 Characteristic nuclear feature of papillary carcinoma (Diagnostic Pathology and Molecular Genetics of the Thyroid: A comprehensive Guide for Practicing Thyroid Pathology, *Wolters Kluwer/Lippincott Williams & Wilkins*, 2009 with permission)

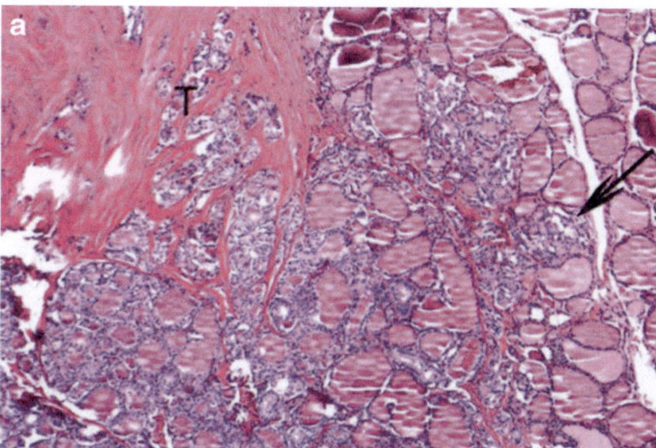

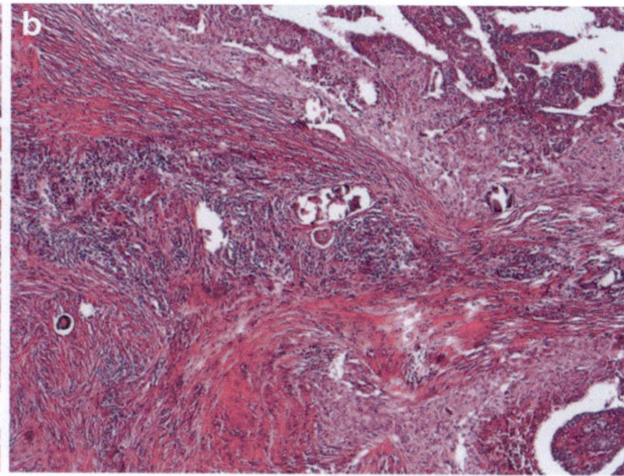

Fig. 9.5 Papillary carcinoma with prominent fibrosing bands (Diagnostic Pathology and Molecular Genetics of the Thyroid: A comprehensive Guide for Practicing Thyroid Pathology, *Wolters Kluwer/Lippincott Williams & Wilkins*, 2009 with permission)

and crowding. To make a diagnosis of oncocytic papillary carcinoma distinction, the nuclear feature should be diffuse and unequivocal.

Instrumentation and Frozen Preparation

FNA and frozen sections are known to induce nuclear changes mimicking papillary carcinoma. Fortunately these changes are usually focal and confined to the areas showing the other associated changes such as hemorrhage, infarction, fibrosis, and vascular proliferation. It is therefore important to shun those areas in the evaluation of nuclear features. Frozen section of thyroid neoplasia is largely discouraged since the evaluation of capsular and/or vascular invasion and nuclear features is compromised.

Key Morphological Features of Follicular Carcinoma

- Encapsulation
- Capsular and/or vascular invasion (Figs. 9.6 and 9.7)

Discussion

In stark contrast to the emphasis on nuclear features in diagnosing thyroid papillary carcinomas, both nuclear and cellular features are virtually ignored in the distinction between follicular adenomas and carcinomas.

Instead, capsular or vascular invasion has been promulgated as the only criterion. Therefore, those follicular lesions with worrisome morpho-

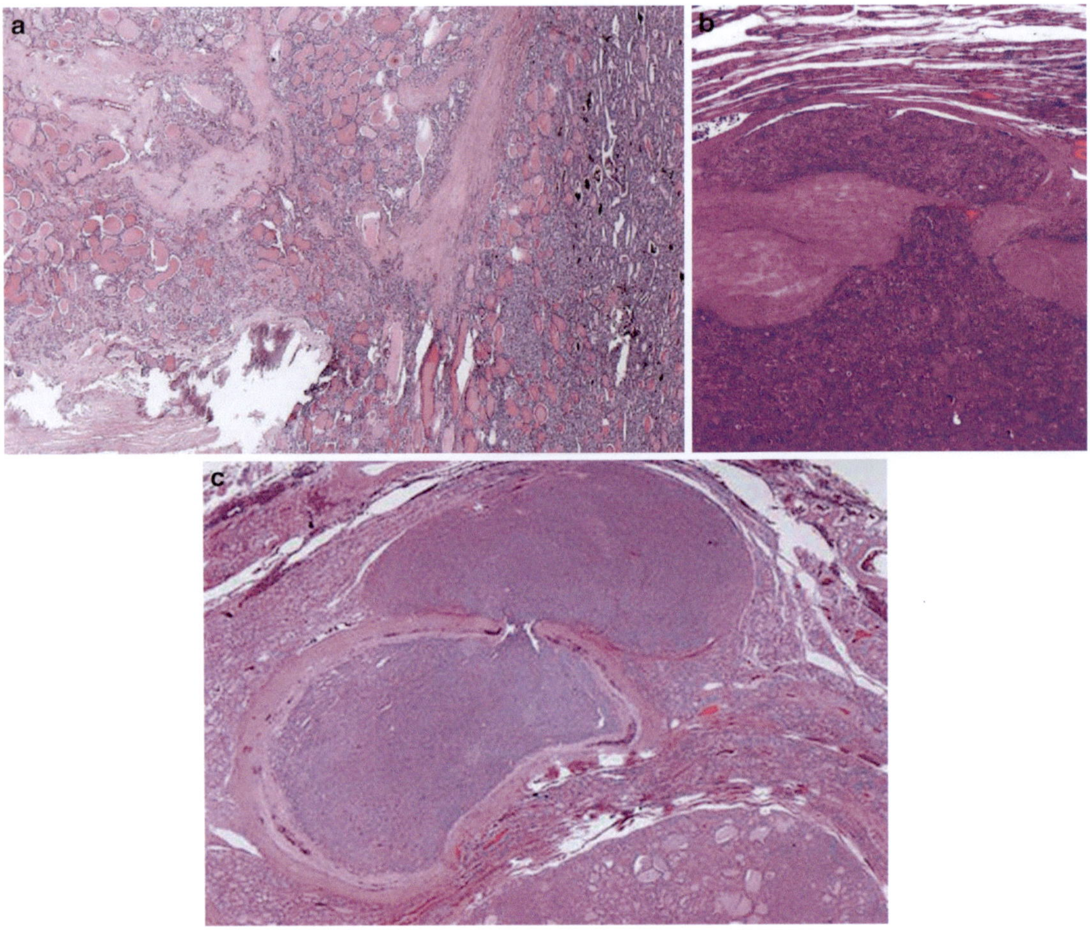

Fig. 9.6 Follicular carcinoma. Capsular invasion (Diagnostic Pathology and Molecular Genetics of the Thyroid: A comprehensive Guide for Practicing Thyroid Pathology, *Wolters Kluwer/Lippincott Williams & Wilkins*, 2009 with permission)

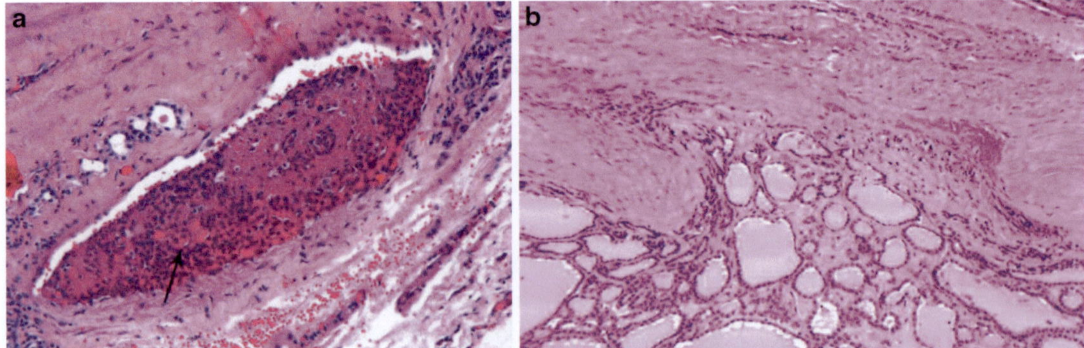

Fig. 9.7 Follicular carcinoma. Vascular invasion (Diagnostic Pathology and Molecular Genetics of the Thyroid: A comprehensive Guide for Practicing Thyroid Pathology, *Wolters Kluwer/Lippincott Williams & Wilkins*, 2009 with permission)

logical changes but short of solid evidence for invasion should be called adenomas. The worrisome changes include necrosis, increased mitotic figures, high cellularity, nuclear atypia, spindle shape, and even thick capsule with entrapped benign cells. Like follicular adenomas with bizzare nuclei, those follicular lesions behave in a benign fashion. Necrosis and mitotic activity have limited use in thyroid pathology. The first use of them is in the differentiating well-differentiated carcinomas (papillary and follicular) from poorly differentiated carcinomas which can present with papillary and follicular patterns and even nuclear features characteristic of papillary carcinomas. They are separated out by frequent necrosis, mitotic activity, and convoluted nuclei. The other use is separating widely invasive follicular carcinomas and medullary carcinomas from anaplastic carcinomas. The latter is characterized by high-grade nuclei, brisk mitotic figures, and necrosis.

While partial capsular invasion has been accepted by some experts, the stringent through-and-through criterion is endorsed by most of the experts [3]. By definition, capsular invasion requires penetration of the full thickness of the tumor capsule (not the thin capsule of the gland) [6]. The rationale behind adopting such a stringent criterion is to sieve out pseudoinvasion. For example, during the capsular formation of follicular adenoma, benign follicles might be entrapped by the fibrous tissue. In evaluating a small nodule outside the main tumor, a connection of the invasive front to the main tumor mass should be traceable. If deeper sectioning reveals no connection through a defect in the capsule, the nodules are more likely to be a separate lesion. The through-and-through criterion also avoids calling the folding of capsule (due to sectioning) capsular invasion.

The invasion most commonly manifests as a mushroom- or hooklike structure. When the tumor becomes widely invasive, the tumor capsule might not be easily recognized. In a manner similar to that of lung adenocarcinomas, the invasive fronts of the follicular carcinomas are rimmed by fibrotic tumor stroma preventing direct contact with the normal tissue [3].

Similarly, strict criteria should be adhered to in the evaluation of vascular invasion in follicular lesions. Because the normal thyroid gland and follicular neoplasms have a very rich endocrine vascular network with little fibrous tissue between the epithelial cells and blood vessels and the endothelial layer is thin and fenestrated, pseudovascular invasion is a common occurrence [7, 8]. Therefore, vessels in the capsule or immediately beyond the capsule should be selected for evaluation. To be called vascular invasion, the tumor clusters must be attached to the vascular wall and covered with a layer of endothelial cells.

Follicular carcinomas are thought to be a well-differentiated malignancy of the thyroid gland, and their clinical outcome correlates well with the extent of invasion irrespective of the degree of morphological differentiation toward normal follicles [3]. When papillary carcinomas are brought into the picture for contemplation, one could not help wondering why these two well-differentiated entities possess contrasting features. For instance, follicular carcinomas have thick capsules but only minimal amount of mesenchymal stroma. Even when the tumor cells have penetrated through the capsule, tumor cells do not come into direct contact with thyroid parenchyma. When the tumor metastasizes, follicular carcinoma cells prefer blood vessels even though abundant lymphatics are present [9]. Papillary carcinomas, on the other hand, lack encapsulation but contain a conspicuous fibrose stroma and infiltrative borders. For tumor dissemination, they favor lymphatics for dissemination. Let alone the characteristic nuclear features discussed in the previous section.

Moreover, follicular and papillary carcinomas seem to thrive in different bioenergetic states [10–12]. Follicular carcinomas have unchanged GLUT-1 level and express no caveolin-1, whereas in papillary carcinomas GLUT-1is overexpressed at both protein and mRNA levels and caveolin-1 is expressed in both tumor and stromal cells. Presumably, little cancer stroma metabolic coupling exists for follicular carcinomas as there is little stroma to start with and the cells are more reactive to TSH which could affect glucose uptake by GLUT-1 translocation and angiogenesis. Papillary carcinomas on the other hand are more likely to take advantage of their abundant stroma in forging a metabolic alliance for tumor growth. In this coupling the glycolytic stromal cells generate high levels of lactate to support mitochondrial oxidative phosphorylation in the adjacent tumor cells. However, if the coupling indeed exists, (an) unconventional mechanism(s) should be involved because in many other types of cancers, loss of caveolin-1 rather than overexpression of it allows autophagy and mitophagy with resultant aerobic glycolysis in the stromal cells [13, 14].

The fetal cell carcinogenesis theory and cytogenetics offer a plausible explanation for the contrasting features of the two entities. According to the fetal cell carcinogenesis theory, follicular carcinoma cells are better differentiated than papillary carcinoma cells with the former deriving from prothyrocytes and the latter thyroblasts [15]. The presence of RET/PTC rearrangement and BRAF mutations prevent the thyroblasts from differentiation and the PAX8–PPAP*r* rearrangement hinders the maturation of prothyrocytes into thyrocytes. The thyroblast-like cells in papillary carcinomas apparently retain some important features of fetal thyroblasts which face the daunting challenge of navigating the mesenchyme and reaching the final destination of the lower neck from the base of prospective tongue. In doing so, the migrating thyroblasts need to develop a close working relationship with the fetal mesenchyme and yet hold themselves together. This feature is accomplished presumably through a collective cell migration mechanism in which cell-to-cell adhesion does not have to be compromised [16]. Thus, the characteristic features of the papillary carcinomas such as infiltrative behavior, abundant accompanying stromal response, and propensity for lymphatics in dissemination can be explained by their retained thyroblastic properties. In line with the theory, papillary carcinoma cells express on fFN, vimentin, and claudin-10, all of which are negative in follicular carcinomas [11, 15].

Capsule formation is apparently a later event during the organogenesis. It coincides with vasculogenesis, cell growth, maturation into prothyrocytes and thyrocytes, and loss of cell motility. It is presumable that through a similar mechanism to that operating in the organogenesis of other highly specialized organs such as the liver, lungs, and kidneys, the maturing follicular cells break up with the mesenchyme and diminish the presence of it in the parenchyma to the minimum (except for a rich network of capillaries surrounding each follicle and a peripheral capsule). In line with the fetal cell carcinogenesis theory, follicular carcinoma cells are more responsive to TSH and have more TPO activity than papillary carcinomas [17–19]. They still maintain the capability to induce sinusoidal angiogenesis and capsule formation and manifest a pushing border (decreased mobility) and blood vessel preference for dissemination [20, 21].

Differential Diagnosis

Follicular Adenoma

They lack unequivocal capsular or vascular invasion even though they can show many concerning features which in other tissues are frequently construed as evidence of malignancy. The presence of them should alert the pathologist to search for signs of invasion by submitting more sections and getting deeper levels.

The awareness of neuroendocrine atypia in the form of adenoma with bizarre nuclei helps alleviate one's concern for possible anaplastic carcinoma in which highly atypical cells present in sheets with associated frequent mitotic and tumor necrosis.

Nodular Goiter

Believed to arise from mature thyrocytes as a result of complex interplay between susceptible genes and environmental factors, nodular goiters usually are multiple nodules with no or only a partial capsule. In contrast to the uniform monotonous growth pattern of the follicular neoplasms with minimal fibrosis, they are characterized by variously shaped and sized follicles composed of cells with variable cell shapes and frequent fibrosis and hemorrhage. Sanderson pollsters and even papillary infoldings can be seen in large follicles.

Papillary Carcinoma

Typical papillary carcinomas are easily differentiated from follicular carcinomas due to their contrasting features. Three variants of papillary carcinoma, however, are potentially troublesome.

As discussed in the papillary carcinoma section, the encapsulated follicular variant probably represents a borderline or precursor lesion. While many of them have characteristic nuclear features, in some cases the changes are focal. In these cases, areas lacking the features are intermixed with typical areas. This is in contrast to papillary carcinomas arising in a follicular adenoma or hyperplastic nodule in which the carcinomatous component presents as a well-circumscribed focus separated from the background lesion.

The diffuse follicular variant resembles follicular neoplasms in many ways.. They show a predominantly small follicular pattern with inconspicuous fibrosis and infrequent psammoma bodies. The tumor cells prefer to spread via the vascular rather than lymphatic route.

Strict adherence to the nuclear criteria steers toward the right diagnosis.

Rare cases of the macrofollicular subtype can be easily missed because they are encapsulated and contain large follicles with abundant colloid, and sometimes the characteristic nuclear features are present focally.

Key Morphological Features of Medullary Carcinoma

- Plethora of cytological and histological appearance, often in one single tumor
- Salt–pepper nuclear texture (Fig. 9.8)

Discussion

Medullary carcinoma of the thyroid gland represents a unique neuroendocrine tumor characterized by its protean cytological and architectural features [22]. This plethora of cytological and histological presentations even surpasses what is seen in papillary carcinomas, and they are usually seen in one single tumor. Medullary carcinoma cells can be round, ovoid to polyhedral, spindle, and plasmacytoid. Typically, cytoplasm is finely granular; however, clear cells and mucin-secreting, oncocytic, and even melanin-containing cells can be present. The typical neuroendocrine nuclear feature is often appreciated. Growth patterns include solid sheets, nests separated by fibrous stroma which frequently contain amyloid material, and calcifications and papillary, follicular/glandular structures.

The tumor cells are positive for calcitonin and CEA providing a very useful tool in the differential diagnosis.

Differential Diagnosis

C Cell Hyperplasia

The distinction is mainly between C cell hyperplasia and micromedullary carcinoma. Micromedullary carcinoma is differentiated from C cell hyperplasia by breakage of follicular basement membrane. One important clue to the presence of basement membrane breach is fibrosis around nests.

Metastatic Tumors

Primary and metastatic neuroendocrine tumors other than medullary carcinoma are rare in the thyroid gland. When the question arises, immunostainings for CEA and calcitonin can be helpful. Metastatic renal cell carcinomas can resemble medullary carcinoma, both architecturally and cytologically, and require utilization of immunostainings for vimentin and calcitonin.

Follicular Carcinoma

Some medullary carcinoma cells have follicular formations or oncocytic changes, thus mimicking follicular carcinoma. When follicular carcinomas present as solid or trabecular growth pattern or clear cells with inconspicuous colloid, medullary carcinoma enters into the differential diagnosis. The presence of neuroendocrine nuclear feature, prominent stroma with amyloid material and calcifications, and lack of a thick capsule cinch the diagnosis. In difficult cases, calcitonin and thyroglobulin immunostainings might be needed.

Papillary Carcinoma

Medullar carcinomas resemble papillary carcinomas in many ways. They lack encapsulation but contain a prominent fibrose stroma. Papillary or pseudopapillary, follicular structures and even nuclear inclusions can be present. Interestingly, tumor cells show propensity for both lymphatic and vessels in dissemination. However, to be called papillary carcinoma, more nuclear features are needed as discussed in the section for papillary carcinomas.

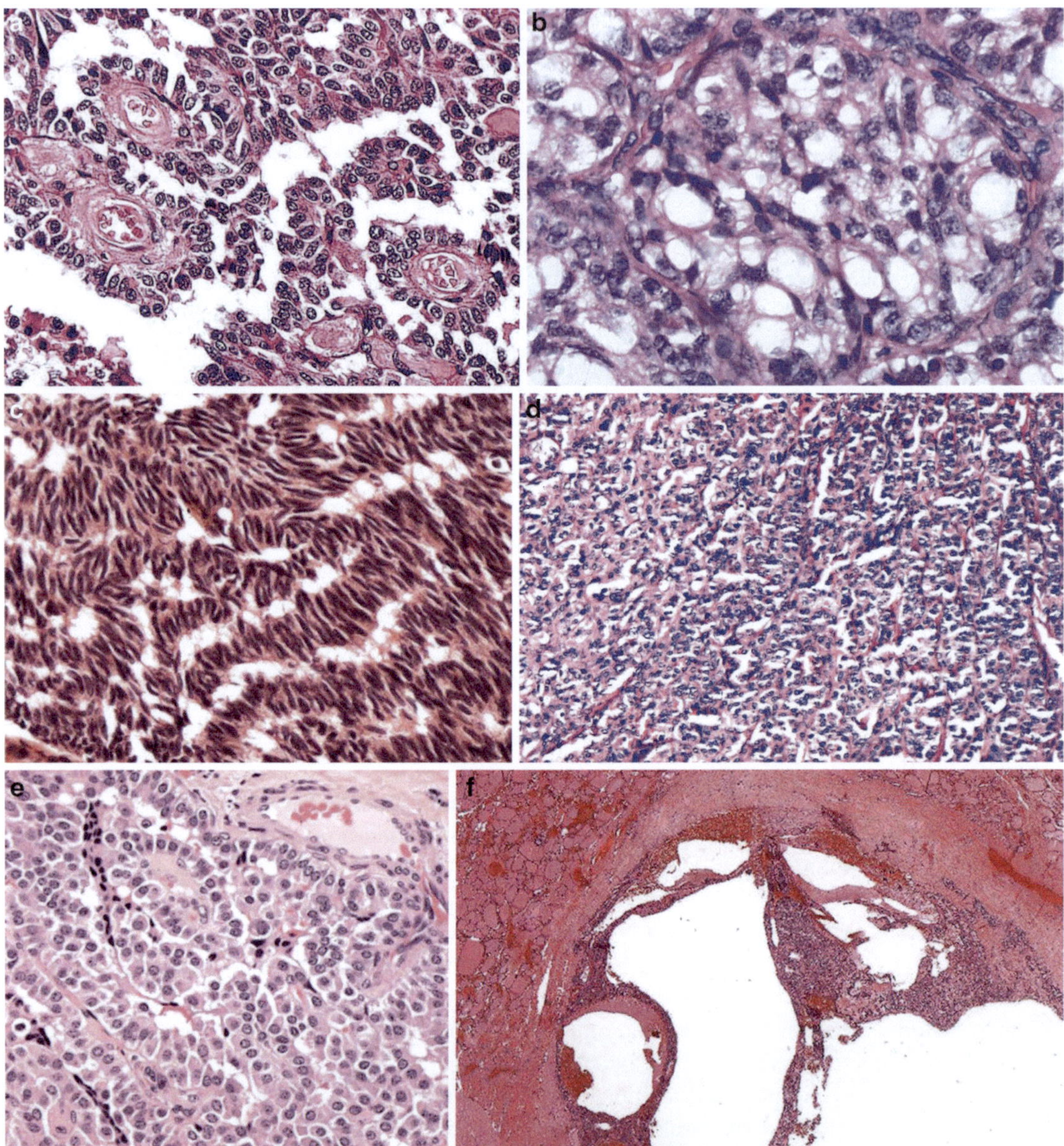

Fig. 9.8 Medullary carcinoma. Different growth patterns (Diagnostic Pathology and Molecular Genetics of the Thyroid: A comprehensive Guide for Practicing Thyroid Pathology, *Wolters Kluwer/Lippincott Williams & Wilkins*, 2009 with permission)

Anaplastic Carcinoma

Anaplastic carcinomas of the thyroid superficially resemble medullary carcinomas in that they also manifest a wide variety of cellular and architectural appearances which are often seen within the same tumor. They are characterized, however, by high-grade nuclear feature, extensive necrosis, brisk mitotic activity, and a widely infiltrative pattern.

Salivary Gland

Review of Pertinent Histology and Physiology

The major salivary glandular unit consists of the acinus, intercalated duct, striated duct, and excretory duct. The overall pattern of the salivary gland unit is a bilayered structure made up by luminal and abluminal cells. The abluminal cells in the first two parts are myoepithelial in nature and in the last two parts are basal. The luminal cells can also be divided into two types: serous and mucinous with the proportion of each type varying at different parts.

Salivary gland epithelial cells have a slow turnover rate (>60 days). It is believed that under normal conditions, the adult epithelial cells are generated through autologous cell division. The progenitor/stem cells are activated only in situations when massive injury has occurred [23]. The salivary gland is known for its vigorous regeneration capabilities. This capability might be accounted for by its secretion of a plethora of growth factors, particularly epithelial growth factor (EGF), and the presence of multiple types of stem/progenitor cells at different parts of the glandular unit. Epithelial stem cells have also been identified in the stroma on the other side of the basement membrane [24]. The salivary glands are highly innervated and the nerve tissue plays an important role in the organogenesis [24]. The multiple populations of stem cells show neural stem cell intermediate filament (nestin) and neuronal markers such as glial fibrillary acid protein (GFAP), neurofilament (NF), and protein gene product 9.5 (PGP9.5).

Overview of Salivary Gland Tumors

Salivary gland tumors include a wide range of morphologically different entities, benign or malignant. The 2005 WHO classification lists 10 benign and 23 malignant epithelial entities [25, 26]. Several unique features of the salivary gland tumors are discussed here to call attention to their differences from the mammary gland tumors which are also legion.

First, most salivary gland epithelial malignancies belong to one of the few specific histotypes for which no in situ component is identified. The specific cytological and architectural features associated with each histotype and the lack of in situ entities allow their quick recognition in small biopsies and situations where stromal/parenchymal invasion is focal and/or insidious. Most breast carcinomas instead fall into the invasive ductal carcinoma, not otherwise specified (NOS), which develops from an in situ component.

Secondly, most salivary epithelial malignancies are composed more than one cell type with the other cell being either myoepithelial or basal in differentiation even though the differentiation sometimes become evident only by immunohistochemistry or at ultracellular level [27–29]. Therefore, immunostainings for myoepithelial cells have little diagnostic utility here. Conversely, most breast carcinomas lack myoepithelial differentiation and immunostainings are very useful in their distinction from benign lesions.

Thirdly, salivary gland epithelial malignancy resembles sarcomas in that they can be transformed from a benign lesion (not an in situ component) and low-grade tumors can progress and even dedifferentiate to a higher grade [28, 29]. In contrast, breast cancers develop from well-documented carcinoma in situ entities. The low-grade and high-grade breast carcinoma families are distinct groups with different molecular changes analogous to the low-grade and high-grade papillary urothelial carcinomas in the bladder.

Lastly, given the fact that most common benign salivary adenomas (with exception of papilloma) are not confined to a ductal wall and no in situ component has been identified for the vast majority of salivary carcinomas, it is tempting to infer that most of the tumor-initiating cells are probably stem/progenitor cells residing outside the basement membrane. For instance, even though the carcinomatous component can be seen adjacent to benign ductal structures in mucoepidermoid carcinomas, no in situ component has been reported [29]. Mammary stem cells reside within the basement membrane. Carcinomas in situ can reach sizable masses before invasion occurs.

Diagnosis of Salivary Malignancies

In this book, we focus on four most common specific histotypes of epithelial malignancy: mucoepidermoid carcinoma, adenocystic carcinoma, PGLA, and acinic cell carcinoma. Their diagnosis is based on their unique histocytological presentations. The adenocarcinoma, not otherwise specified, and carcinoma ex pleomorphic adenoma are discussed in the differential diagnosis of adenoid cystic carcinoma. For the other uncommon malignancies (probably through transformation) which have a benign counterpart, identification of stromal/parenchymal invasion constitutes the sole criterion for malignancy. Examples include basal cell adenocarcinoma, myoepithelial carcinoma, cystadenocarcinoma, and even carcinoma ex pleomorphic adenoma. Importantly, invasion in salivary gland pathology is defined as involvement of the stroma and/or adjacent parenchyma without specification of the status of basement membrane.

Key Morphological Features of Low-Grade Mucoepidermoid Carcinoma

- Three distinct cell types (mucinous, squamoid, and intermediate)
- Prominent cystic structures lined by mucinous and squamoid cells (Figs. 9.9 and 9.10)

Discussion

Mucoepidermoid carcinomas represent the most common subtype of salivary epithelial malignancy [30–32] and are largely well circumscribed and even encapsulated. Most contain characteristic MECT1-MAML2 fusion oncogene derived from translocation t(11;19) (q21:p13). They are characterized by three types of epithelial cells: mucinous, epidermoid, and intermediate. In most tumors, the intermediate cells are the predominant cell type. Low-grade tumors contain predominant cystic structures lined by bland mucinous and epidermoid cells [33]. The epidermoid cells are usually scattered among the other two types, even though they can partially line some cystic spaces and form small nests. Importantly, when nest-like structures are formed, they are usually surrounded by intermediate cells. Authentic keratin forming cells are rare and they occur only in tumors with prominent inflammatory infiltration. They should not be not confused with oncotic cells.

Differential Diagnosis

Inverted Papilloma

Intraductal papillomas have complex papillary structures composed of cuboidal to columnar cells inside a duct. Inverted ductal papillomas are well-circumscribed papillary masses in the lamina propria and are composed of columnar and squamous cells. They lack intermediate cells, cystic formation, and infiltration of the adjacent tissue.

Sialometaplasia

Sialometaplasia contains nests of benign squamous cells and ductal epithelial cells arranged in a lobular pattern with regular smooth edges. Neither cystic nor intermediate cell components are present.

Cystadenoma and Carcinoma

These rare entities consist of multiple single cystic structures lined by mucinous cells and less commonly squamous cells. Luminal papillary structures are frequent in unicystic lesions. Multiple cysts are separated by a small amount of fibrous tissue. Typically, they intermediate cells and solid/island growth even though small islands can be seen in the cyst wall or intraluminal projections.

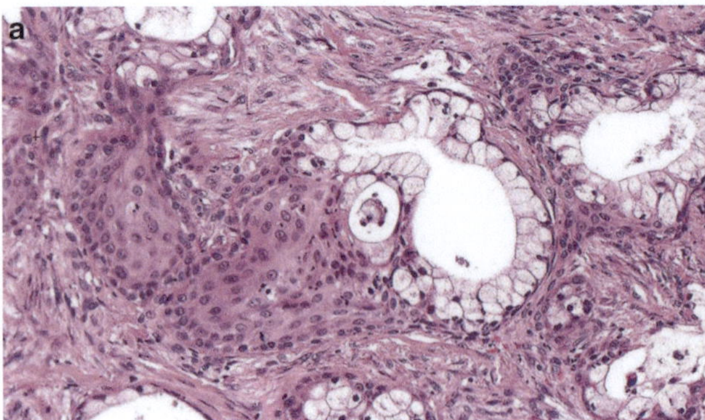

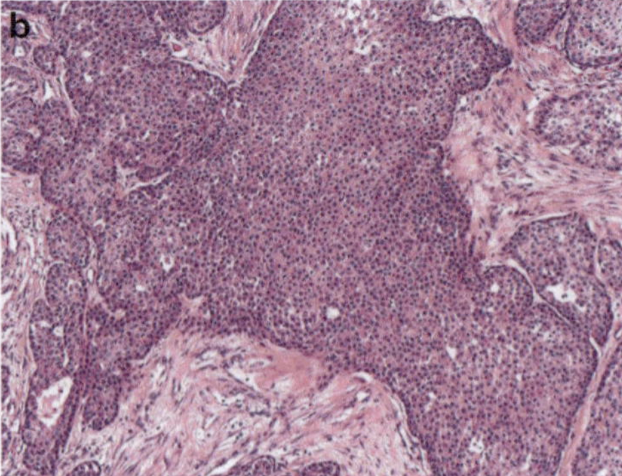

Fig. 9.9 Low-grade mucoepidermoid carcinoma. Squamoid cell, mucinous cells, and intermediate cells (Tumors of the Salivary Glands, *Armed Force Institute of Pathology/American Registry of Pathology*, 2008 with permission)

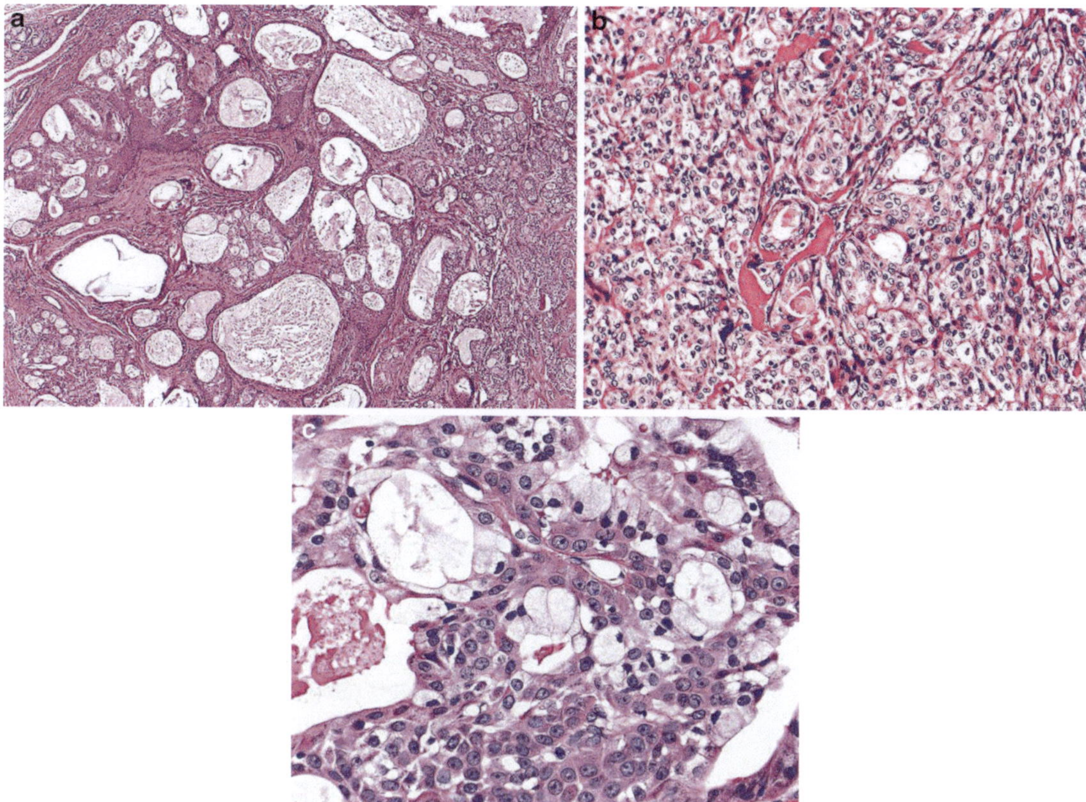

Fig. 9.10 Low-grade mucoepidermoid carcinoma. Abundant cystic formations (**a**), intermediate cells (**b**), and cyst lined by mucinous and squamoid cells (**c**) (Tumors of the Salivary Glands, Armed Force Institute of Pathology/American Registry of Pathology, 2008 with permission)

Pleomorphic Adenoma

Pleomorphic adenomas can have squamous metaplasia and mucin-containing cells. The cellular zone of pleomorphic adenoma can be mistaken for intermediate cells. However, the tumor contains characteristic myxoid and chondromyxoid stroma and lacks cystic formation. Additionally, the squamoid cells in mucoepidermoid carcinoma do not form discrete nests and show only focal keratinization.

Squamous Cell Carcinoma and Adenosquamous Carcinoma

Primary squamous cell carcinoma is very rare in the salivary gland and it typically lacks mucin-containing and intermediate cells. Importantly, the residual benign ductal structures should not be mistaken as neoplastic. The tumor lacks cystic structures which are characteristic of low-grade tumors, the epidermoid cells in mucoepidermoid carcinoma have only focal keratinization, and well-formed squamoid nests are rare. In difficult cases, immunostaining for CK7 can help make the distinction since most mucoepidermoid carcinomas show positivity for the marker, whereas squamous cells are negative for it.

Adenosquamous cell carcinoma lacks intermediate cells and cystic structures. It also lacks the intimacy between the squamous and glandular components, even though there are always regions where two components are separate. Also as in squamous cell carcinoma, the squamous cells have diffuse keratinization.

Key Morphological Features of Classical Adenoid Cystic Carcinoma

- Cribriform and tubular structures composed of biphasic cells with monophasic angulated, myoepithelial predominance
- Abundant basement membrane and amorphous extracellular material (Figs. 9.11 and 9.12)

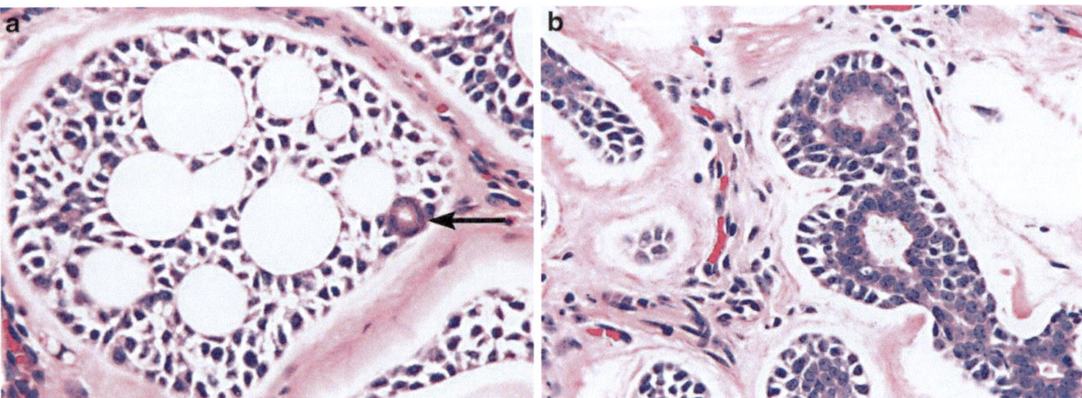

Fig. 9.11 Adenoid cystic carcinoma. Cribriform structures composed of biphasic cells. Angulated myoepithelial cells. Ductal formation (*arrow*) (Tumors of the Salivary Glands, *Armed Force Institute of Pathology/American Registry of Pathology*, 2008 with permission)

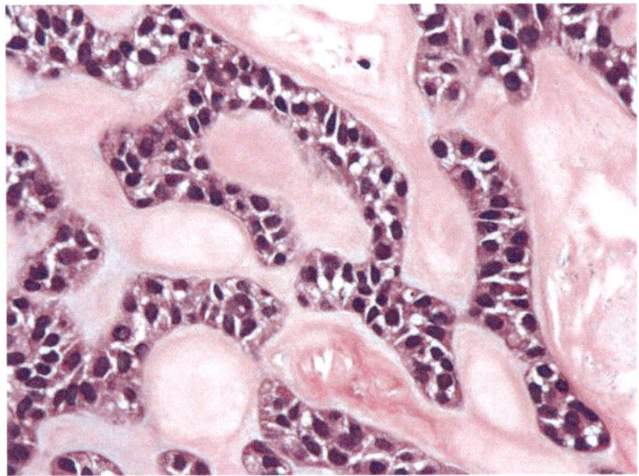

Fig. 9.12 Adenoid cystic carcinoma. Abundant basement membrane and extracellular material (Tumors of the Salivary Glands, *Armed Force Institute of Pathology/American Registry of Pathology*, 2008 with permission)

Discussion

Representing the second most common salivary malignancy, adenoid cystic carcinoma is characterized by a biphasic proliferation of ductal and myoepithelial cells in three major histological patterns: tubular, cribriform, and solid [34, 35].

Tumors with tubular and cribriform structures are considered classical and belong to the intermediate grade malignancy category according to the three-tier grading system. Prominent solid growth pattern puts the tumor in the high-grade category. Interestingly the cribriform spaces and tubular lumen are filled with basement membrane and other extracellular matrix material. These spaces are lined by luminal epithelial cells which apparently are not the source of the material. Instead, these luminal spaces are in continuity with the tumor stroma indicating the pseudoluminal nature of the spaces.

The epithelial cells are bland and become conspicuous in the tubular structures which are clearly surrounded by myoepithelial cells. The myoepithelial cells have distinct cell borders with clear or eosinophilic cytoplasm. Characteristically, the nuclear size is uniform, whereas the shape varies with many of them being angulated and irregular.

Grossly, adenocystic carcinomas are infiltrative and poorly circumscribed in appearance except for small lesions. The tumor is notoriously known for its propensity for extension along nerve tract, accounting for frequent recurrence.

Molecular studies have implicated involvement of the 6q region in the pathogenesis of adenoid cystic carcinoma. Immunohistochemically, the tumor cells are positive for c-kit and the epithelial cells show reactivity for EMA.

Differential Diagnosis

Pleomorphic Low-Grade Adenocarcinoma

Present mainly in minor salivary glands, the tumor represents one of the most important mimickers of adenoid cystic carcinoma as it can have cribriform and tubular structures as well a propensity for perineural invasion. However, pleomorphic low-grade adenocarcinoma has more other histopathological presentations including targetoid growth pattern as seen in lobular carcinomas of the breast. The tumor cells are bland looking and there is no apparent dual cell population.

Pleomorphic Adenoma

Pleomorphic adenoma is usually easily differentiated from adenoid cystic carcinoma since it has characteristic myxochondroid stroma material. Even though both of them contain biphasic cell components, the myoepithelial cells are blended in with the stroma in the former. In adenoid cystic carcinoma, the tumor cells are clearly separated from the stromal material.

Pleomorphic adenoma can have focal areas resembling adenoid cystic carcinoma. In these areas, the epithelial proliferation forms ductal structures surrounded by a layer of myoepithelial cells. The cells are bland unless affected by infarction in which adenoid cystic carcinoma is simulated. In adenoid cystic carcinoma, the myoepithelial cells are typically angulated. In difficult cases, immunostaining for c-kit can help.

Basal Cell Adenoma and Adenocarcinomas

Basal cell adenoma and adenocarcinoma typically do not form cribriform structures, and they rarely contain tubules. Even though biphasic structures lined by myoepithelial cells can be seen, they are inconspicuous. Typically, the tumor cells are small, uniform with round to ovoid nuclei, and palisading is present at the interface with stroma.

Key Morphological Features of Pleomorphic Low-Grade Adenocarcinoma

- A wide range of architectural and cytological features in one tumor
- Uniformly bland cells (Figs. 9.13 and 9.14)

Discussion

The tumor is characterized by a plethora of architectural patterns which include tubules, cribriform formations, trabeculae, sheets and nests, and single cells [36]. Typically, the center of the tumor is composed of solid sheets and nests, whereas single cells predominate at the periphery in a targetoid fashion. Unlike those seen in adenoid cystic carcinoma and epithelial–myoepithelial tumors, the tubules are lined by one layer of cuboidal cells only. In general, the tumor cells are uniformly bland and can show oncocytic, clear cell, and even mucinous changes. Immunohistochemically, they are positive for Bcl-2 and both luminal epithelial and myoepithelial cell markers.

Differential Diagnosis

Adenoid Cystic Carcinoma

Pleomorphic low-grade adenocarcinoma resembles adenoid cystic carcinoma in many aspects so that it is considered by some authorities as a variant of the latter. However, the former lacks the characteristic angulated nuclei, basement membrane, and other extracellular matrix material. It also lacks a prominent cribriform component and a conspicuous dual cell population.

Pleomorphic Adenoma

Pleomorphic adenoma can have myriad of histological presentations. It is characterized by the presence of chondromyxoid material, and the tubular structures are oftentimes not surrounded by myoepithelial cells. The tumor does not infiltrate the parenchyma, stroma, and nerves.

Adenocarcinoma, Not Otherwise Specified (NOS), Carcinoma ex Pleomorphic Adenoma

Adenocarcinoma, not otherwise specified, represents a group of salivary tumors with glandular structures and infiltrative growth pattern but lacks well-defined distinct features as those specific subtypes. Low-grade tumors are composed of bland cells with well-formed glandular spaces. Whereas they lack the myriads of histological presentations as seen in pleomorphic low-grade adenocarcinomas, tumor cells can take on many morphological forms (columnar, cuboidal, polygonal, plasmacytoid, clear, and oncocytic). Dual cellular structures are unusual. The tumor also shows propensity for perineural and vascular invasion. The tumor stroma seems to be more collagenous.

A diagnosis of carcinoma ex pleomorphic adenoma requires the presence of benign and malignant carcinomatous components. If the carcinomatous is still confined to the tumor capsule, it is usually called carcinoma in situ. Most of the carcinomas in this setting are adenocarcinoma, NOS, and can be graded as such.

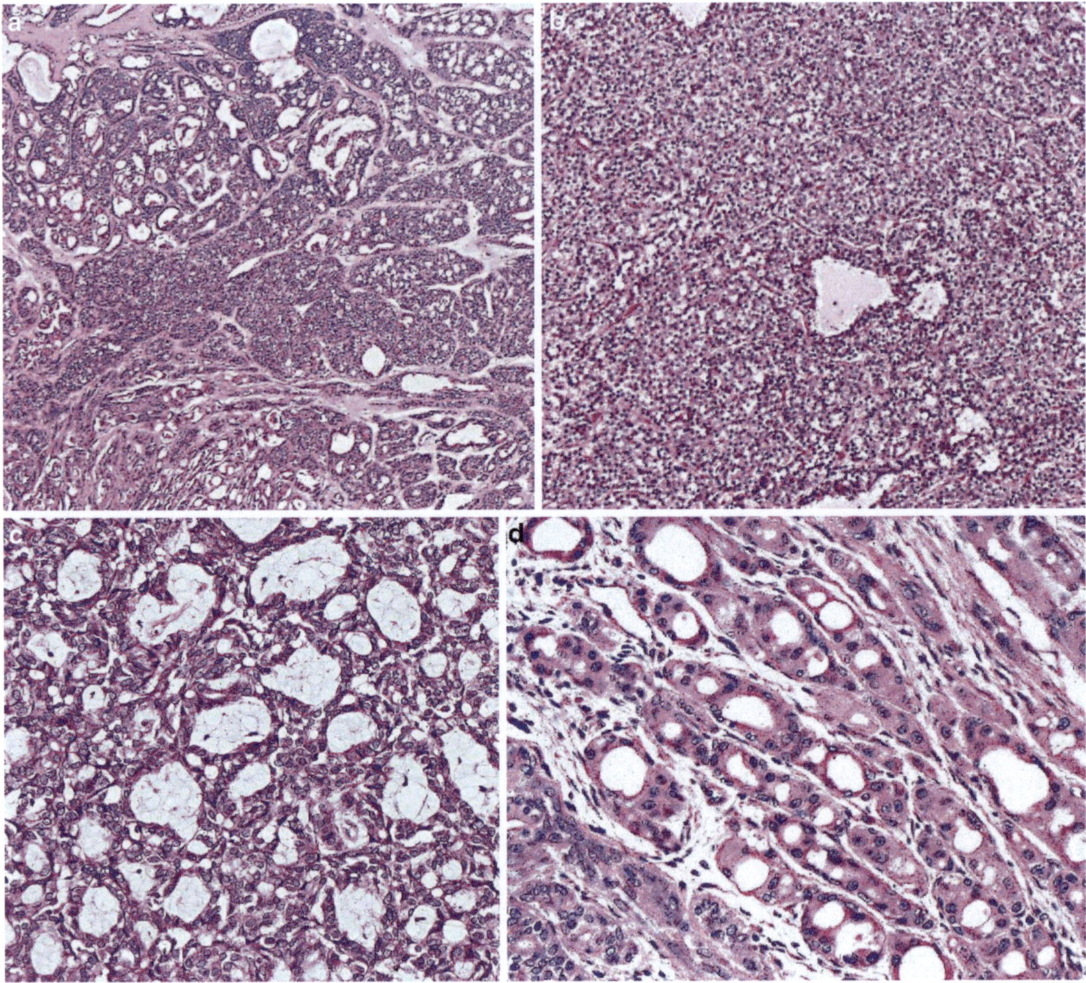

Fig. 9.13 Pleomorphic low-grade adenocarcinoma. A variety of architectural presentations (Tumors of the Salivary Glands, *Armed Force Institute of Pathology/American Registry of Pathology*, 2008 with permission)

Key Morphological Features of Acinic Cell Carcinoma

- Well-circumscribed nodules
- At least a fraction of cells with serous differentiation (Figs. 9.15, 9.16, and 9.17)

Discussion

Traditionally acinic cell carcinoma has been considered a low-grade malignancy. Grossly, the tumor is well circumscribed and sometimes seems to be encapsulated.

Acinic cell carcinoma of the salivary gland is the only salivary gland malignancy that manifests serous cell differentiation [33]. However, in many cases, this differentiation manifests in only a fraction of tumor cells. In contrast to their pancreatic counterpart, acinic cell carcinoma of the salivary gland can assume many different growth patterns and cellular types. The growth patterns include solid, microcystic, follicular, and papillary structures. Acinic, intercalated ductal, nonspecific glandular, clear, hobnail, and mucin-containing cells have been reported. Intercalated cells are the prominent cellular component in a significant fraction of tumors. Vacuolated cells are frequently seen and sometimes become the predominant cell type. It is for these reasons that the tumor is often misdiagnosed as adenocarcinoma, not otherwise specified.

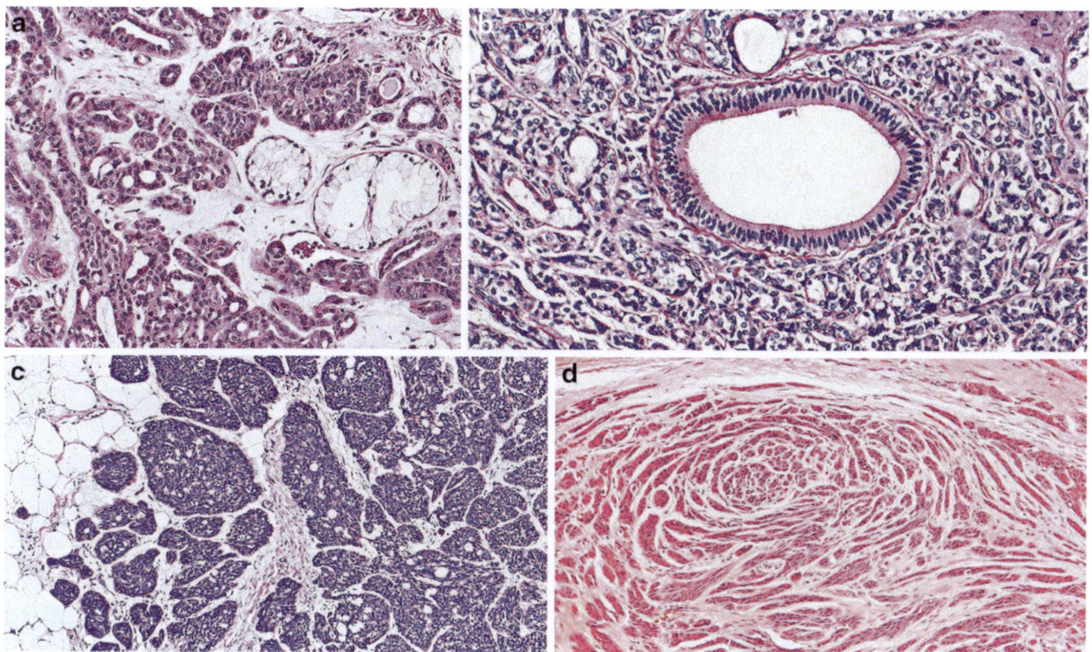

Fig. 9.14 Pleomorphic low-grade adenocarcinoma. More achitectural presentations (Tumors of the Salivary Glands, *Armed Force Institute of Pathology/American Registry of Pathology*, 2008 with permission)

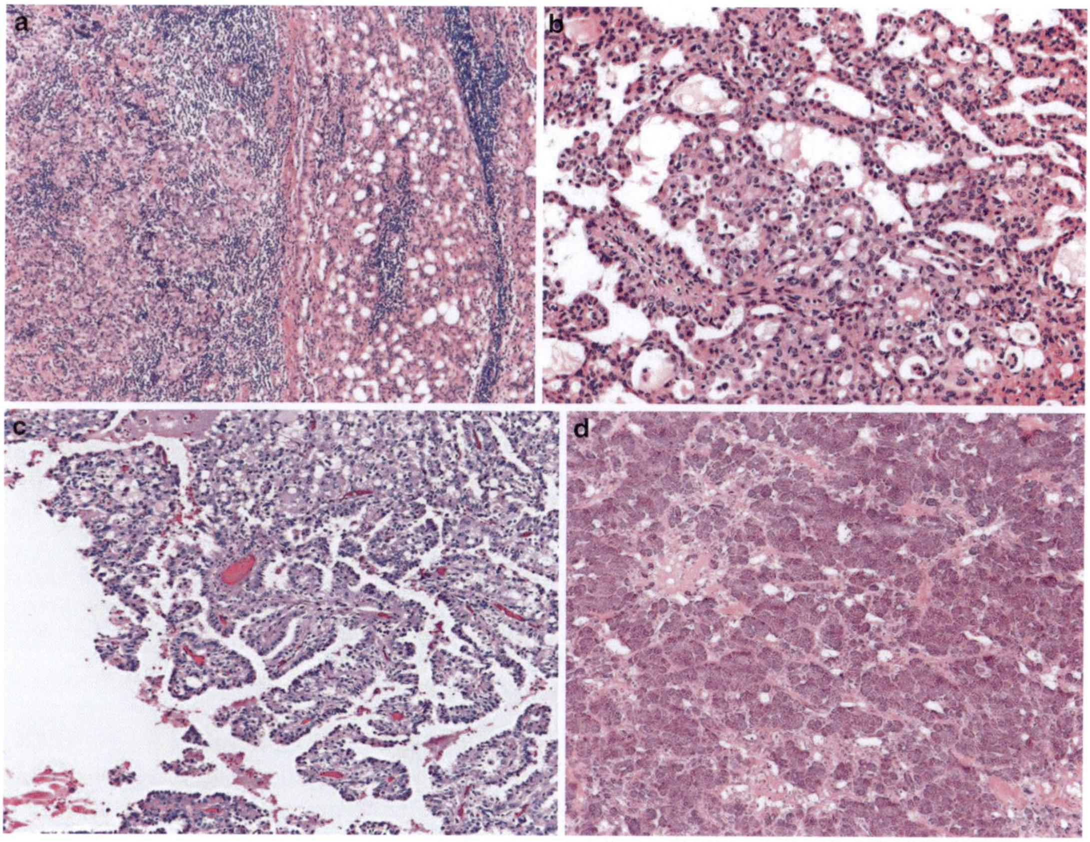

Fig. 9.15 Acinic cell carcinoma. Different architectural presentations (Tumors of the Salivary Glands, *Armed Force Institute of Pathology/American Registry of Pathology*, 2008 with permission)

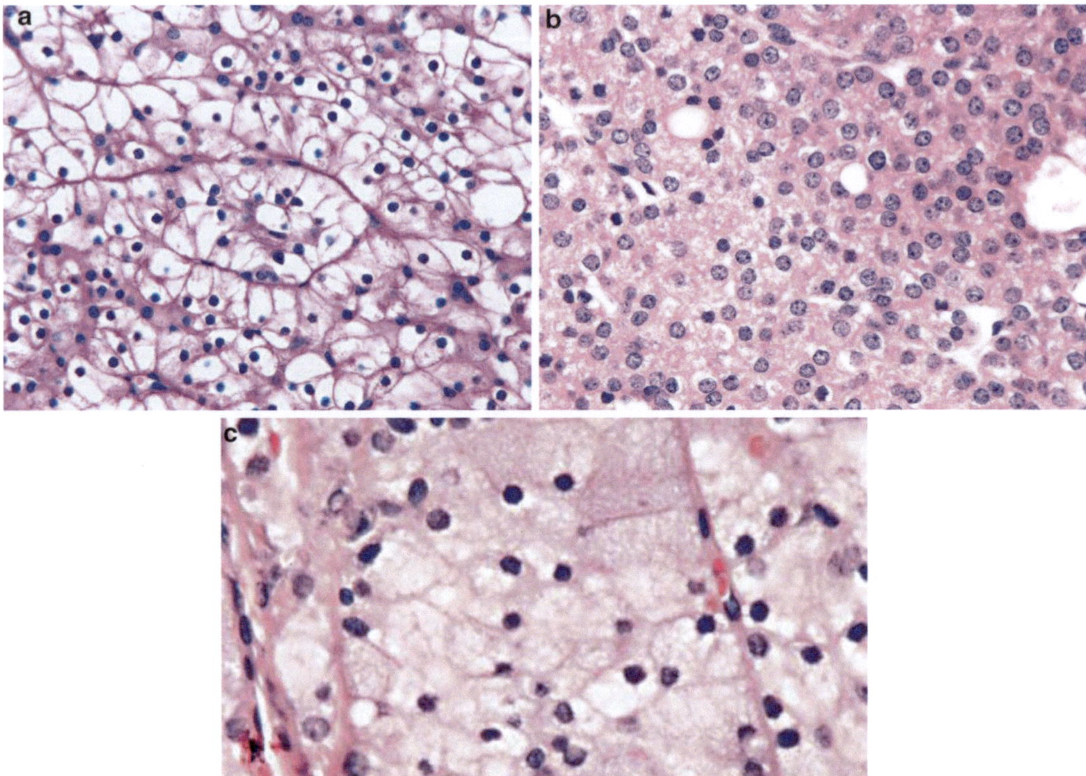

Fig. 9.16 Acinic cell carcinoma. Different cytological presentations (Tumors of the Salivary Glands, *Armed Force Institute of Pathology/American Registry of Pathology*, 2008 with permission)

Recognition of acinic cell differentiation is not as easy as that for pancreatic tumors. They are polygonal cells with conspicuous borders. The nuclei are uniformly small with inconspicuous nucleoli. The cellular granules can be fine or coarse. In addition, the cytoplasmic basophilia is not as characteristic as that of the pancreatic acinic cells. Thus, occasionally, it takes an immunostaining or special staining to reveal the cell nature.

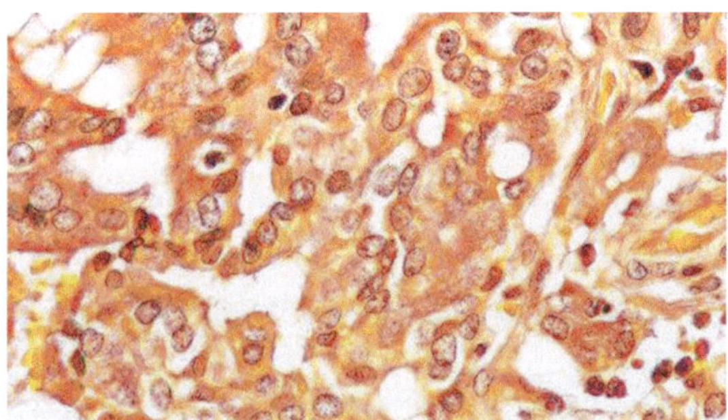

Fig. 9.17 Acinic cell carcinoma. PAS stain highlights granules (Tumors of the Salivary Glands, *Armed Force Institute of Pathology/American Registry of Pathology*, 2008 with permission)

Differential Diagnosis

Pleomorphic Low-Grade Adenocarcinoma

The tumor resembles acinic carcinoma in that it presents in multiple cytological ad histological patterns. It lacks well circumscription and even encapsulation. Instead, the tumor is infiltrative with propensity for perineural invasion and targetoid cellular distribution at the periphery. CK 7 has been reported to differentiate the two entities as the low-grade tumor cells are positive for CK7.

Mucoepidermoid Carcinoma

Low-grade mucoepidermoid carcinoma has prominent cystic structures and causes confusion with the microcystic variant acinic cell carcinoma. It has characteristic three-cell population with intermediate cells being the predominant. The tumor lacks well circumscription and lobulation.

Other Entities With Papillary, Follicular, and Cystic Patterns

As salivary gland acinic cell carcinoma can have a variety of histological and cytological presentations, it is important that those common lesions with similar morphological features are considered in the differential diagnosis. They might include papillary cystadenocarcinoma, thyroid follicular lesions, and even clear cells tumors such as myoepithelioma, clear cell oncocytoma, and metastatic renal cell carcinoma. Immunohistochemical or special stains might be needed in these situations.

Thymus

Key Morphological Features of Atypical Thymoma

(Also called well-differentiated thymic carcinoma, WHO B3 thymoma)

- Round or epithelioid cells forming sheets with an organoid appearance
- Small population of immature T cells (Figs. 9.18 and 9.19)

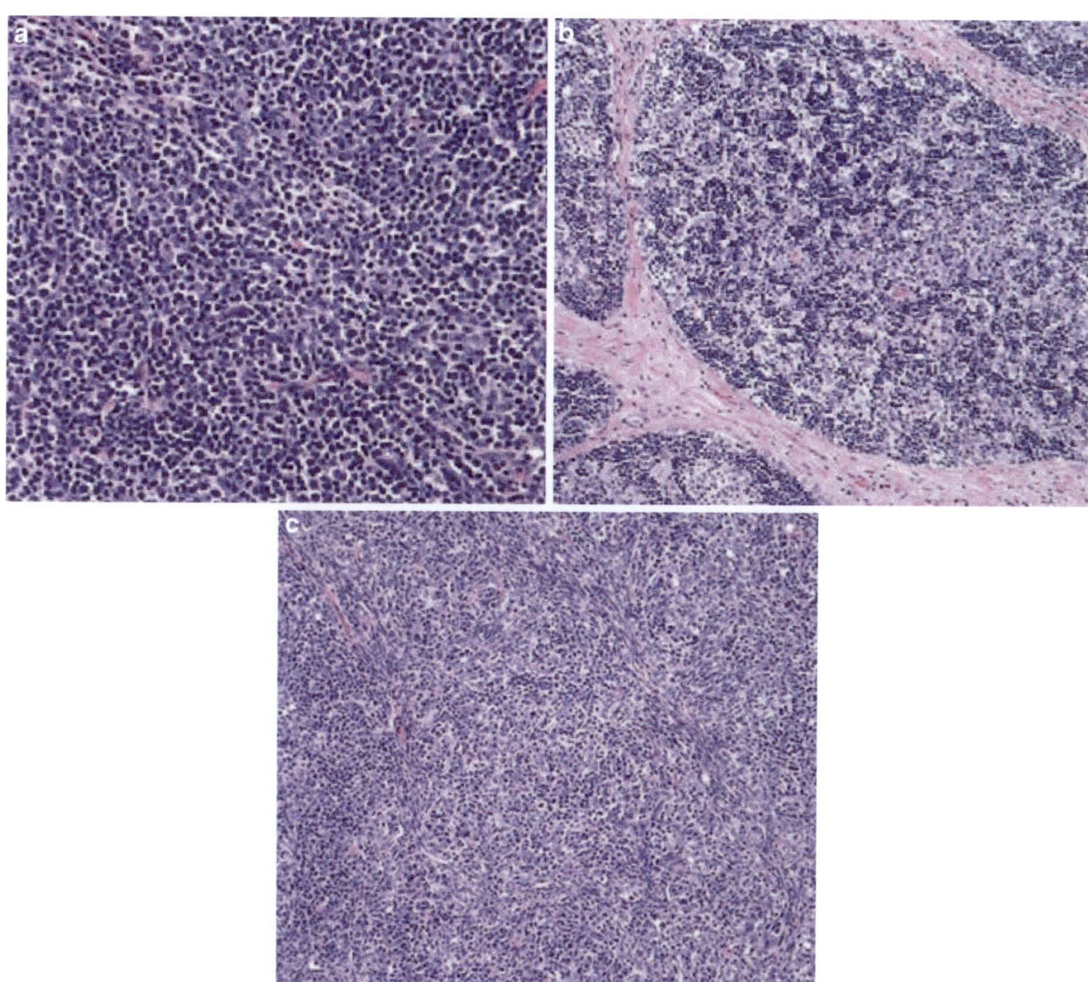

Fig. 9.18 Atypical thymoma. Sheets and lobular arrangement of bland round/epithelioid cells

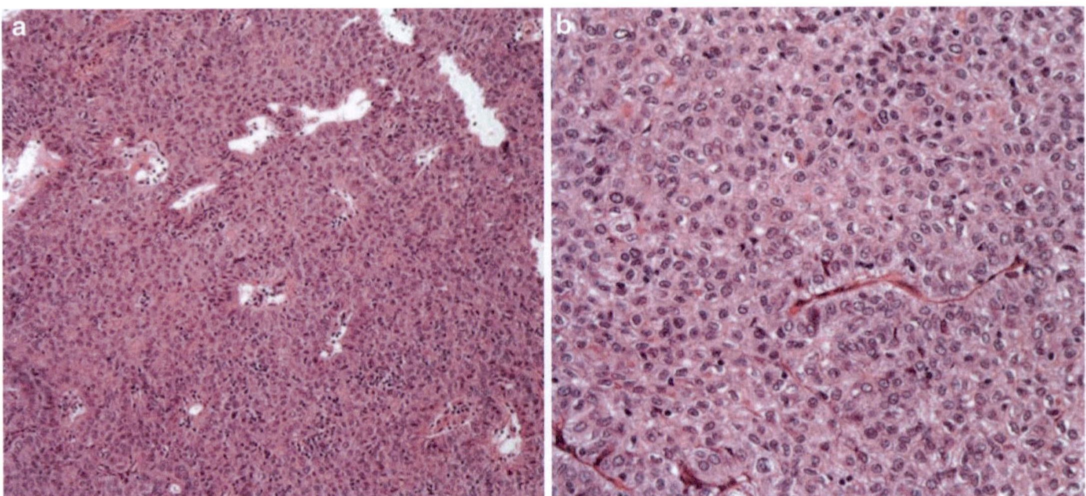

Fig. 9.19 Atypical thymoma. Sheets of round or epithelioid cells with scattered lymphocytes

Discussion

As a vital organ for T cell education, the normal thymus is structured in lobules, each of which is composed of two morphologically distinct areas: the cortex and medulla. Through complex interactions with the thymic epithelial cells, the neural crest-derived mesenchyme plays an important role in the organogenesis participating in the formation of the capsule, septae, and perivascular spaces/blood/thymus barrier and the reticular arrangement of epithelial cells into cortical and medullary compartments [37, 38].

All thymomas are encapsulated and have an organoid appearance, and they can be considered as different maturational stages of the thymic epithelial progenitor cells with the type B3 representing the least mature type [39]. For type B thymomas, there is an inverse relationship between the tumor grade and the size of the immature T cell population. Therefore, type B3 thymoma cells have obtained increased proliferation potential to form sheets with a markedly reduced population of immature T cells indicating a significantly impaired symbiotic relationship (functionality) between the neoplastic thymic epithelial cells (TEC) and immature T lymphocytes [40]. With increasing thymoma grade, there is also a concurrent increase in microvessel density. This increase in microvessel density corresponds to increased PDGF production by thymoma cells [41]. It seems that thymoma cells still employ the same angiogenic mechanism as the normal fetal thymic tissue since the PDGFR-positive mesenchymal cells are involved in the formation of the capsule, septae, and thymic blood barrier and regulation of endothelial function [42].

Thymic carcinomas as defined by the WHO scheme lack encapsulation, organoid arrangement of epithelial cells, and a population of immature T cells [43, 44]. Underlying these morphological features is the total breakdown of the epithelial–mesenchymal and epithelial–lymphocytic cross talks which are the cornerstone of the delicate thymic microenvironment essential for the normal function of the thymus. The clinical dissociation between thymic carcinomas and paraneoplastic autoimmune diseases reflects the loss of T cell nurturing capability in carcinoma cells. However, this does not stop them from attracting mature lymphocytes. The lymphocytes are usually accompanied by eosinophils and plasma cells. Moreover, the lymphocytes in thymic carcinomas lack the intimacy with the epithelial cells evidenced in thymomas (exception: rare lymphoepithelioma-like variant). They are instead largely restricted to the fibrous stroma [45]. Furthermore, without healthy epithelial–mesenchymal interaction, the carcinoma cells rely heavily on hypoxia–VEGF pathway for angiogenesis [46, 47] and no perivascular spaces are formed.

Differential Diagnosis

Thymic Carcinoma

The nonkeratinizing squamous cell carcinomas need to be differentiated from type B3 thymoma, particularly when the latter contains some squamoid areas and frequent Hassall corpuscles. The most important feature of the former is the lack of organoid pattern. Even though desmoplastic fibrous tissue may be abundant, it is distributed randomly with little resemblance to the normal thymic septae. Second, the carcinomatous cells are Cd5 and CD70 positive and usually have more cytological atypia with an overt infiltrative pattern. Inflammatory cells can be frequently encountered. However, they are more often present in the tumor stroma rather than in the parenchyma. The inflammatory cells include eosinophils and plasma cells which are rare in thymomas. In lymphoepithelioma-like carcinomas, the inflammatory cells can intimately admix with epithelial cells. They are, however, mature B and T cells.

The differentiation of the B3 thymoma from a rare variant of basaloid carcinoma can be difficult since the latter has many features of thymomas such as encapsulation and perivascular spaces [48]. In general, the tumor cells show more cytological atypia and immunostainings for immature T cells (TdT, CD1a, and CD99) could help in making the distinction. Thymic squamous cell carcinomas are positive for CD5 and CD70.

Type B1 and B2 Thymomas

B 1 thymomas are differentiated from B3 thymomas by their resemblance to the normal functional thymus in the former. They have a rich lymphocytic component with predominant cortical-like areas.

B2 thymomas still contain a predominance of lymphocytes even though no apparent medullary differentiation is evident. Paradoxically, the cells are more atypical than type B3 tumor cells (2005 WHO criteria). Due to the predominance of the lymphocytic component, no sheetlike or squamoid growth pattern is evident even though both can show focal infiltrative growth pattern.

References

1. Kakudo K, et al. Encapsulated papillary thyroid carcinoma, follicular variant: a misnomer. Pathol Int. 2011;62(3):155–60.
2. Liu Z, et al. Encapsulated follicular thyroid tumor with equivocal nuclear changes, so-called well-differentiated tumor of uncertain malignant potential: a morphological, immunohistochemical, and molecular appraisal. Cancer Sci. 2011;102(1):288–94.
3. Nikiforov YE, Ohori PN. Chapter 11. Papillary carcinoma. In: Nikiforov YE, Biddinger PW, Thompson LDR, editors. Diagnostic pathology and molecular genetics of the thyroid. Baltimore/Philadelphia: Lippincott Williams & Wilkins; 2009. p. 160–213.
4. Baloch ZW, LiVolsi VA. Etiology and significance of the optically clear nucleus. Endocr Pathol. 2002;13(4):289–99.
5. Rezk S, et al. beta-Catenin expression in thyroid follicular lesions: potential role in nuclear envelope changes in papillary carcinomas. Endocr Pathol. 2004;15(4):329–37.
6. Nikiforov YE, Ohori PN. Chapter 10. Follicular carcinoma. In: Nikiforov YE, Biddinger PW, Thompson LDR, editors. Diagnostic pathology and molecular genetics of the thyroid. Baltimore/Philadelphia: Lippincott Williams & Wilkins; 2009. p. 132–59.
7. Mete O, Rotstein L, Asa SL. Controversies in thyroid pathology: thyroid capsule invasion and extrathyroidal extension. Ann Surg Oncol. 2009;17(2):386–91.
8. Mete O, Asa SL. Pathological definition and clinical significance of vascular invasion in thyroid carcinomas of follicular epithelial derivation. Mod Pathol. 2011;24(12):1545–52.
9. Lin X, et al. Follicular thyroid carcinoma invades venous rather than lymphatic vessels. Diagn Pathol. 2010;5:8.
10. Yasuda M, et al. Glucose transporter-1 expression in the thyroid gland: clinicopathological significance for papillary carcinoma. Oncol Rep. 2005;14(6):1499–504.
11. Aldred MA, et al. Papillary and follicular thyroid carcinomas show distinctly different microarray expression profiles and can be distinguished by a minimum of five genes. J Clin Oncol. 2004;22(17):3531–9.
12. Kim D, Kim H, Koo JS. Expression of caveolin-1, caveolin-2 and caveolin-3 in thyroid cancer and stroma. Pathobiology. 2012;79(1):1–10.
13. Sotgia F, et al. Understanding the Warburg effect and the prognostic value of stromal caveolin-1 as a marker of a lethal tumor microenvironment. Breast Cancer Res. 2011;13(4):213.
14. Sotgia F, et al. Caveolin-1 and cancer metabolism in the tumor microenvironment: markers, models, and mechanisms. Annu Rev Pathol. 2011;7:423–67.
15. Takano T. Fetal cell carcinogenesis of the thyroid: theory and practice. Semin Cancer Biol. 2007;17(3):233–40.

16. Fagman H, Nilsson M. Morphogenesis of the thyroid gland. Mol Cell Endocrinol. 2010;323(1):35–54.
17. Mitchell JC, Parangi S. Angiogenesis in benign and malignant thyroid disease. Thyroid. 2005;15(6):494–510.
18. Gerard AC, et al. Correlation between the loss of thyroglobulin iodination and the expression of thyroid-specific proteins involved in iodine metabolism in thyroid carcinomas. J Clin Endocrinol Metab. 2003;88(10):4977–83.
19. Takamatsu J, et al. Peroxidase and coupling activities of thyroid peroxidase in benign and malignant thyroid tumor tissues. Thyroid. 1992;2(3):193–6.
20. Hama Y, et al. Three-dimensional structure of the micro-blood vessels in thyroid tumors analyzed by immunohistochemistry coupled with image analysis. Thyroid. 1999;9(9):927–32.
21. Katoh R, et al. Confocal laser scanning microscopic observation of angioarchitectures in human thyroid neoplasms. Hum Pathol. 1999;30(10):1226–31.
22. Biddinger PW. Chapter 114. Medullary carcinoma. In: Nikiforov YE, Biddinger PW, Thompson LDR, editors. Diagnostic pathology and molecular genetics of the thyroid. Baltimore/Philadelphia: Lippincott Williams & Wilkins; 2009. p. 249–302.
23. Okumura K, Shinohara M, Endo F. Capability of tissue stem cells to organize into salivary rudiments. Stem Cells Int. 2012;2012:502136.
24. Knox SM, et al. Parasympathetic innervation maintains epithelial progenitor cells during salivary organogenesis. Science. 2010;329(5999):1645–7.
25. Guzzo M, et al. Major and minor salivary gland tumors. Crit Rev Oncol Hematol. 2010;74(2):134–48.
26. Leivo I. Insights into a complex group of neoplastic disease: advances in histopathologic classification and molecular pathology of salivary gland cancer. Acta Oncol. 2006;45(6):662–8.
27. Nagao T, et al. Immunohistochemical analysis of salivary gland tumors: application for surgical pathology practice. Acta Histochem Cytochem. 2012;45(5):269–82.
28. Cheuk W, Chan JK. Advances in salivary gland pathology. Histopathology. 2007;51(1):1–20.
29. Ellis GL, Auclair PL. In: Silverberg SG, editor. Tumors of the salivary glands, AFIP atlas of tumor pathology. Washington, DC: American Registry of Pathology in collaboration with the Armed Forces Institute of Pathology; 2008. Chapter 5: malignant epithelial neoplasms.
30. Bhaijee F, et al. New developments in the molecular pathogenesis of head and neck tumors: a review of tumor-specific fusion oncogenes in mucoepidermoid carcinoma, adenoid cystic carcinoma, and NUT midline carcinoma. Ann Diagn Pathol. 2011;15(1):69–77.
31. Ettl T, et al. Salivary gland carcinomas. Oral Maxillofac Surg. 2012;16(3):267–83.
32. Seethala RR. Histologic grading and prognostic biomarkers in salivary gland carcinomas. Adv Anat Pathol. 2011;18(1):29–45.
33. Ellis GL, Auclair PL. Chapter 5. Malignant epithelial neoplasms. In: Tumors of the salivary glands. Silver Spring: ARP Press; 2008. p. 173–438.
34. Seethala RR. An update on grading of salivary gland carcinomas. Head Neck Pathol. 2009;3(1):69–77.
35. Liu J, et al. Molecular biology of adenoid cystic carcinoma. Head Neck. 2011;34(11):1665–77.
36. Schwarz S, et al. Morphological heterogeneity of oral salivary gland carcinomas: a clinicopathologic study of 41 cases with long term follow-up emphasizing the overlapping spectrum of adenoid cystic carcinoma and polymorphous low-grade adenocarcinoma. Int J Clin Exp Pathol. 2011;4(4):336–48.
37. Gordon J, Manley NR. Mechanisms of thymus organogenesis and morphogenesis. Development. 2011;138(18):3865–78.
38. Nowell CS, Farley AM, Blackburn CC. Thymus organogenesis and development of the thymic stroma. Methods Mol Biol. 2007;380:125–62.
39. Inoue M, et al. Correlating genetic aberrations with World Health Organization-defined histology and stage across the spectrum of thymomas. Cancer Res. 2003;63(13):3708–15.
40. Alves NL, et al. Thymic epithelial cells: the multitasking framework of the T cell "cradle". Trends Immunol. 2009;30(10):468–74.
41. Cimpean AM, et al. Platelet-derived growth factor and platelet-derived growth factor receptor-alpha expression in the normal human thymus and thymoma. Int J Exp Pathol. 2011;92(5):340–4.
42. Foster K, et al. Contribution of neural crest-derived cells in the embryonic and adult thymus. J Immunol. 2008;180(5):3183–9.
43. Moran CA, Suster S. The World Health Organization (WHO) histologic classification of thymomas: a reanalysis. Curr Treat Options Oncol. 2008;9(4–6): 288–99.
44. Travis WD, Brambilla E, Muller-Hermelink HK, Harris CC. Pathology and genetics of tumors of the lung, pleura, thymus and heart, World Health Organization classification of tumours. Lyon: IARC Press; 2004.
45. Shimosato Y, Mukai K, Matsuno Y. Tumors of the mediastinum, AFIP atlas of tumor pathology series 4. Silver Spring: ARP Press; 2010. Chapter 2: thymoma.
46. Tomita M, et al. Correlation between tumor angiogenesis and invasiveness in thymic epithelial tumors. J Thorac Cardiovasc Surg. 2002;124(3):493–8.
47. Kojika M, et al. Immunohistochemical differential diagnosis between thymic carcinoma and type B3 thymoma: diagnostic utility of hypoxic marker, GLUT-1, in thymic epithelial neoplasms. Mod Pathol. 2009;22(10):1341–50.
48. Shimosato Y, Mukai K, Matsuno Y. Chapter 3. Thymic carcinoma. In: Tumors of the mediastinum. Silver Spring: ARP Press; 2010. p. 115–56.

10 Mammary Gland

The Low-Grade Breast Neoplasia Family

Key Morphological Features of Low-Grade Ductal Carcinoma In Situ (DCIS)

- Cribriform, papillary formation with uniform round or columnar cells
- Regular cell placement with preserved cell polarity around lumens (Fig. 10.1)

Key Morphological Features ofClassical Lobular Carcinoma In Situ (LCIS)

- Lobular extension (>½ of a lobule)
- Small, uniform, loosely cohesive small cells (Fig. 10.2)

Key Morphological Features of Columnar Cell Lesion (CCL) and Flat Epithelial Atypia (FEA)

- Dilated cystic structures
- Monomorphic cell population with preserved cellular polarity (Figs. 10.3 and 10.4)

Discussion

Review of Pertinent Mammary Gland Development and Histology

The postnatal development of the mammary gland is a very complicated process orchestrated mainly by the concerted efforts of systemic steroids, peptide hormones, as well as local growth factors [1–3]. In the process which can span up to 50 years, the gland goes through four tightly regulated stages: ductal morphogenesis, lobuloalveolar development during pregnancy, synthesis and secretion of milk proteins and lipids at lactation, and involution following weaning. In addition, the ductal and lobular structures also undergo cyclic changes (proliferation and apoptosis) corresponding to the menstrual phases. Derived from the terminal end buds (TEB), the adult mammary functional and histological unit, terminal duct lobular unit (TDLU), is the site where most breast lesions arise. Upon close review of the TDLU, one could discern three distinct parts of the unit with each of them having their corresponding benign and neoplastic simulators (Fig. 10.1).

The ductal part:

Ductal hyperplasia → DCIS → invasive ductal carcinoma

The lobular (acinar) part:

Adenosis, lobular hyperplasia (lactation) LCIS → invasive lobular carcinoma

X. Sun, *Well-Differentiated Malignancies: New Perspectives*, Current Clinical Pathology,
DOI 10.1007/978-1-4939-1692-4_10, © Springer Science+Business Media New York 2015

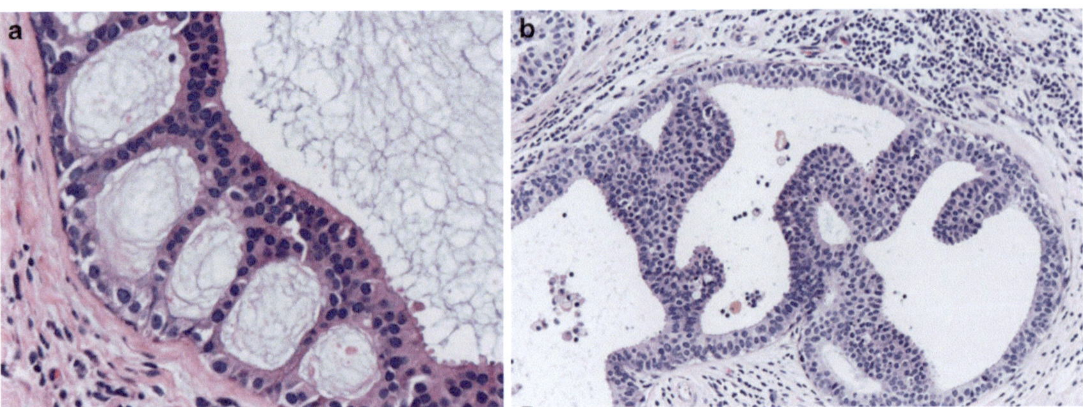

Fig. 10.1 Low-grade ductal carcinoma in situ. Cribriform and papillary structures composed of uniformly bland cells (Breast Pathology, *Elsevier/Saunders*, 2012 with permission)

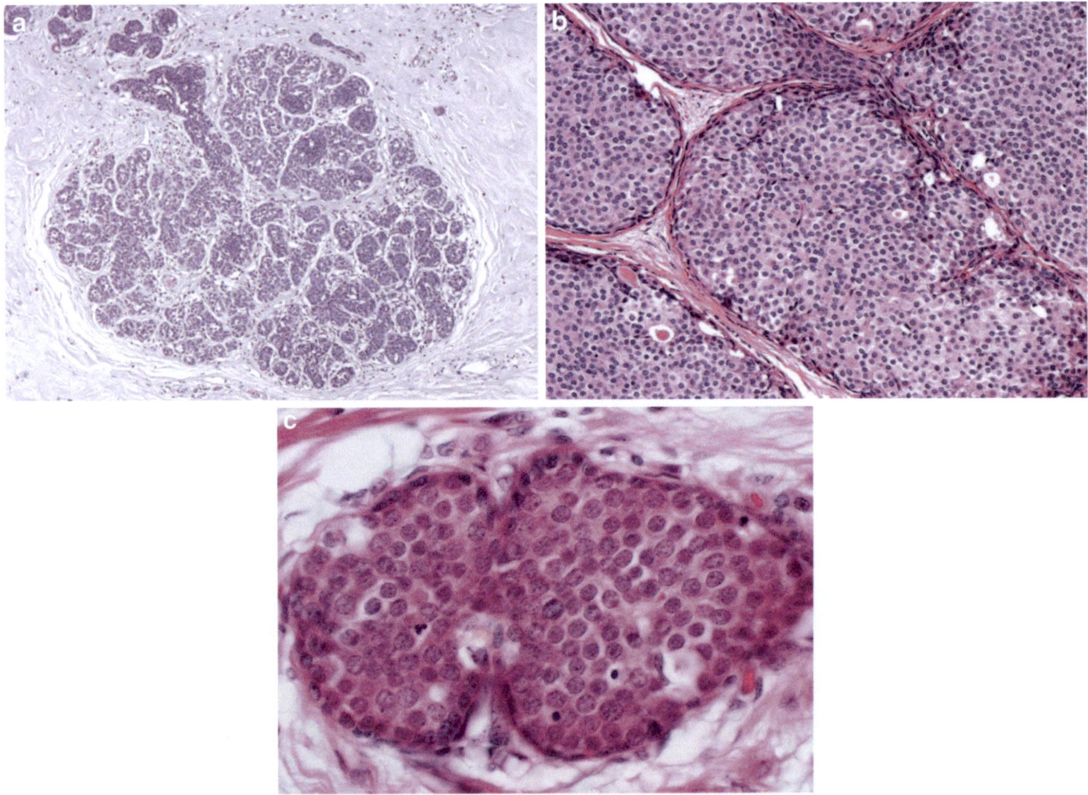

Fig. 10.2 Lobular carcinoma in situ. Expanded lobules composed of uniformly bland cells (Breast Pathology, *Elsevier/Saunders*, 2012 with permission)

The junction part:

Tubular adenosis and blunt duct adenosis, columnar cell lesion/flat cell atypia → tubular carcinoma

In breast pathology, the designations "lobular," "ductal," and "tubular" only denote the neoplastic cell differentiation rather than the actual tumor site. Understandably, the in situ component of one type can progresses into or associate with another type of invasive carcinoma.

A well-developed myoepithelial layer lines almost the whole gland system except for a short segment of the collecting duct at the nipple orifice.

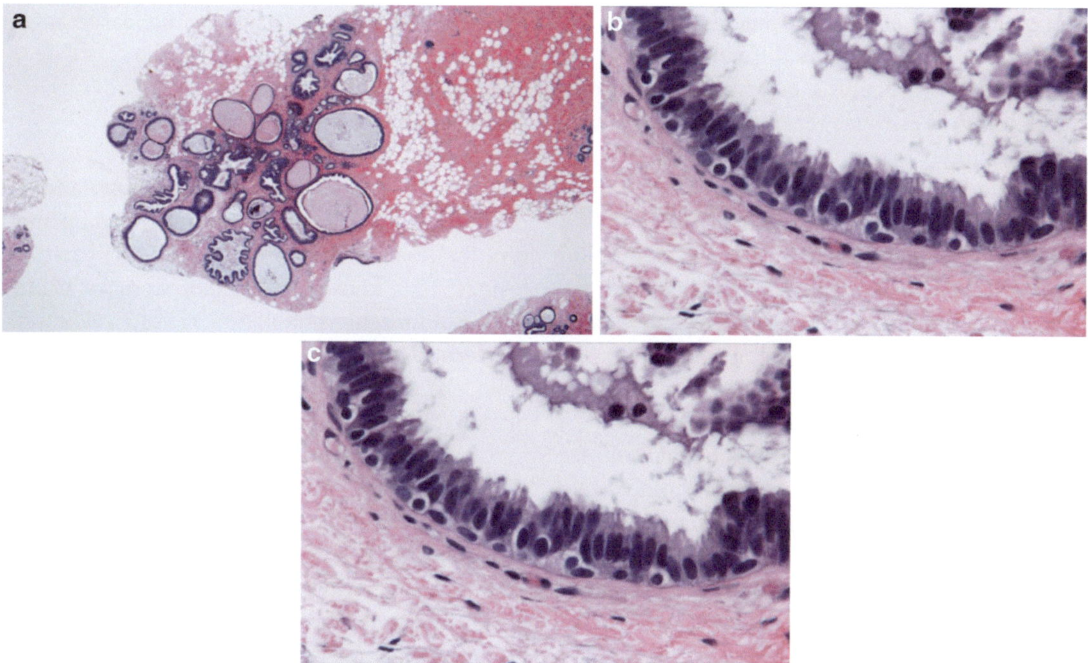

Fig. 10.3 Columnar cell lesion. Dilated cystic structures composed of uniformly bland columnar cells (Breast Pathology, *Elsevier/Saunders*, 2012 with permission)

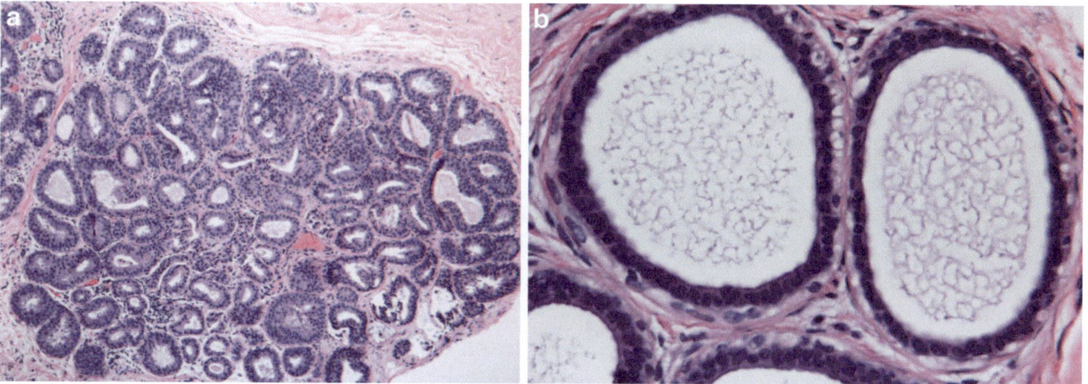

Fig. 10.4 Flat cell lesion. Dilated cystic structures lined by uniformly bland flat cells (Breast Pathology, *Elsevier/Saunders*, 2012 with permission)

This layer plays a very important chaperone role in the organogenesis and functions of the gland (see more discussion in the invasive carcinoma section).

The Low-Grade Concept and Cellular Changes

The concept of low-grade breast neoplasia family has gained increasing recognition in recent years. Included in this family are low-grade ductal carcinoma in situ (DCIS), lobular carcinoma in situ (LCIS), columnar cell lesion (CCL), flat epithelial atypia (FEA), and low-grade invasive carcinoma. This family shares characteristic deletion of 16q and gains of 1q and 16p [4–6]. The preinvasive lesions in this family are characterized by two morphological features: a bland and monomorphic cell population and presence of a peripheral myoepithelial layer. Compared to benign proliferative lesions (ductal hyperplasia in particular), the neoplastic precursor cells are actually more mature and differentiated toward luminal cells probably as a result of increased proliferation of estrogen receptor (ER) expressing cells which rely on autocrine growth factors.

The low-grade precursor lesions are clonal proliferations of apparent luminal cells or transit amplifying cells in which the differentiation switch toward myoepithelial is inactivated [7, 8]. This clonal proliferation of mildly defective cells accounts for the cellular monotony and blandness of low-grade precursor lesions. This cellular feature tends to get neglected if the stereotypic picture of dysplasia (increased N/C ratio and cellular polymorphism) predominates in the mind's eye of the pathologist. This feature is particularly important in their distinction from florid ductal hyperplasia which has many features of dysplasia. An analogy exists in lymph nodes where a low-grade B cell lymphoma contains a monomorphic cell population, whereas reactive cells are polymorphic and even alarmingly atypical.

LCIS cells have lost their adhesion molecule E-cadherin and thus are loosely cohesive, whereas the molecule expression is preserved in DCIS, CCL, and FEA accounting for their cellular cohesiveness and maybe even polarity. This important feature is often used in the distinction between pleomorphic lobular carcinoma from high-grade ductal carcinoma and in the diagnosis of cancerization of lobules by DCIS cells. In cancerization, neoplastic cells involve the lobules and replace the normal luminal cells. On the other hand, lobular carcinoma cells can involve ductules in a pagetoid spread pattern in which the neoplastic cells manage to drive a wedge between the ductular luminal and myoepithelial cells. They can even form small acinar structure along the ductal lumen (clover leaf pattern).

The myoepithelial cells present at the periphery are not part of the monoclonal proliferation. Rather they represent remnants of TDLUs which have been occupied by neoplastic cells. The clonal epithelial cells have gained the capacity to break away from the inhibitory control of myoepithelial cells but are still restricted by the barrier composed of myoepithelial cells and the basement membrane. Evidence is emerging that the seemingly normal myoepithelial cells are altered at least functionally [9, 10].

Papillary DCIS and DCIS Involving Papilloma

The overemphasis of a uniform cell population in distinction between carcinoma in situ and benign proliferation can be problematic for papillary lesions. It is known that some papillary DCISs have a dimorphic population [11–13]. The second group of cells stands out because of their abundant pale cytoplasm. Their basally located nuclei reinforce the impression that a layer of myoepithelial cells are present. Attention to other features such as thin, delicate fibrovascular core and cell polarity and judicious use of myoepithelial markers can help avoid an underdiagnosis.

When a papilloma is involved by low-grade DCIS, the myoepithelial layer within the tumor is oftentimes attenuated as in papillomas, particularly those with superimposed ductal hyperplasia. In both situations, a myoepithelial layer is still present in the peripheral ductal wall. To identify the DCIS area, attention to cellular uniformity and blandness takes precedence. The neoplastic cells can grow on the scaffold of a preexisting papilloma which might be affected by ductal hyperplasia, rendering evaluation for papillary structure and myoepithelial cell less useful. In ambiguous cases, a stain for CK5/6 stain or estrogen receptor (ER) can be used. Hyperplastic ductal cells show a typical mosaic pattern for CK5/6 which is negative for neoplastic cells. The neoplastic cells are diffusely and strongly positive for ER which shows only focal and weak positivity for hyperplastic cells.

Papillary carcinomas are frequently mistaken for papillary DCIS. They lack, however, myoepithelial cells not only at the periphery but also inside the tumor mass.

Differential Diagnosis

For DCIS

Usual Ductal Hyperplasia (UDH) and Atypical Ductal Hyperplasia (ADH)

UDH represents a non-monoclonal syncytial proliferation of glandular epithelial proliferation characterized by irregular arrangement of a heterogeneous group of cells which differ not only in cell size, shape, orientation, and staining property but also in differentiation. This difference in differentiation (maturation) can be highlighted with high molecular weight keratin stain which shows a mosaic expression. DCIS cells are negative for the stain, and instead they show diffuse ER staining. ADH is defined as a monoclonal epithelial proliferation which contains a component with features of UDH or residual ductal epithelium. Other authorities use the term to describe a small DCIS (<2 mm in size).

Collagenous Spherulosis

Collagenous spherulosis can be seen in a wide range of benign breast lesions. It contains characteristic lumina filled with basement membrane and other extracellular matrix material. The luminal material is produced by myoepithelial cells which line the lumina. The myoepithelial cells are typically elongated and spindle. Cribriform DCIS cells are uniformly round cells with polarity. In difficult cases, a stain for myoepithelial cells would suffice.

The problem is confounded when spherulosis is involved by LCIS cells. Since the carcinomatous cells are uniformly round, they resemble cribriform DCIS to perfection. Immunostaining for E-cadherin would help make the distinction.

LCIS

Both low-grade DCIS and LCIS belong to the same low-grade family and derive from the small breast functional and histological units, TDLU. It is understandable that they can not only coexist side by side but have some overlapping involvement patterns as mentioned in the discussion. DCIS and LCIS not only coexist but also show overlapping involvement patterns as discussed above. In general, loose cellular cohesion, presence of intracellular vacuoles, and solid growth pattern favor LCIS, whereas cellular cohesion, extracellular lumen formation, and cellular polarity around the lumina are indicators of ductal differentiation. In questionable cases, immunostaining for E-cadherin helps make the right diagnosis.

Gynecohyperplasia

Gynecomatoid hyperplasia can show micropapillary formation. Like in ductal hyperplasia, it contains a heterogeneous proliferation of cells and lacks the cellular uniformity and regularity characteristic of micropapillary DCIS.

Invasive Carcinoma

See the invasive carcinoma section.

For LCIS

Artificial Discohesion and Lactational Changes, Myoepithelial Proliferation, and Intraepithelial Histiocytes

Artificial discohesion of lobular cells due to poor fixation can result in an overdiagnosis of LCIS. There is, however, no lobular expansion.

Focal lactational changes can simulate LCIS as a result of cellular vacuoles. The affected lobules usually are just one to two cells thick, and the cells are swollen with abundant cytoplasm and frayed luminal borders.

LCIS cells can sometimes have clear cell metaplasia. Therefore, the distinction from adenosis with myoepithelial hyperplasia might need the use of E-cadherin immunostaining.

The pagetoid spread of LCIS can be simulated by intraepithelial histiocytes. The histiocytes, however, contain foamy cytoplasm and lack cytoplasmic lumina.

Lobular Hyperplasia and Atypical Lobular Hyperplasia

Lobular hyperplasia is not a frequently used term in surgical pathology probably because the mammary lobular structures only reach their full structural and physiological potentials during lactation. Atypical lobular hyperplasia refers to a lesion with partial involvement of acini by cells with similar morphological features of LCIS. The criterion is less than 50 % of with or without acinar distention.

DCIS

See DCIS differential diagnosis.

Invasive Carcinoma

See invasive carcinoma section.

For CCL and FEA

Benign Cysts

Benign cysts are lined by attenuated, cuboidal, and apocrine cells. They lack cellular uniformity, regularity, and polarity characteristic of CLL and FEA.

Apocrine Lesion

When CCL and FEA show apocrine cytoplasm, they need to be differentiated from apocrine metaplasia and hyperplasia. Apocrine lesions lack cellular uniformity and contain prominent nucleoli and more abundant cytoplasm. In a difficult case, immunostaining for ER and BScl-2 could help. CLL and FEA cells typically show diffuse positivity for them.

DCIS and UDH

When CCL proliferation creates mounds, differentiation from micropapillary DCIS is in order even though the distinction is most likely of no diagnostic significance. CCL cells have pencillate nuclei and the micropapillae lack a club-shaped and Roman bridge-like structures characteristic of micropapillary DCIS.

The ductal hyperplasia cells can form micropapillae. They are, however, slender with neither cellular uniformity and polarity nor bridge arch structures.

Key Morphological Features of Low-Grade Invasive Ductal Carcinoma

- Well-formed glands, papillary or cribriform structures in nonlobular presentation
- Lack of a peripheral myoepithelial layer (Fig. 10.5)

Key Morphological Features of Low-Grade Invasive Lobular Carcinoma

- Uniform discohesive cells in a single cell file, trabeculae, and sheets in fibrous stroma
- Lack of a peripheral myoepithelial layer (Figs. 10.6 and 10.7)

Discussion

In contrast to malignant salivary tumors, most of which belong to one of those well-characterized morphological subtypes, the vast majority of breast cancers are invasive ductal carcinomas with heterogeneous microscopic appearances (invasive ductal carcinoma, NOS). The rest of them are made up by invasive lobular carcinomas and those rare special subtypes. As with the precursor lesions, the ductal and lobular and tubular designations connote tumor cell differentiation toward the three parts of the TDLU rather than the site of origin. The special subtypes are singled out because of their distinct histomorphological presentations and/or associated clinical outcomes. The tubulolobular carcinoma subtype is characterized by having distinct areas of both ductal and lobular features.

Invasive mammary carcinomas are defined as epithelial proliferations which have gained the capacity to penetrate the basement membrane with resultant stromal and/or parenchymal invasion. Histological evaluation of invasion, however, is not always straightforward with breast cancers. Some breast cancers invade as nodules or papillary, and even cribriform structures and oftentimes little or no desmoplastic reaction is elicited. Classical lobular carcinomas tend to invade in an inconspicuous Indian file pattern. On the other hand, some benign breast lesions appear to have infiltrative borders, and when involved by those precursor lesions, they mimic low-grade invasive carcinomas to perfection. In this section, we elaborate on the concept of using myoepithelial cell as a valuable indicator for basement membrane breakdown and stromal invasion. While this approach works the best with low-grade breast cancers, it can also be applied to epithelial malignancies of higher grades with a few caveats.

Mammary Myoepithelial Cells: The Important Chaperone

The mammary gland myoepithelial cells are spindle or elongated shaped with pale cytoplasm and arranged in parallel with the long axis of ducts and ductule and in a basket-like structure around the lobules. Their long cytoplasmic processes

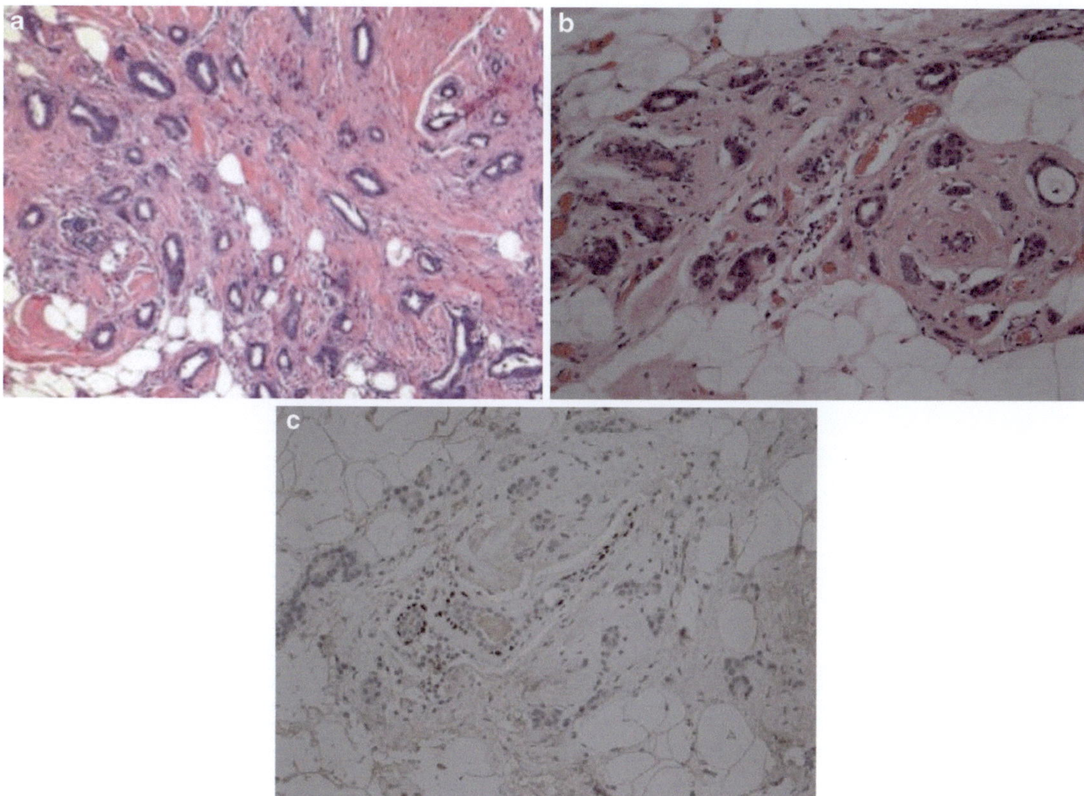

Fig. 10.5 Invasive well-differentiated ductal carcinoma. Lack of myoepithelial cells (**c**, p63 stain) (Journal of Clinical Pathology, *American Society of Clinical Pathology*, 2013 with permission)

wrap around the luminal cells resulting in a distinct cellular intermediary layer between the basement membrane and luminal ones. The myoepithelial cell contacts the former by hemidesmosomes and the latter desmosomes. They are adhered to each other through intermediate or gaps and other adhesive molecules.

The myoepithelial cells are derived from the bipotent mammary stem/progenitor cells under the regulation by oxytocin [7]. Compared to the luminal cells, they have a low cell turnover rate. Immunohistochemically, they are positive for smooth muscle actin (SMA), CK5/6, p63, and other high molecular weight keratin, but negative for ER and PR. They also stain negatively for vimentin which is characteristic of myofibroblasts on the other side of the basement membrane.

In addition to their well-known function in milk ejection during lactation, the myoepithelial cells play a very important role in all the postnatal development stages [9, 10, 14]. On one hand, they participate in the branching, elongation of ductules, and formation of new acini by sculpting through the existing basement membrane and adjacent stroma and laying down new basement membrane material for the new growths to cling to. On the other hand, they produce morphogens and growth factors for luminal cell growth and differentiation. It is highly likely that this important chaperone-like role also includes some check and balance mechanisms (factors) for the normal luminal cell growth and functioning. It is thus no wonder that the myoepithelial cells are somewhat involved in the pathogenesis of almost all the mammary epithelial lesions, benign or malignant.

Role of Myoepithelial Cells in Mammary Gland Tumorigenesis

Many lines of evidence have indicated that differentiated myoepithelial cells possess important tumor suppressor functions through inducing tumor cell apoptosis, disruption of tumor–stroma

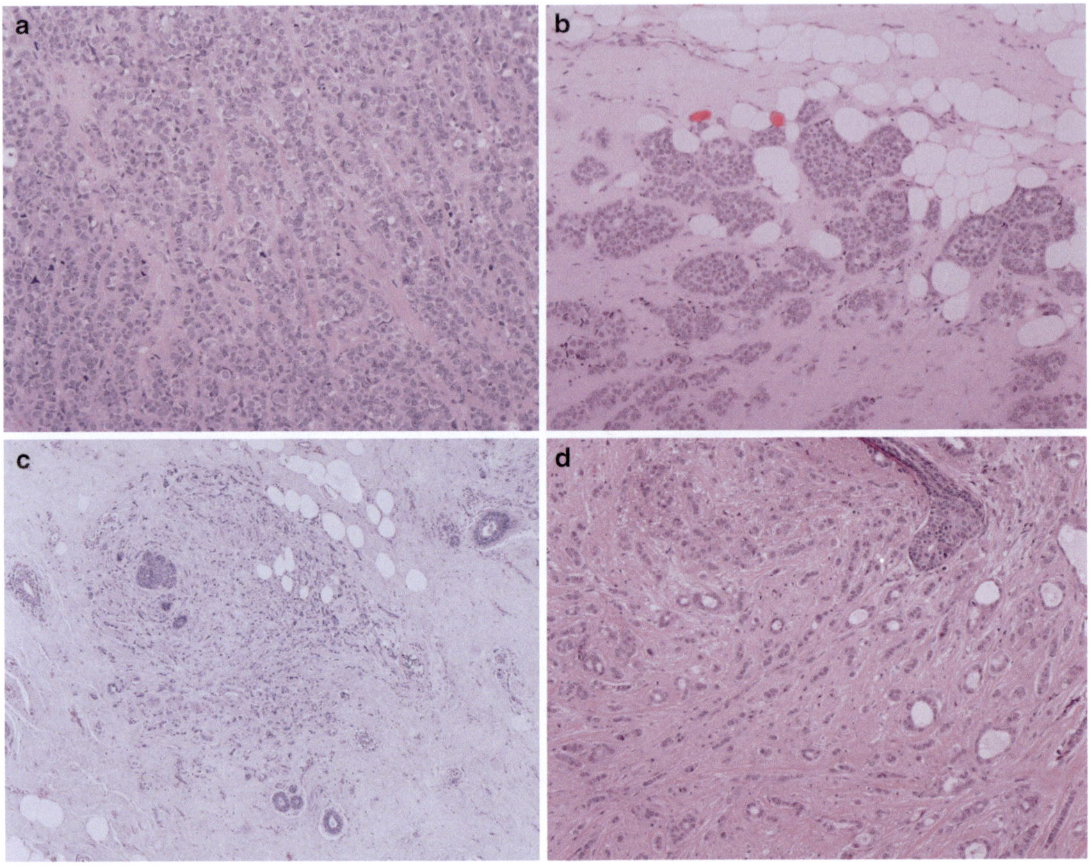

Fig. 10.6 Invasive lobular carcinoma. Uniform discohesive cells in different growth patterns (Breast Pathology, *Elsevier/Saunders*, 2012 with permission)

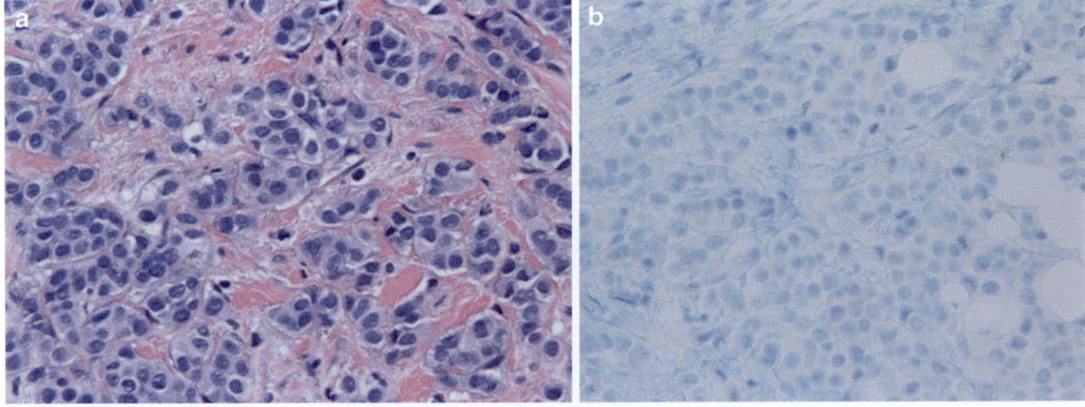

Fig. 10.7 Invasive lobular carcinoma. Cells are negative for E-cadherin (**b**)

interactions, and inhibition of angiogenesis and tumor invasion [9, 10, 14].

It is long known that all benign and precursor lesions have myoepithelial cells at the periphery with microglandular adenosis being the only exception. Invasive carcinomas, on the other hand, lack a chaperoning myoepithelial layer. The mechanism underlying their disappearance remains unclear. Invasive mammary carcinomas are derived from precursor lesions which have only one layer of myoepithelial cells at the periphery. The myoepithelial cells represent the remnant of involved TDLUs rather than a component of the neoplastic proliferation. The low-grade mammary epithelial carcinomas have virtually no myoepithelial cells both within and at the periphery of the tumor mass. Conversely, a small fraction of high-grade tumors can show scattered cells expressing myoepithelial markers. This difference indicates that different pathogenic mechanisms are probably at play. The low-grade lesions are likely to derive from luminal cells or transit amplifying cells which lack capability for myoepithelial cell differentiation [15–18]. When the cells gain the strength to break away from the physical barrier of myoepithelial layer and basement, the tumor becomes invasive. Like their in situ counterparts, the invasive cells show no myoepithelial differentiation. High-grade malignancies, on the other hand, probably derive from the adult stem cells or bipotent stem cells in which the cellular myoepithelial differentiation machinery is not completely shut off yet, allowing random (scattered) myoepithelial differentiation [17–19]. Importantly, these cells are randomly distributed with no tendency to concentrate at the periphery or form connections with other similarly phenotypic cells. In support of this view, recent data suggest that the claudin-low subtype (molecular classification) might arise from the myoepithelial progenitor [8].

Pitfalls with Myoepithelial Markers

The current belief holds that as long as there are some peripheral myoepithelial cells (positive for at least two markers), a lesion should be considered noninvasive. This is in stark contrast to the situation with salivary gland tumors where immunochemical evaluation of the myoepithelial cells is of little practical significance as most benign and malignant salivary gland tumors are composed of more than one cell type with one of them showing myoepithelial and/or basal cell differentiation.

The traditional myoepithelial markers have been increasingly replaced by more sensitive and specific ones including calponin, SMA heavy chain (SMA-HC), and p63. In the practice of evaluating myoepithelial cells in lieu of invasion, it is highly recommended that a panel of at least two of them is employed and the interpreting pathologist should become aware of several potential pitfalls associated with these stains [20].

Pitfall 1. Myofibroblasts are positive for both calponin and SMA. The periductal linear stromal staining can be confused as the presence of a myoepithelial layer. However, myofibroblasts are negative for p63. Their smooth linear arrangement is in contrast to the bumpy arrangement of myoepithelial cells on the basement membrane.

Pitfall 2. Microvessels are positive for both calponin and SMA-HC. This pitfall is particularly pertinent for papillary lesions which are highly vascularized. Attention to their location and shape of immunostaining cells as well correlation with p63 staining help avoid this pitfall.

Pitfall 3. Over 10 % of invasive carcinomas can show p63 positivity. While most of them are high-grade ductal carcinomas, low-grade adenosquamous carcinoma is an exception. The squamous component can express diffuse positivity for p63, but not for SMA-HC and calponin. In high-grade carcinomas with positivity for p63, the cell morphology and location are very important clues. The positive cells are randomly scattered and rarely form pairs.

Pitfall 4. It is important to realize that many benign breast lesions can have an attenuated myoepithelial layer. In difficult cases where there is only minimal residual myoepithelial cell staining, attention to the morphological features (such as confluence and irregularity) as well as adjacent glands is recommended. Sometimes a stain for basement membrane might be helpful to confirm that minimal myoepithelial staining is real.

Pitfall 5. Three other rare subtypes of mammary carcinomas are known to stain positive for myoepithelial markers. They include adenocystic carcinoma, adenomyoepithelial and myoepithelial carcinomas, and even medullary carcinoma. Fortunately, their character-

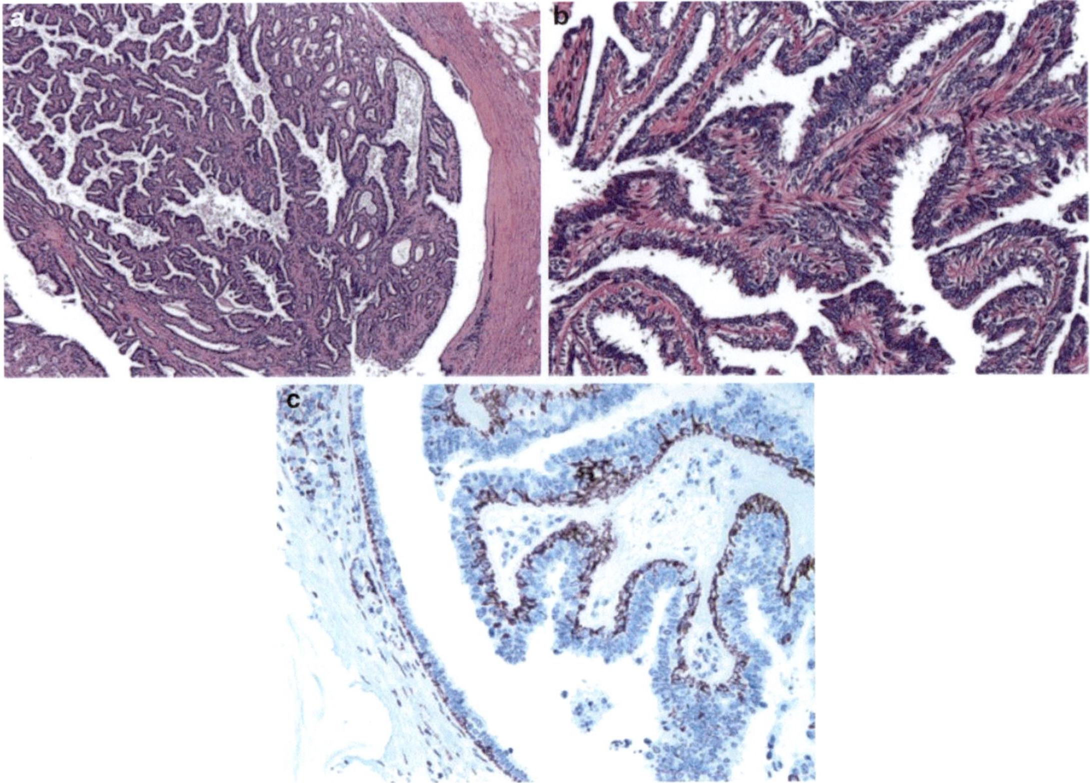

Fig. 10.8 Papilloma with conspicuous myoepithelial cells (Histopathology, *John Wiley&Sons, Inc*, 2008 with permission)

istic histological presentations as well as the location of positive cells easily set them apart from benign and precursor lesions.

Papillary Carcinoma

In breast pathology, papillary structures can be seen in a variety of lesions ranging from papillary hyperplasia, papilloma, DCIS involving papilloma (atypical papilloma), papillary DCIS, and invasive papillary carcinoma (Figs. 10.8, 10.9, and 10.10). Pure invasive papillary carcinomas are very rare. Oftentimes, papillary structures are present as an in situ component in association with classical invasive ductal carcinomas. Understandably, invasive papillary carcinomas are usually mistaken for papillary DCIS (difference other than myoepithelial cells). The encapsulated papillary carcinomas and solid papillary carcinomas are probably rare variants of invasive papillary carcinoma which invade through expansion or represent unique entities in transit between carcinoma in situ and frankly invasive carcinoma. Presumably, their circumscription and slow clinical progression result from a resistant fibrotic stroma or aging tumor cells with limited invasive capability. Both entities are present in the elderly women in their seventies and eighties.

The micropapillary variant is a separate entity from papillary carcinoma because of its associated poor prognosis like its counterparts in other organs.

Differential Diagnosis

For Ductal Carcinoma

Sclerosis Adenosis, Radial Scar

While characterized by a lobulocentric proliferation of small glands with variable compression and distortion by fibrous stroma, sclerosing adenosis can have an infiltrative appearance, particularly when the adjacent fat tissue is involved. The compressed and distorted glands can further

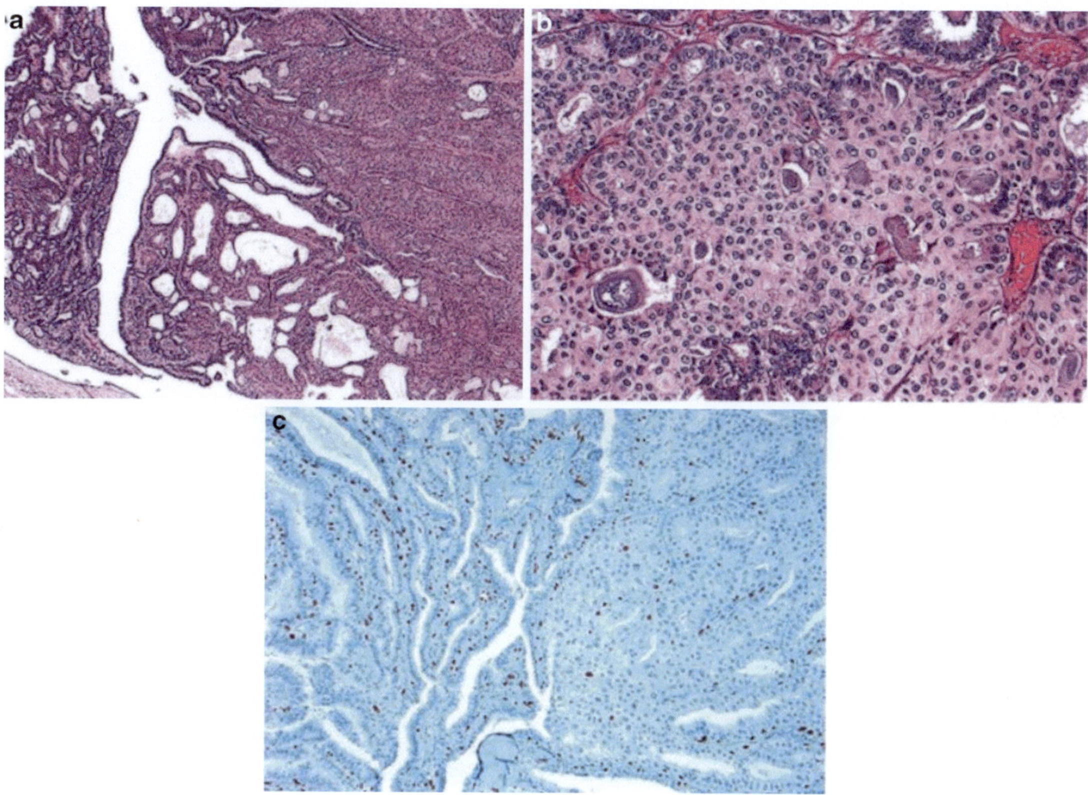

Fig. 10.9 Low-grade ductal carcinoma in situ involving a papilloma. Note greatly reduced number of myoepithelial cells in the abnormal area (Histopathology, *John Wiley&Sons*, Inc, 2008 with permission)

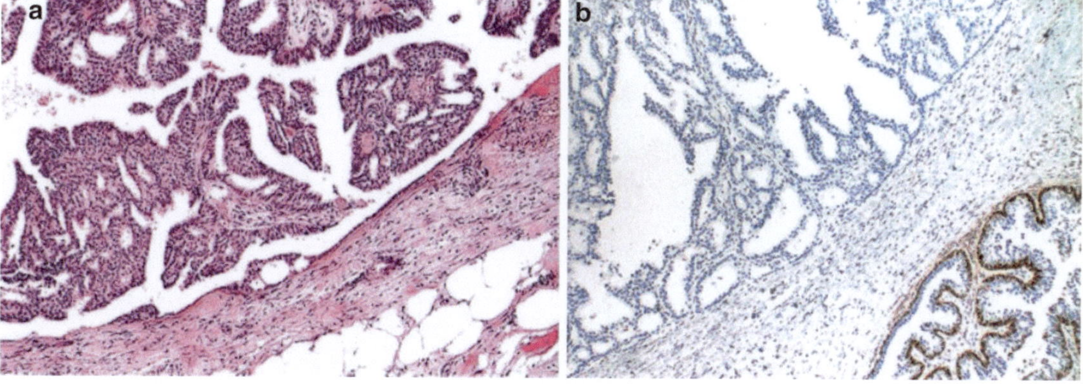

Fig. 10.10 Papillary carcinoma. No myoepithelial cells (Histopathology, *John Wiley&Sons*, Inc, 2008 with permission)

reinforce the impression of invasion (Figs. 10.11 and 10.12) Attention to the lobulocentric appearance and judicious use of myoepithelial cell markers can help.

Radial scars contain a central fibroelastic core, radially arranged glands in an intermediary zone, and a seemingly infiltrative periphery which shows other proliferative changes and even pre-

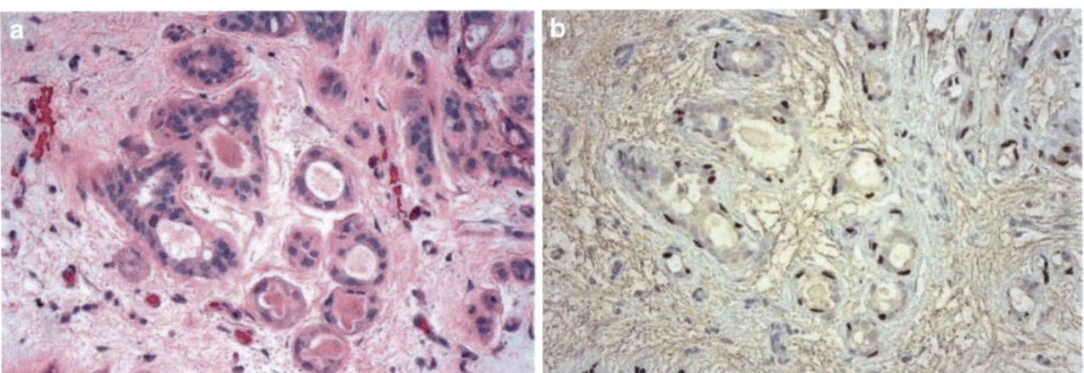

Fig. 10.11 Sclerosing adenosis. Irregular glandular structures lined by myoepithelial cells (SMM-HC) (American Journal of Surgical Pathology, *Wolters Kluwer/Lippincott Williams & Wilkins*, 2003 with permission)

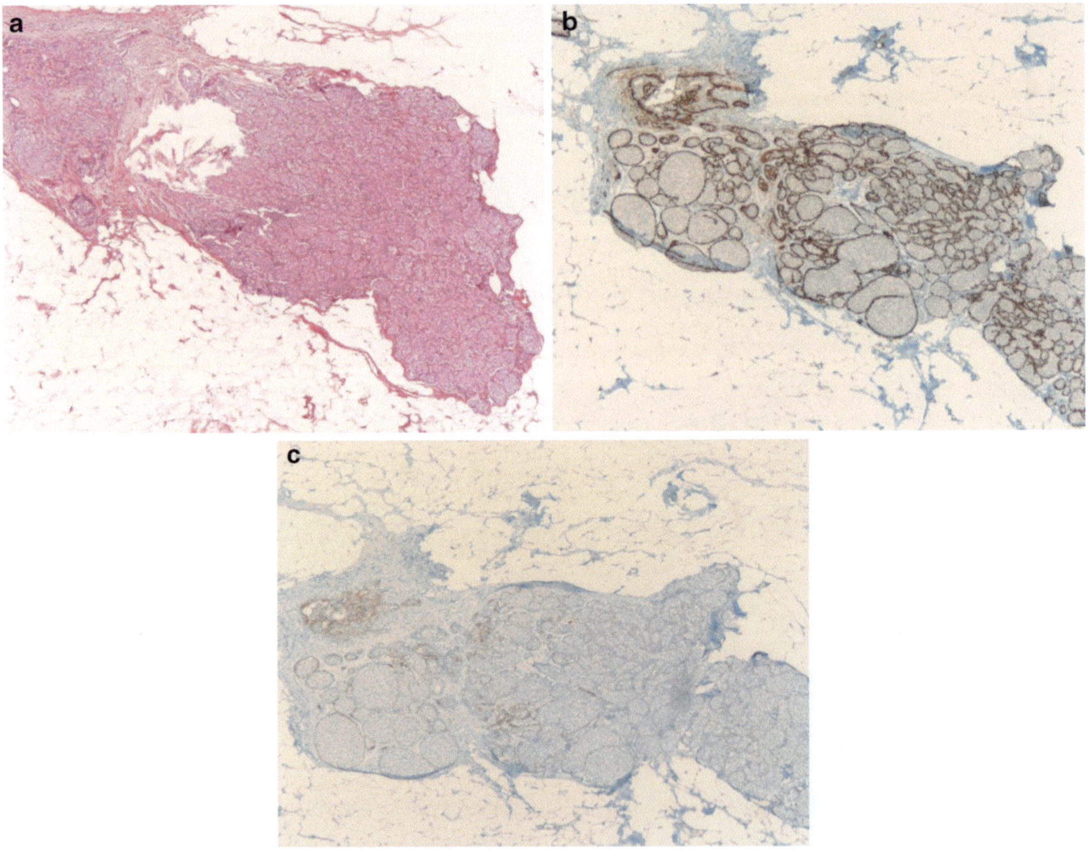

Fig. 10.12 Lobular carcinoma in situ involving sclerosing adenosis which is lined by myoepithelial cells (p63 stain). Tumor cells are negative for E-cadherin (**c**) (Archives of Pathology and Laboratory Medicine, *American Society of Clinical Pathology*, 2013 with permission)

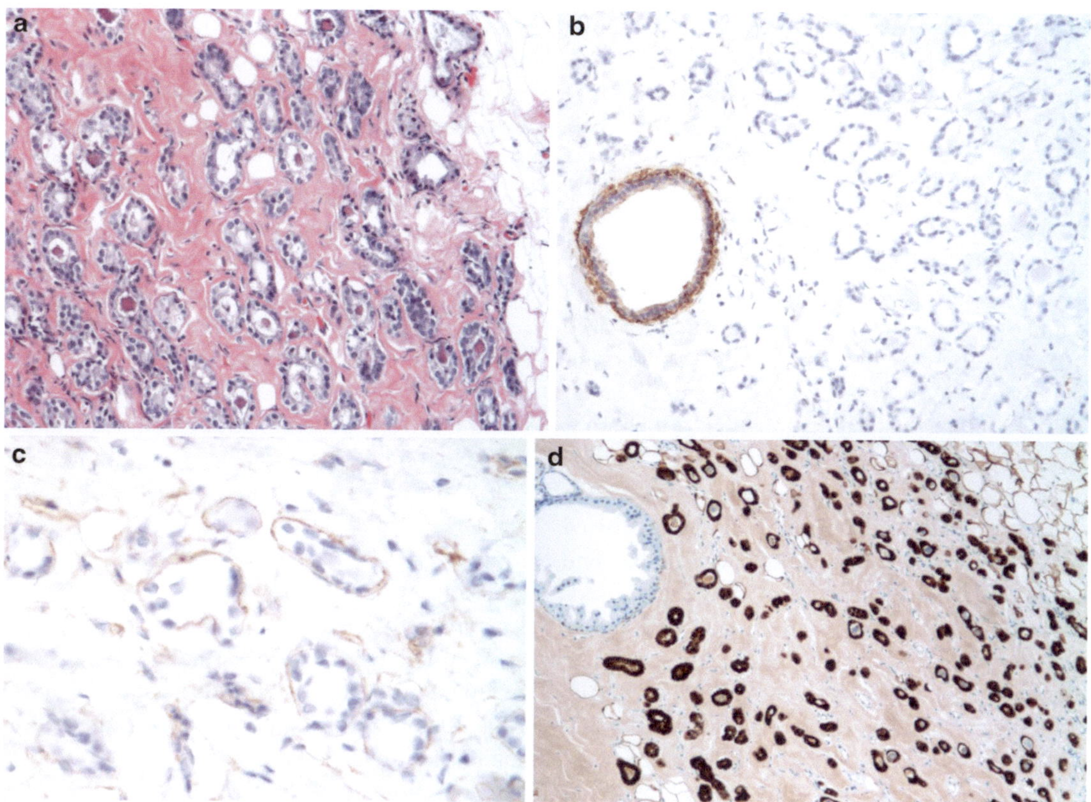

Fig. 10.13 Microglandular adenosis without myoepithelial rimming. Cells are positive for S100 (Archives of Pathology and Laboratory Medicine, *American Society of Clinical Pathology*, 2013 with permission)

cursor lesions. The radial arrangement of glands which are usually angulated is unlike the haphazardly distributed malignant glands. In difficult cases, a myoepithelial panel can be applied. The benign compressed glands are enshrouded with myoepithelial cells even though they might become attenuated.

Microglandular Adenosis and Secretory Adenosis

Microglandular adenosis represents the only benign mammary epithelial lesion which lacks a layer of accompanying myoepithelial cells (Fig. 10.13). It is composed of small uniformly round glands made of bland cells. However, it assumes no lobular growth pattern. Instead, the small round glands infiltrate the surrounding stroma and adipose tissue. The cells are negative for ER, PR, EMA, HER2/neu, and GCDFP-15, but positive for S100, (epithelial growth factor receptor) EGFR, and cathepsin D [21]. Presumably, microglandular adenosis represents a distinct proliferation of bipotent stem cells in response to increased local EGF secretion. This lack of response to oxytocin and steroids results in a cellular growth pattern unlike any other benign mammary epithelial proliferations [22]. Alternatively, microglandular adenosis might arise from luminal cells rescued from physiological involution by local EGF secretion. The failure of myoepithelial cells to survive the involution allows for its infiltrative growth behavior [22].

Secretory adenosis has similar morphological feature to microglandular adenosis. However, it contains luminal secretion and a layer of myoepithelial cells.

Tubular Adenosis

Tubular adenosis has a haphazard arrangement of elongated and angulated glands. When involved by ductal carcinoma in situ, it simulates invasive carcinoma to perfection. However, it contains a myoepithelial layer separating it from tubular carcinoma. Tubular adenosis also lacks comma-like shape and apical snouts characteristic of tubular carcinoma.

Nipple Duct Adenoma, Syringomatous Adenoma

Typical nipple adenomas are composed of ductal hyperplasia and adenosis-like proliferations with relative circumscription. However, when involved by marked fibrosis, they can manifest a pseudoinfiltrative pattern. Attention to the presence of myoepithelial cells and the location of the tumor help steer one away from a diagnosis of invasive carcinoma.

Syringomatous adenomas can be confused with low-grade adenosquamous carcinomas and tubular carcinomas because of their highly infiltrative patterns, irregular often teardrop-shaped glands, and occasional solid and cystic areas. The glands are composed to two cell layers with the outer layer showing no apparent myoepithelial differentiation. The infiltration can be seen into the subareolar tissue and sometimes along nerve fibers. They are differentiated from low-grade adenosquamous carcinoma by its location in the nipple or subareolar region. Adenosquamous carcinomas are peripherally located, and they are usually accompanied by other epithelial lesions and perhaps a desmoplastic stroma. The tubules in tubular carcinomas have only one layer of cells and are usually associated with low-grade DCIS, but not a squamous component.

Myoepithelial Lesions

Pure myoepithelial cell tumors are very rare in the breast. Histopathologically, they do not enter the diagnosis of low-grade epithelial carcinomas because they present as nodular mass with spindle, clear cells, and plasmacytoid and epithelioid cells.

Adenomyoepitheliomas represent the other end of the spectrum of intraductal epithelial proliferation with papillomas being at one end. They typically manifest biphasic tubular structures (both luminal and myoepithelial cells) with either of them being predominant. Mitotic activities and even necrosis can been seen in the myoepithelial component and are not signs of malignant transformation. Malignant transformation is defined as having infiltrative borders and can be in the form of myoepithelial carcinoma, leiomyosarcoma, or undifferentiated malignancy. Neoplastic myoepithelial cells can have variable staining patterns for the markers, and some cells can be devoid of reactivity completely.

Adenoid cystic carcinomas are very rare in the breast and they have characteristic morphological features (prominent epithelial–myoepithelial component, cribriform and tubular structures, and characteristic stroma material) which allow for their easy differentiation from low-grade invasive ductal carcinomas. The tumor cells are positive for p63 and other myoepithelial markers.

For Lobular Carcinoma

Inflammatory Cells

In some lobular carcinomas, the tumor cells can be largely overlooked and dismissed as scattered inflammatory cells on low power examination due to their discohesiveness and lack of stromal reaction. Inflammatory cells, however, are not arranged in a linear or targetoid pattern and lack occasional intracytoplasmic vacuoles.

Lymphoma

Lymphomas enter into the differential diagnosis when invasive lobular carcinoma cells present in trabeculae or sheets. Low-grade B cell lymphoma cells typically show evident nuclear atypia and lack intraluminal vacuoles. In a difficult case, an immunostaining for CD45 helps clinch a diagnosis.

For Papillary Carcinoma

Papillary Hyperplasia, Papilloma

Papillary hyperplasia is a form of ductal hyperplasia which can be differentiated from a papilloma by the lack a fibrovascular core (a vascular stalk only) and a hierarchical branching pattern.

Papillomas can be associated with sclerosis and adenosis (ductal adenoma) which might result in the obliteration of papillary structures and angulation of glands in a fibroblastic background, creating a pseudoinfiltrative impression. Papillomas can show necrosis and epithelial displacement due to instrumentation or torsion around the fibrovascular stalk. It is important that the displaced epithelium should not be overcalled as an invasive component when seen in breast stroma or lymphovascular lumens.

Both lesions are underlined by myoepithelial cells within the lesion and at the periphery. Papillary carcinomas lack myoepithelial cells.

Papillary DCIS and Atypical Papilloma (DCIS Involving) Papilloma

These two concepts are frequently confused for each other. Actually, they are two different entities with different morphologies. Papillary DCISs have thin, delicate papillae composed of uniformly cuboidal to columnar cells with polarity. The neoplastic cells can be one to several cells thick, but they lack an underneath myoepithelial layer, even though, however, a layer of myoepithelial cell is still present at the periphery of the involved space.

When a papilloma is involved by DCIS, the neoplastic cells are usually round and form a solid, cribriform, or micropapillary pattern. The thick and fibrotic papillary scaffold of a papilloma remains. Myoepithelial cells are usually attenuate or absent in the involved areas. To differentiate the DCIS component from ductal hyperplasia superimposed on the papilloma, immunostaining for CK5/6 and ER can be employed. The hyperplastic cells show a mosaic staining pattern but only focal and weak staining for ER. DCIS cells show a reverse staining pattern.

Micropapillary Carcinoma

The micropapillae in micropapillary carcinomas lack a fibrovascular core and appear to be suspended in clear spaces. The tumor cells have moderate to severe nuclear grade and in two thirds of cases are associated with micropapillary or cribriform DCIS (with higher nuclear grade than the low-grade family). Apparently, during the progression to invasive carcinoma, the cell polarity apparatus is compromised to result in reversed cell polarity and detachment from stroma. The reversed polarity can be illustrated by immunostaining for EMA and MUC-1.

The Mammary Gland Stroma

Key Morphological Features of Borderline Phyllodes Tumor

- Prominent leaflike structures with intracanalicular growth pattern
- Heterogeneous stromal expansion with moderate cellular atypia and mitotic activity (10/10 HPF) (Fig. 10.14)

Discussion

Like the purely epithelial proliferations, both fibroadenomas and phyllodes tumors are also derived from the basic breast functional and structural units, TDLU. Both of them, however, contain a conspicuous proliferation component of the specialized intralobular mesenchyme.

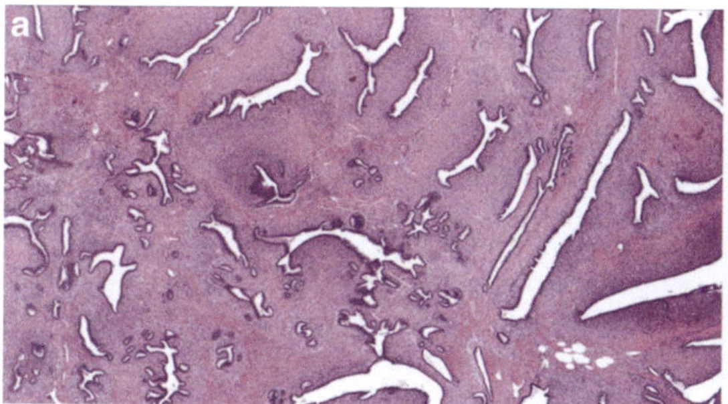

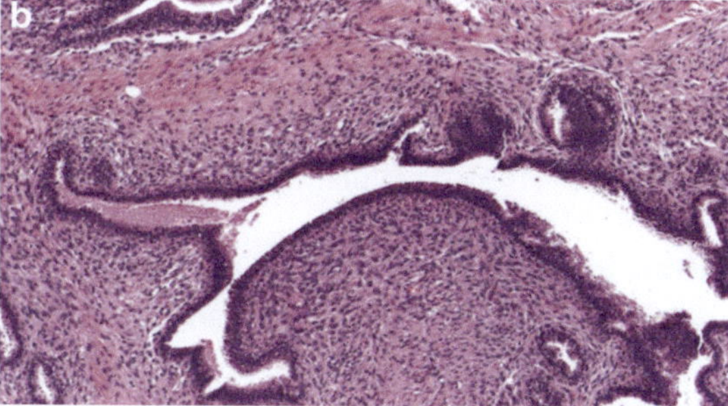

Fig. 10.14 Borderline phyllodes tumor. Leaflike structures with intracanalicular growth pattern. Periductal condensation and cellular atypia are evident (Breast Pathology, *Elsevier/Saunders*, 2012 with permission)

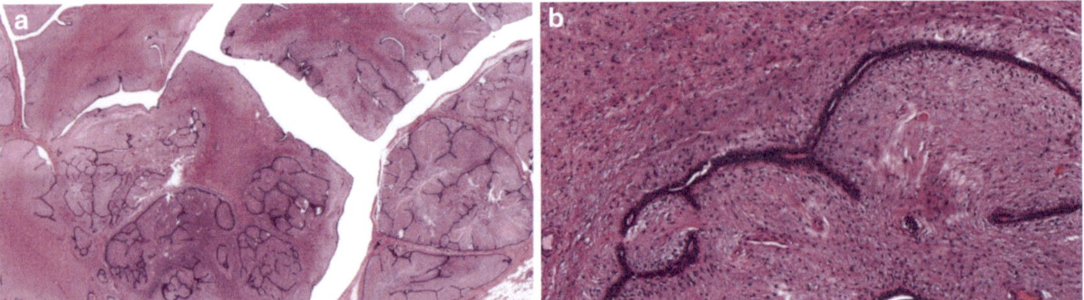

Fig. 10.15 Benign phyllodes tumor without periductal condensation of spindle cells (Breast Pathology, *Elsevier/Saunders*, 2012 with permission)

It is believed that fibroadenomas are hyperplastic in both the epithelial and stromal components, whereas the stromal proliferation in phyllodes tumors is clonal [23, 24].

By definition, borderline phyllodes tumors exhibit intermediate features between benign and malignant phyllodes tumors. In general they have moderate cellularity, cellular atypia, and mitotic activities with circumscribed or infiltrative borders. Importantly, periductal stromal condensation is present in all phyllodes tumors and therefore cannot be considered a feature of malignancy or borderline malignancy even though it is an important diagnositic feature of adenosarcomas in the female reproductive system. Exception: a very rare entity of periductal sarcoma of the breast has periductal stromal condensation, but no leaflike structures [23].

Instead, stromal overgrowth constitutes a sign of malignancy here [24]. Defined as stroma proliferation without accompanying epithelial cells, it signifies the breakdown of the coupling between epithelium and intralobular stroma which is maintained in benign and borderline phyllodes tumors. The stromal growth in borderline tumors is also characterized by heterogeneous cellularity. Benign phyllodes have homogenous stromal cellularity.

Differential Diagnosis

Cellular Fibroadenoma and Benign Phyllodes Tumor

Cellular fibroadenomas can have an intracanalicular growth pattern and high cellularity. They lack long leaflike structures projecting into spaces, periductal stromal condensation, and stromal mitoses.

Benign phyllodes tumors generally have a pushing border, with mild to modest hypercellularity, atypia, and mitotic activities (Fig.10.15).

Spindle proliferation such as fibromatosis, myofibroblastomas, nodular fasciitis, and sarcomas all lack leaflike structures lined by epithelial cells. Even malignant phyllodes tumors have residual leaflike structures present in areas showing no stromal overgrowth.

Spindle cell carcinomas (metaplastic carcinomas) of the breast may have foci of typical invasive ductal carcinoma or DCIS. Pseudoangiomatous stromal hyperplasia has dense collagenous stroma and blood vessel-like clefts lined by myofibroblasts. In areas where cellularity is high, the cells tend to aggregate into fascicles. They can be differentiated from phyllodes tumors by the lack of leaflike structures and periductal stromal condensation.

References

1. Watson CJ, Khaled WT. Mammary development in the embryo and adult: a journey of morphogenesis and commitment. Development. 2008;135(6):995–1003.
2. Gjorevski N, Nelson CM. Integrated morphodynamic signalling of the mammary gland. Nat Rev Mol Cell Biol. 2011;12(9):581–93.
3. Jay R, Harris MEL, Monica Morrow C, Kent O. Chapter 1. Breast anatomy and development. In: Diseases of the breast. 4th ed. Philadelphia: Wolters Kluwer/Lippincott Williams & Wilkins; 2010. p. 1–28.
4. Pare R et al. Breast cancer precursors: diagnostic issues and current understanding on their pathogenesis. Pathology. 2013;45(3):209–13.

5. Abdel-Fatah TM et al. High frequency of coexistence of columnar cell lesions, lobular neoplasia, and low grade ductal carcinoma in situ with invasive tubular carcinoma and invasive lobular carcinoma. Am J Surg Pathol. 2007;31(3):417–26.
6. Abdel-Fatah TM et al. Morphologic and molecular evolutionary pathways of low nuclear grade invasive breast cancers and their putative precursor lesions: further evidence to support the concept of low nuclear grade breast neoplasia family. Am J Surg Pathol. 2008;32(4):513–23.
7. Smalley MJ et al. Regulator of G-protein signalling 2 mRNA is differentially expressed in mammary epithelial subpopulations and over-expressed in the majority of breast cancers. Breast Cancer Res. 2007; 9(6):R85.
8. Zhao X et al. Derivation of myoepithelial progenitor cells from bipotent mammary stem/progenitor cells. PLoS One. 2012;7(4):e35338.
9. Pandey PR, Saidou J, Watabe K. Role of myoepithelial cells in breast tumor progression. Front Biosci (Landmark Ed). 2010;15:226–36.
10. Adriance MC et al. Myoepithelial cells: good fences make good neighbors. Breast Cancer Res. 2005;7(5): 190–7.
11. Esposito NN. Chapter 13. Papilloma and papillary lesions. In: Dabbs D, editor. Breast pathology. Philadelphia: Saunders/Elsevier; 2012. p. 252–62.
12. Rosen PP, Hoda SA. Chapter 4. Benign papillary tumors. In: Breast pathology: diagnosis by needle core biopsy. Philadelphia: Wolter Kluwer Health/ Lippincott Williams & Wilkins; 2010. p. 27–51.
13. Rosen PP, Hoda SA. Chapter 11. Papillary carcinoma. In: Breast pathology: diagnosis by needle core biopsy. Philadelphia: Wolter Kluwer Health/Lippincott Williams & Wilkins; 2010. p. 171–86.
14. Gudjonsson T et al. Myoepithelial cells: their origin and function in breast morphogenesis and neoplasia. J Mammary Gland Biol Neoplasia. 2005;10(3):261–72.
15. Raouf A et al. The biology of human breast epithelial progenitors. Semin Cell Dev Biol. 2012;23(5):606–12.
16. Bombonati A, Sgroi DC. The molecular pathology of breast cancer progression. J Pathol. 2011;223(2): 307–17.
17. Kaimala S, Bisana S, Kumar S. Mammary gland stem cells: more puzzles than explanations. J Biosci. 2012; 37(2):349–58.
18. Tiede B, Kang Y. From milk to malignancy: the role of mammary stem cells in development, pregnancy and breast cancer. Cell Res. 2011;21(2):245–57.
19. Haupt B, Ro JY, Schwartz MR. Basal-like breast carcinoma: a phenotypically distinct entity. Arch Pathol Lab Med. 2010;134(1):130–3.
20. Bhargava R, Dabbs D. Chapter 11. Diagnostic immunohistology of the breast. In: Dabbs D, editor. Breast pathology. Philadelphia: Saunders/Elsevier; 2012. p. 189–232.
21. Clark BZ, Dabbs D. Chapter 14. Adenosis and microglandular adenosis. In: Dabbs D, editor. Breast pathology. Philadelphia: Saunders/Elsevier; 2012. p. 263–85.
22. Watson CJ, Kreuzaler PA. Remodeling mechanisms of the mammary gland during involution. Int J Dev Biol. 2011;55(7–9):757–62.
23. Shin SJ, Rabban JT. Chapter 31. Mesenchymal neoplasms of the breast. In: Dabbs D, editor. Breast patholog. Philadelphia: Saunders/Elsevier; 2012. p. 596–641.
24. Rosen PP, Hoda SA. Chapter 23. Mesenchymal neoplasms. In: Breast pathology: diagnosis by needle core biopsy. Philadelphia: Wolter Kluwer Health/ Lippincott Williams & Wilkins; 2010. p. 274–302.

Index

X. Sun, *Well-Differentiated Malignancies: New Perspectives*, Current Clinical Pathology,
DOI 10.1007/978-1-4939-1692-4, © Springer Science+Business Media New York 2015

C

D

E

S